Ribes · Luna · Ros
Learning Diagnostic Imaging

R. Ribes · A. Luna · P. R. Ros (Eds.)

Learning Diagnostic Imaging

100 Essential Cases

With Contributions by

L. Alcala Mata · M. Alvarez Benito · F. Bravo-Rodriguez · J. Camps Herrero
P. Daltro · R. Diaz-Aguilera · S. Espejo · E. Feliu · L. C. Hygino Cruz Jr.
J. Lopez Mora · A. Luna Alcala · S. Mejia · R. do A. Nogueira · M. T. C. Porto
M. Potolicchio · A. C. Rebollo Aguire · R. Ribes · S. E. Rossi · P. Segui
J. A. Vallejo Casas · J. C. Vilanova

With 347 Figures in 397 Separate Illustrations, 50 in Color

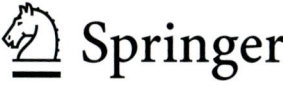 Springer

Ramon Ribes, MD, PhD
Interventional Radiology and MR Units
Reina Sofia University Hospital
14005 Cordoba
Spain

Antonio Luna, MD
Chief, MR Unit
Clinica Las Nieves
Sercosa
23007 Jaen
Spain

Pablo R. Ros, MD, MPH
Chairman, Department of Radiology
Sant Pau Hospital
Autonomous University
08025 Barcelona
Spain
and
Professor, Department of Radiology
Harvard Medical School
Brigham & Women's Hospital
75 Francis St.
Boston MA 02115
USA

ISBN 978-3-540-71206-0   e-ISBN 978-3-540-71207-7

DOI 10.1007/978-3-540-71207-7

Library of Congress Control Number: 2007943071

Cover design: Frido Steinen-Broo, eStudio Calamar, Spain
Layout: Verlagsservice Teichmann, 69256 Mauer, Germany

Printed on acid-free paper

9 8 7 6 5 4 3 2 1

springer.com

Preface

In my first days as a Radiology resident I remember myself in dire need of a book in which I could begin to study the specialty. In those days I was thirsty for radiological knowledge and was recommended a classic manual on conventional chest X-ray which was the very same the oldest radiologist of the staff had studied when he was a beginner. Unfortunately the book I was recommended covered less than 5% of the specialty as it is conceived nowadays.

"Learning Diagnostic Imaging. A Teaching File" is intended to provide medical students, residents of Radiology, and anybody else beginning to be involved in the radiological world, with a useful tool that gives them a quick and comprehensive overview of Radiology. With this book, written in a user-friendly format, Radiology residents, nurses, technicians, and medical students would see their first radiological images in a sort of introduction of what will become their professional activities in the rest of their lives.

One of the main problems that Radiology residents face throughout their residency is that in rounds and clinical sessions they receive information they cannot apprehend because they lack the essential background needed to integrate what they are taught. For example, when, in a radiological session, a resident is looking at an angiogram and has no prior interventional radiology education, he/she inevitably misses the opportunity of learning by being exposed to a great deal of information without the necessary tools to assimilate it. Whenever a mammogram is shown at the radiological session, a first year resident, who has no prior training on breast imaging, knowing beforehand that he is not supposed to be asked about it, loses interest in the subject and it is likely that his mind drifts away until the next case is shown. In clinical sessions, the level of concentration of residents is optimal only in the cases they have prior education on.

With this book, residents independently of their year of residency, would count on the foundations of the specialty as a whole and optimize their time in rounds and clinical sessions. Although initially aimed at Radiology residents, the book would be useful, on the one hand, for medical students, Radiology nurses and technicians and, on the other hand, for senior radiologists and residents and referring physicians of other specialties. As a way of example, the breast imaging senior radiologist would have a basic overview of cardiac imaging at his disposal in just a few pages that otherwise would be impossible for him because no mammographer is supposed to be interested in classic cardiac imaging books as no cardiovascular radiologist has any interest in breast imaging manuals.

The scarcity of books of this sort is easily understandable taking into account that Radiology is divided up in many subspecialties that constitute a universe of their own. To convey an overall view of the specialty is extremely difficult nowadays and will be even more difficult in the future because, due to the fragmentation of the specialty, the old-days only Radiological session, which was attended by the whole Department, has been replaced by a myriad of subspecialty sessions that, by definition, cannot be attended by the entire Radiology Department.

Cordoba, November 22, 2007   RAMON RIBES

Contents

8 Nuclear Medicine

Juan Antonio Vallejo Casas and Angel C. Rebollo Aguirre
Luisa Maria Mena Bares (Contributor) 179

9 Pediatric Radiology

Pedro Daltro, L. Celso Hygino Cruz Jr., Renata do A. Nogueira,
and Miriam T. C. Porto 205

10 Ultrasound Imaging

Pedro Segui and Simona Espejo 231

Contributing Authors

LIDIA ALCALA MATA
Radiology Resident
Department of Radiology
Ciudad de Jaen Hospital
Jaen
Spain

MARINA ALVAREZ BENITO
Chief, Breast Unit
Reina Sofia University Hospital
Cordoba
Spain

F. BRAVO-RODRIGUEZ
CT and MR Units
Reina Sofia University Hospital
Cordoba
Spain

JULIA CAMPS HERRERO
Chief, Radiology Department
Hospital de la Ribera
Alzira, Valencia
Spain

PEDRO DALTRO
CDPI
Pediatric Radiology
Rio de Janeiro
Brazil

ROCIO DIAZ-AGUILERA
Radiology Department
Hospital Alto Guadalquivir
Jaen
Spain

SIMONA ESPEJO
CT and MR Unit
Radiology Department
Reina Sofia University Hospital
Cordoba
Spain

ELOISA FELIU
MR (Magnetic Resonance)
Inscanner
Alicante
Spain

L. CELSO HYGINO CRUZ Jr.
Neuroradiology
CDPI
Rio de Janeiro
Brazil

ANTONIO LUNA ALCALA
Chief, MR (Magnetic Resonance)
Clinica Las Nieves
Sercosa
Jaen
Spain

SERGIO MEJIA
Chief, Cardiology Department
Xanit International Hospital
Benalmadena
Malaga
Spain

JOAQUINA LOPEZ MORA
Centro de Diagnostico Dr. E. Rossi
Affiliated to Buenos Aires University
Buenos Aires
Argentina

Renata do A. Nogueira
Pediatric Radiology CDPI
Rio de Janeiro
Brazil

Miriam T. C. Porto
Pediatric Radiology CDPI
Rio de Janeiro
Brazil

Marcelo Potolicchio
Ultrasound Section
DADISA
Cadiz
Spain

Angel C. Rebollo Aguirre
Nuclear Medicine Department
Virgen de las Nieves Hospital
Granada
Spain

Ramon Ribes
Interventional Radiology and MR Units
Reina Sofia University Hospital
Cordoba
Spain

Santiago E. Rossi
Centro de Diagnostico Dr. E. Rossi
Affiliated to Buenos Aires University
Buenos Aires
Argentina

Pedro Segui
Ultrasound Unit
Radiology Department
Reina Sofia University Hospital
Cordoba
Spain

Juan Antonio Vallejo Casas
Department of Nuclear Medicine
Reina Sofia Hospital
Cordoba
Spain

Joan C. Vilanova
Department of Magnetic Resonance
Clinica Girona
Girona
Spain

Contributors

Sandra Baleato
Department of Magnetic Resonance
Clinica Girona
Girona
Spain

Melcior Sentis Criville
Breast and Gynecology Units
Fundacio Parc Tauli, Sabadell
Barcelona
Spain

Maria Martinez Galvez
Chief, Radiology Department
Hospital de Torrevieja
Alicante
Spain

Luisa Maria Mena Bares
Resident, Nuclear Medicine Department
Reina Sofia Hospital
Cordoba
Spain

Breast Imaging

MARINA ALVAREZ BENITO and JULIA CAMPS HERRERO
MELCIOR SENTIS CRIVILLE and MARIA MARTINEZ GALVEZ (Contributors)

Introduction

A breast imaging unit performs a variety of diagnostic techniques and image-guided interventional procedures. Mammography, ultrasound, galactography, and magnetic resonance imaging (MRI) are some of the most widely used modalities in breast imaging. Common image-guided interventional procedures in the breast are percutaneous biopsies guided by stereotaxy, ultrasound, or MRI, preoperative marking of non-palpable lesions, and the injection of radioactive substances in sentinel node biopsy.

The widespread use of mammography as a screening method for breast cancer in asymptomatic women has introduced many improvements in both the technique itself and in radiologists' reading skills. The BI-RADS (Breast Imaging Reporting and Data System) categories are now widely used in mammographic interpretation and reporting, allowing for uniformity in reports and improving communication between radiologists and clinicians. The latest edition includes a section for breast ultrasound and breast MRI, reflecting the progressively extensive use of these imaging modalities in breast imaging.

After mammography, ultrasound is undoubtedly the most widely used imaging technique in breast imaging: it is the only imaging modality employed in young patients and is a complementary method to mammography in older patients, as well as a crucial technique in image-guided procedures.

Breast MRI has recently been acknowledged to have the highest sensitivity for breast cancer. The main indications for breast MRI are local staging in patients with breast cancer, searching for the primary tumor in cancer of unknown origin, assessing the integrity of breast implants, monitoring the response to neoadjuvant chemotherapy for breast cancer, and screening in high-risk patients. The use of MRI by experienced professionals has been demonstrated to influence the therapeutic approach in breast cancer patients.

One of the most important improvements in recent years is perhaps the introduction of percutaneous breast biopsy procedures. Percutaneous breast biopsies enable histological study of a lesion with lower costs and less morbidity than a surgical biopsy. Various systems, gauges, and methods of approach enable us to biopsy almost any type of breast lesion. Breast interventional procedures are not limited to obtaining material for histologic diagnosis or placing markers for surgical guidance: percutaneous excision or radiofrequency ablation of breast cancers are promising techniques that are currently in the developmental stages.

The diversity of therapeutic approaches to breast cancer, such as breast-conserving surgery, sentinel node biopsy, or systemic treatment with chemotherapy entail important consequences for radiologists, because we are expected to provide accurate information on the size, number, and distribution of tumors, the condition of regional lymph nodes, as well as the outcome of systemic or surgical therapies.

Digital imaging also poses new challenges and opportunities, enabling us to improve our diagnoses through better image quality and the introduction of new imaging algorithms.

In summary, the breast imaging unit is at present a dynamic and wide-ranging section that assumes great responsibilities in the diagnostic and therapeutic process of breast cancer, working together with the rest of the specialist physicians dedicated to breast diseases.

Case 1
■ Ductal Carcinoma in Situ

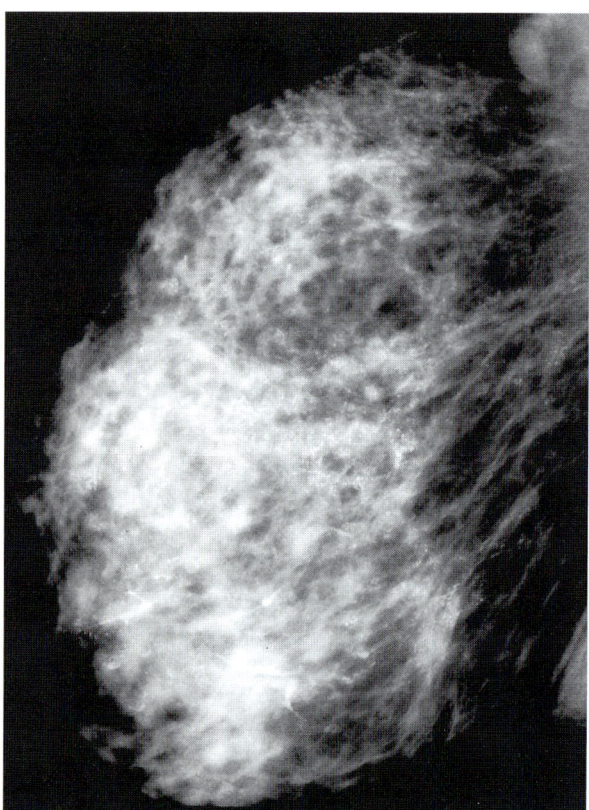

Fig. 1.1.1

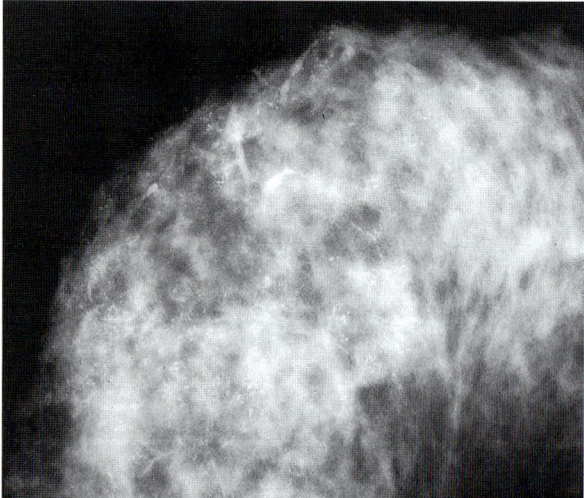

Fig. 1.1.2

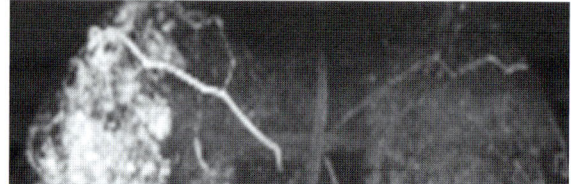

Fig. 1.1.3

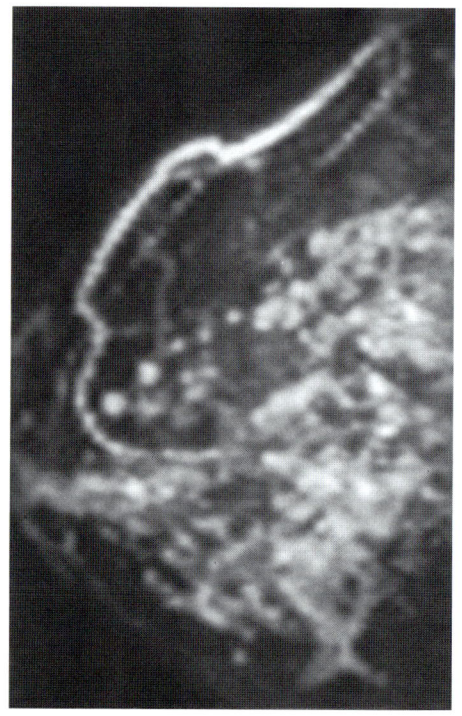

Fig. 1.1.4

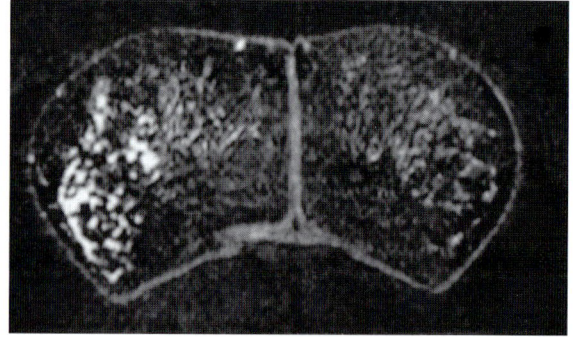

Fig. 1.1.5

A 57-year-old woman presented with spontaneous bloody nipple discharge from the right breast and no palpable abnormalities. The patient had no family history of breast cancer and had already reached menopause but was not on hormone replacement therapy. A mammogram showed extensive microcalcifications in both outer quadrants of the right breast. Ultrasound showed a diffuse area of decreased acoustic through-transmission and an ultrasound-guided biopsy with a 14-gauge needle was performed. Core-biopsy histology revealed a high-grade ductal carcinoma in-situ (DCIS). Axillary ultrasound revealed no suspicious lymph nodes. A breast MRI was then performed to stage the patient's disease and revealed a segmental enhancement distributed in both outer quadrants, but no other suspicious enhancing areas were identified in the rest of either gland. The patient was treated with a right mastectomy due to the extensive and multicentric distribution of the disease and histopathology confirmed high-grade comedo DCIS in all four quadrants and a negative sentinel node biopsy (G3 pTis pN0 pMx).

Comments

Ductal carcinoma DCIS is a malignant intraductal epithelial proliferation that is confined to the duct by its basement membrane. It manifests with a variety of histologic patterns and can be broadly divided into comedo (high-grade) and non-comedo subtypes. Comedo refers to the plug-like appearance of necrotic material that fills the affected ducts. This necrotic debris results in the typical fine, linear branching pattern of calcifications seen on mammography. Granular pleomorphic microcalcifications are uncommon in comedo DCIS. Comedo DCIS is considered to be the more aggressive DCIS subtype and tends to present more malignant cytologic features and behavior than non-comedo DCIS. It has, therefore, a higher probability of microinvasion. Mammography is the imaging test of choice in DCIS; it shows rod-shaped linear, branching or granular calcifications. Microcalcifications can be very unspecific; therefore, all suspicious microcalcifications are biopsied. MRI is an adjunct to mammography that is used to stage the disease extension and is particularly useful in dense breasts, but although the sensitivity of MRI for high-grade DCIS is relatively high (80–90%), low or intermediate grade DCIS show variable degrees of enhancement.

Imaging Findings

Oblique mediolateral and partial craniocaudal mammographic views (Figs. 1.1.1 and 1.1.2) show a dense breast pattern and diffuse granular and branching microcalcifications extending over both outer quadrants. Maximum intensity projections (MIP) of the corresponding breast MRI (Figs. 1.1.3 and 1.1.4) in craniocaudal and lateral views show diffuse enhancement in both outer quadrants. Coronal subtraction MRI image (Fig. 1.1.5) depicts enhancement in the breast that shows nodular and linear morphology patterns, highly suggestive of DCIS.

Case 2
■
Invasive Ductal Carcinoma with MRI Staging

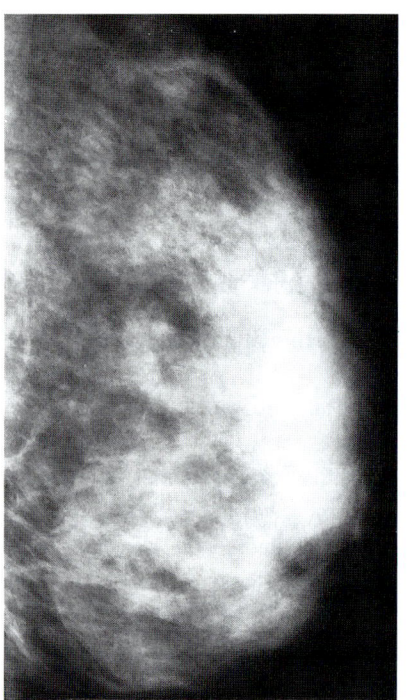

Fig. 1.2.1

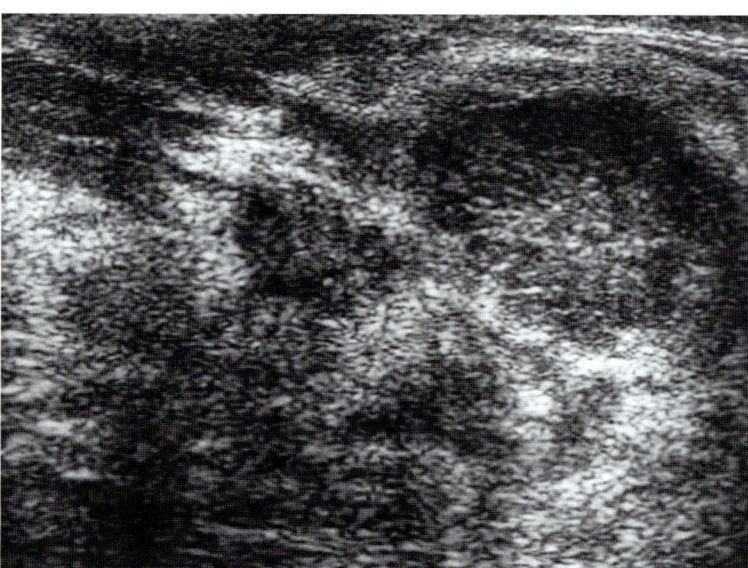

Fig. 1.2.2

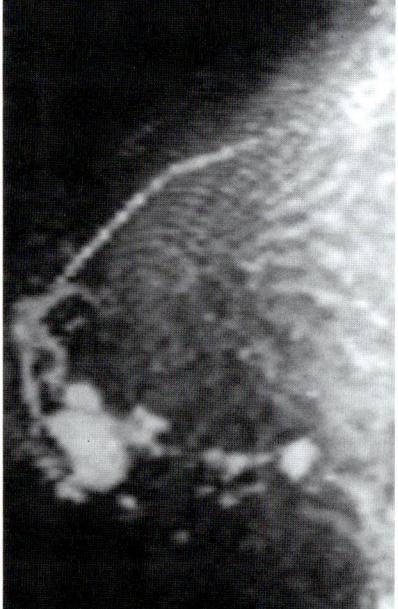

Fig. 1.2.3

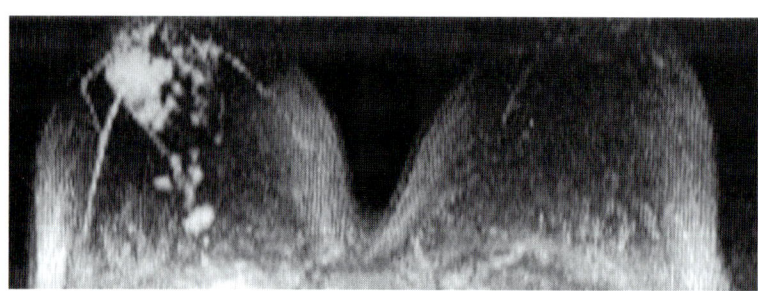

Fig. 1.2.4

A 32-year-old woman without a family history of breast cancer presented with a palpable lump in the lower-outer quadrant of the left breast. Four months earlier, breast ultrasound diagnosed a fibroadenoma in the same location but she had noticed that the palpable lump had become harder and had increased in size. Ultrasound was performed first and showed two ill-defined microlobulated solid masses that were biopsied with a 14-gauge needle because of the morphology and the rapid growth of the palpable lump. Axillary ultrasound showed no suspicious lymph nodes in the left axilla. Mammography showed dense breasts but no other remarkable findings. Core-biopsy histopathology showed an invasive ductal carcinoma (IDC). Breast MRI was performed to stage the disease and a multifocal distribution in the union of both lower quadrants with sparing of the nipple-areola complex was found. The patient underwent breast conserving surgery. Histological study of the surgical specimen confirmed IDC, not otherwise specified, grade II (pT2, pN0, pMx), and all the margins were free of tumor within 10 mm.

Comments

Invasive (or infiltrating) breast cancer can be broadly divided into ductal and lobular subtypes. Invasive ductal carcinoma accounts for the majority (90%) of invasive breast cancers and can be further divided into those "not otherwise specified" (NOS) and "special type" tumors. NOS breast carcinomas account for 50–75% of all invasive breast cancers. Their most distinctive appearance in mammography is that of a spiculated mass, although in women with dense breasts the margins of the tumor may be difficult to identify. Mammography has a 85–90% sensitivity for breast cancer; however, in dense breasts this figure drops to 40–60%. In these cases, palpation and ultrasound play a major role. At ultrasound, IDC shows decreased through-transmission and irregular margins. Breast MRI is increasingly being used to stage invasive breast cancer because its capability to depict tumor angiogenesis is independent of breast density. In expert hands, breast MRI improves breast cancer staging and changes the initial therapeutic approach planned taking only mammography and ultrasound into account in 18–30% of patients.

Imaging Findings

Oblique mediolateral view of the left breast (Fig. 1.2.1) shows a dense breast pattern where no distinct breast masses can be identified. Ultrasound image (Fig. 1.2.2) depicts two solid masses with microlobulated margins. The presence of two adjacent masses raises the possibility of multifocal disease but only MRI (Figs. 1.2.3 and 1.2.4) is able to show the distribution of the multifocal tumor along the union of both lower quadrants, providing more accurate information to guide surgical excision.

Case 3
■ Breast Implant Rupture

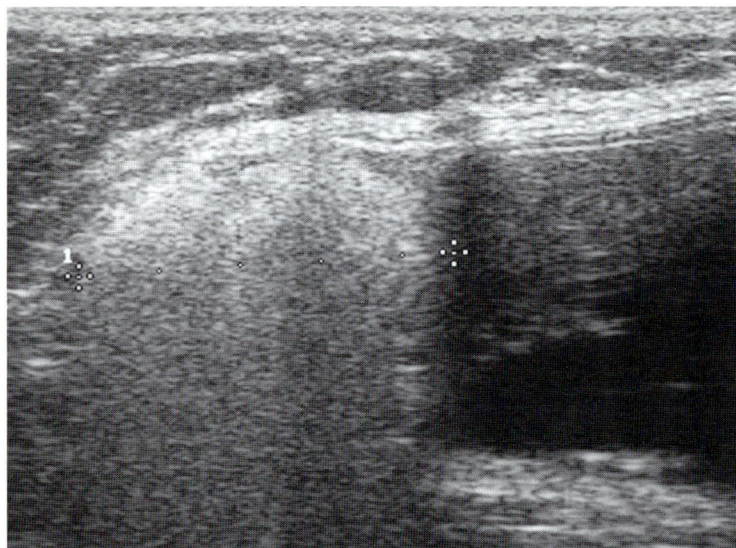

Fig. 1.3.1

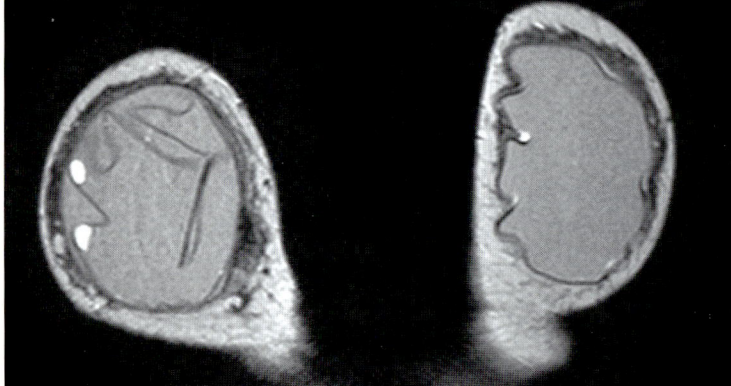

Fig. 1.3.2

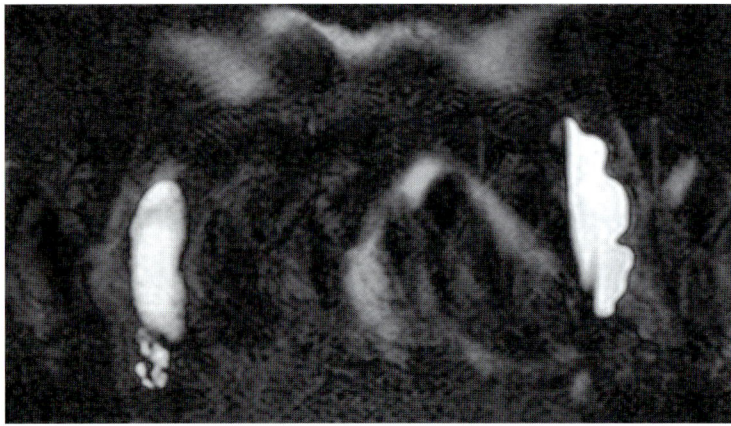

Fig. 1.3.3

A 42-year-old patient presented with pain and a palpable lump in the lower quadrants of the right breast. She had undergone a surgical procedure 10 years prior and had two retropectoral silicone breast implants. Breast ultrasound revealed an area suspicious for extracapsular silicone. Breast MRI was performed and an extracapsular rupture of the right breast implant was confirmed. A new breast implant was surgically implanted.

Comments

Breast implants can be classified as retroglandular or retropectoral depending on their anatomic location. In addition, taking into account the capsule of breast tissue surrounding the implant, breast implant ruptures are divided into intracapsular and extracapsular. This capsule begins to appear immediately after surgery as a natural foreign body reaction. Intracapsular ruptures leave the capsule intact around the implant and there is no extravasation of the implant's contents to the rest of the breast tissue or the lymph nodes. Conversely, extracapsular ruptures produce an extravasation of silicone or saline to the adjacent breast tissue or the lymph nodes. There have been concerns about the possibility of implants producing autoimmune diseases or cancer, but there is no solid evidence for that. Screening mammography is more easily performed in retropectoral implants. Breast MRI is generally accepted as the state-of-the-art technique for evaluating implant integrity, with a sensitivity of 74–100% and a specificity of 63–100%, depending on the technique applied and rupture criteria.

Imaging Findings

In Figure 1.3.1, an ultrasound image shows the "snow storm" sign caused by the presence of extracapsular silicone adjacent to the implant. In Figure 1.3.2, a T2-weighted MRI sequence shows the most certain sign of intracapsular rupture that usually accompanies extracapsular ruptures: the "linguine" sign, caused by the infolding of the implant's capsule within the silicone gel, often arranged parallel to the fibrous capsule. Small hyperintense droplets can be seen trapped between the folds of the ruptured implant capsule and are also a sign of rupture in double-lumen implants, where saline droplets mix with silicone gel. In Figure 1.3.3, a silicone-only MRI sequence, silicone droplets appear hyperintense, adjacent to but outside of the right breast implant in a 6 o'clock position. This is a certain sign of extracapsular rupture.

Case 4
■
Papillary Lesions

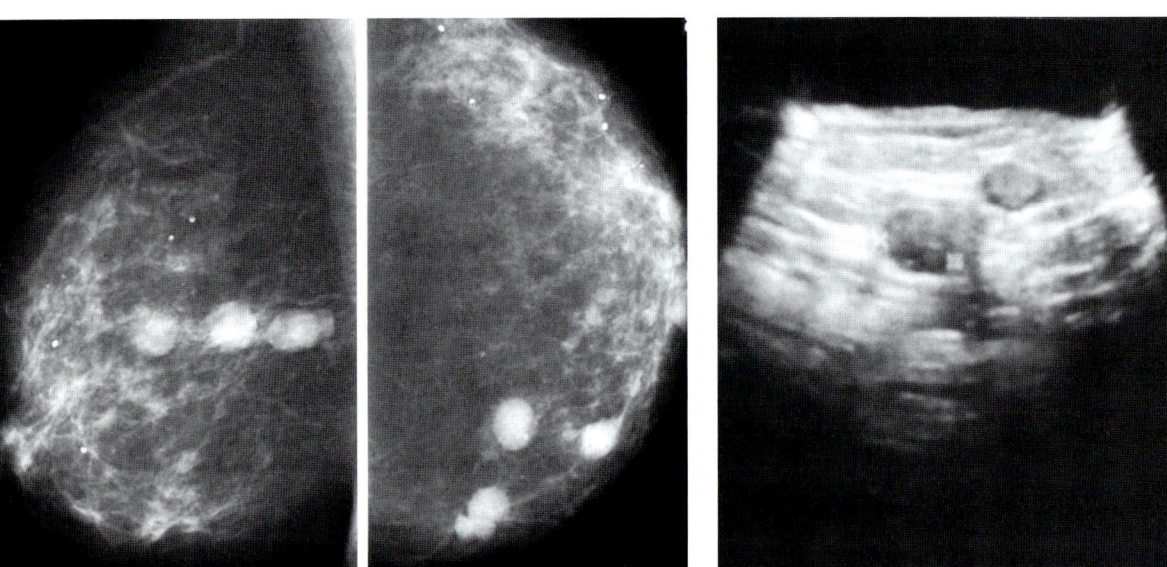

Fig. 1.4.1   Fig. 1.4.2

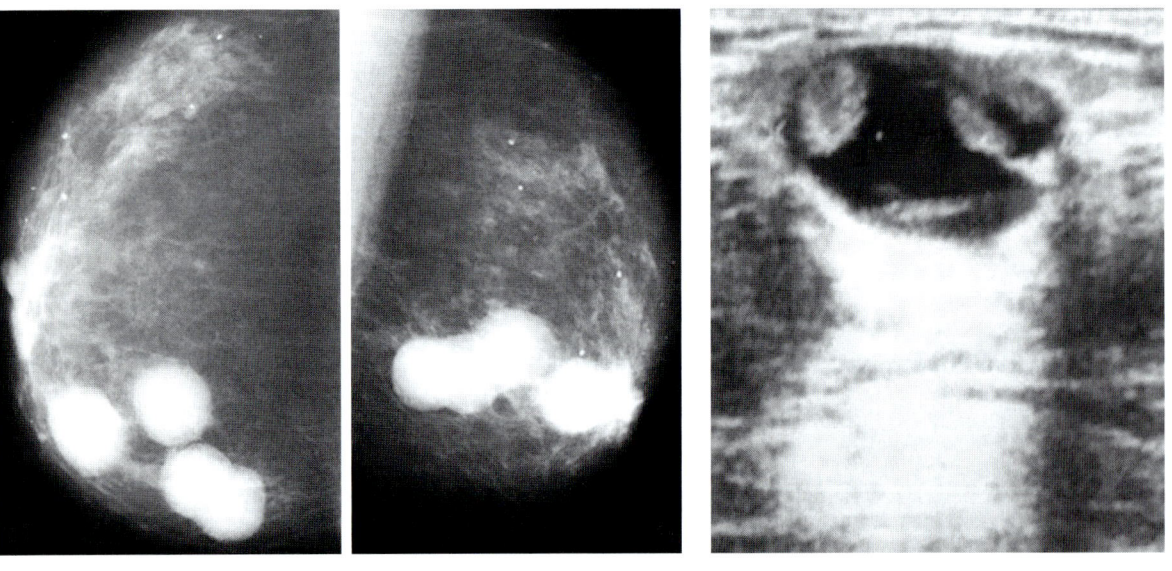

Fig. 1.4.3   Fig. 1.4.4

A 70-year-old woman presented with a right breast lesion adjacent to the nipple-areolar complex.

Physical examination revealed a well-circumscribed, mobile mass of firm consistency.

Bilateral mammography and diagnostic breast ultrasound showed multiple solid nodules with partly ill-defined borders in the right breast. Histological study of ultrasound-guided percutaneous biopsy samples yielded intraductal papilloma, and annual follow-up was recommended.

At follow-up mammography and breast ultrasound 12 months later, an increase in the size of the lesion was observed and surgical biopsy confirmed the existence of intracystic papillary carcinoma.

Comments

Papillary breast lesions constitute a varied and heterogeneous group of lesions, including intraductal papilloma, intracystic carcinoma, and papillary carcinoma, among others.

Except for intraductal papillary lesions, which tend to present clinically with nipple discharge, peripheral papillary lesions tend to appear at midlife, as single or multiple lesions, both synchronically and metachronically. Mammography characteristically shows one or multiple masses, which may be either well- or ill-defined; ultrasound shows mixed lesions with solid and cystic components.

The use of percutaneous biopsy in this type of lesions is controversial because cancer is often underestimated in these lesions with this technique; the false-negative results are probably due to their histological heterogeneity. Although findings of malignant papillary lesion after percutaneous biopsy permits therapeutic planning, surgical biopsy should be proposed in cases with findings of benign papillary lesion.

Some authors think that papillary lesions can evolve to become more aggressive and patients with papillary lesions present a higher probability of developing breast carcinoma. Papillary carcinoma has a better prognosis than other types of ductal carcinoma.

Imaging Findings

Mammography carried out at the time of initial consultation (Fig. 1.4.1) shows multiple rounded and oval-shaped masses with partly ill-defined borders in the right breast. Breast ultrasound (Fig. 1.4.2) confirms their solid nature.

In the 12 month follow-up mammogram and breast ultrasound, an increase in the size of the lesions can be observed. Their ill-defined contours are highlighted in the mammogram (Fig. 1.4.3). The ultrasound image is characteristic, showing mixed lesions, with cystic and solid components (Fig. 1.4.4).

Case 5
■
Microcalcifications

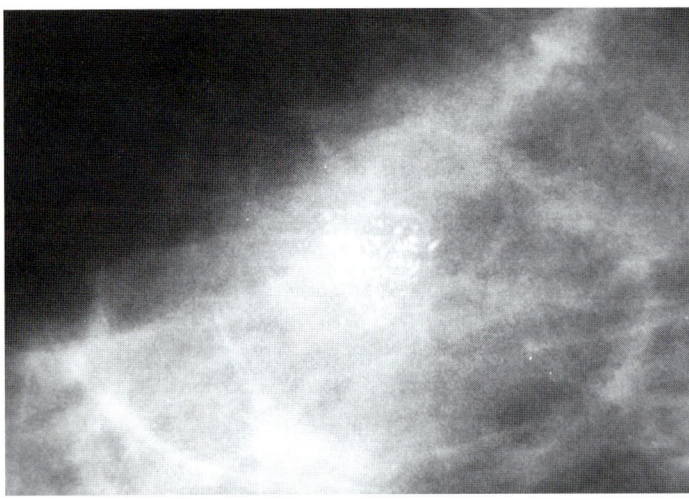

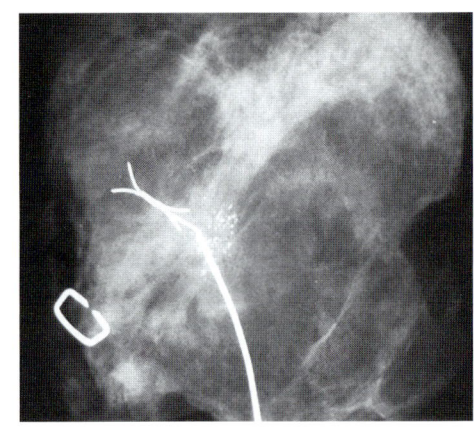

Fig. 1.5.4

Fig. 1.5.1

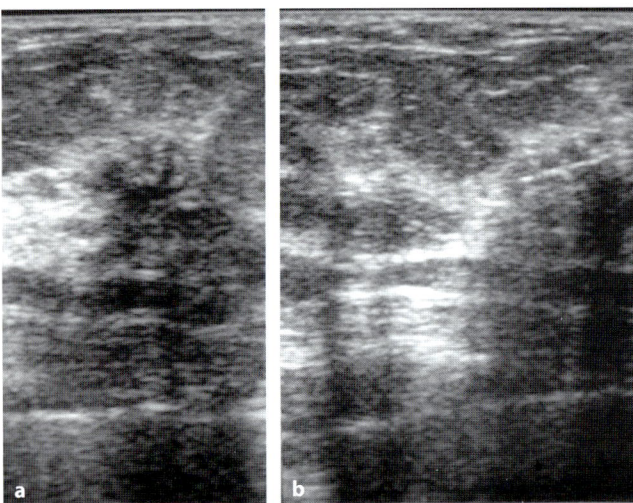

Fig. 1.5.2a,b

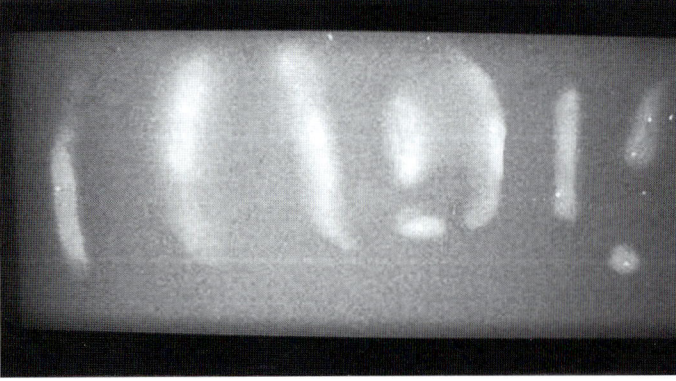

Fig. 1.5.3

A 55-year-old woman with unremarkable history was referred to the breast unit for a newly detected cluster of microcalcifications in the left breast at screening mammography.

Breast ultrasound confirmed the existence of microcalcifications in the upper-outer quadrant of the left breast, visualized as hyperechoic points on a hypoechogenic background. Histological study of material obtained at ultrasound-guided percutaneous biopsy yielded infiltrating ductal carcinoma with an in-situ component. The patient underwent tumorectomy and selective sentinel-node biopsy (SBSN). Definitive pathologic staging was stage I (T1 N0M0).

Programs for early breast cancer detection have favored the diagnosis of small lesions, without lymph-node involvement. In addition to having a more favorable prognosis, these lesions enable less aggressive treatments, such as conservative surgery as opposed to mastectomy or selective sentinel node biopsy instead of lymphadenectomy for axillary staging.

Microcalcifications are one of the forms of presentation of cancer and other breast lesions. The BIRADS system (Breast Imaging Reporting and Data System) recommends classifying them in relation to their morphology (typically benign, amorphous, heterogeneous, pleomorphic, linear, or linear and branching) and distribution (cluster, segmental, linear, regional and diffuse).

Pleomorphic microcalcifications are suspicious for malignancy and are frequently associated to a carcinoma in-situ. Breast microcalcifications are usually biopsied under stereotactic guidance. On breast ultrasound, pleomorphic microcalcifications seen on a hypoechogenic background may signal the existence of an invasive component that calls for ultrasound-guided biopsy.

Magnified view of the upper-outer quadrant of the left breast shows a cluster of pleomorphic microcalcifications (Fig. 1.5.1). Ultrasound shows multiple hyperechogenic points in the left image (Fig. 1.5.2a) that correspond to microcalcifications on a hypoechogenic area. Figure 1.5.2b (right) shows the microcalcifications traversed by a hyperechoic line representing the biopsy needle (Fig. 1.5.2).

It is essential to perform a radiograph of the specimen to confirm the presence of microcalcifications in the biopsy cores (Fig. 1.5.3). Furthermore, a radiograph of the surgical specimen should be carried out if breast-conserving surgery of nonpalpable lesions is performed. Figure 1.5.4 shows the surgical specimen containing the lesions, which are traversed by the needle localization wire; all have acceptable margins and one is marked with a surgical clip.

Case 6
■
Architectural Distortion

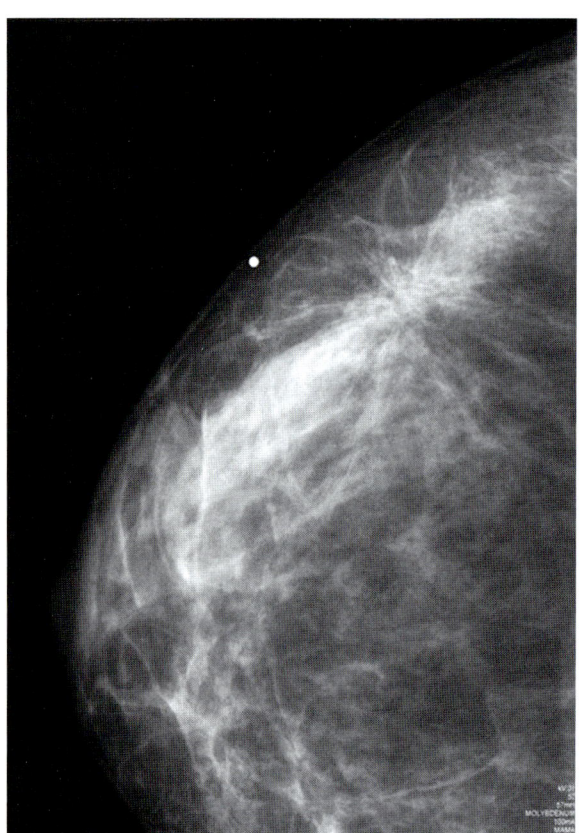

Fig. 1.6.1

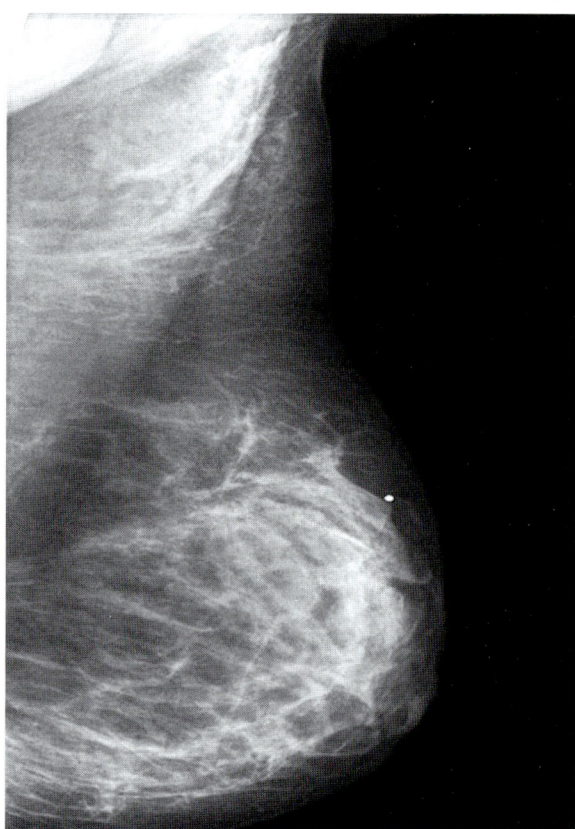

Fig. 1.6.2

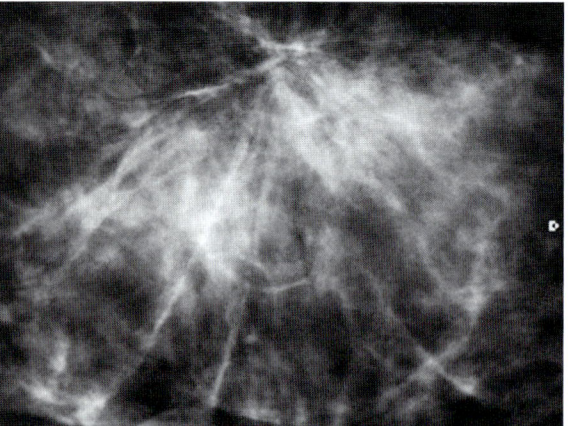

Fig. 1.6.3

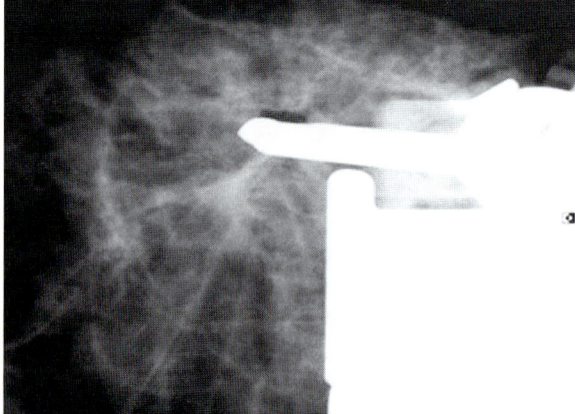

Fig. 1.6.4

A 25-year-old woman presented with a retroareolar mass. Breast ultrasound was initially performed and showed multiple bilateral circumscribed solid masses and a hypoechoic area in the upper-outer quadrant of the right breast.

The diagnostic study was completed with mammography, in which an image of architectural distortion in the upper-outer quadrant of the right breast could be observed. Histological study of material obtained by stereotactic-guided vacuum-assisted percutaneous biopsy found a radial scar, and this finding was confirmed in the surgical biopsy specimen some weeks later.

Comments

In patients younger than 35, or younger than 30 with a family history of breast cancer, breast ultrasound should be the first diagnostic test when there is a palpable abnormality. This test should be complemented with a mammogram when ultrasound does not show any abnormality or shows a suspicious lesion.

Architectural distortion is one type of mammographic presentation of breast pathologies. It is often a subtle finding, described as the reorganization of the mammary tissue toward an eccentric point from the nipple. There are strands of tissue that converge toward a point forming a typical "star" or "whirlwind" shape.

Approximately 50% of cases are malignant, and it is impossible to predict its benign or malignant nature by imaging tests alone. Biopsy should be performed in cases of architectural distortion without previous surgery, injury, or biopsy, although the performance of a percutaneous biopsy in these lesions is controversial, since underestimation of the lesion or false-negative results can be obtained.

Larger gauge needles, such as those used in vacuum-assisted biopsy, improve the accuracy of the technique in comparison to core needle biopsy. Some authors claim that when a minimum of 12 cylinders are obtained with these systems, surgical biopsy can be avoided in the absence of atypia.

Imaging Findings

Craniocaudal and oblique mammographic views of the right breast show architectural distortion or alteration in the distribution of the mammary tissue in the upper-outer quadrant; linear tracts converge toward a point forming the typical "star" shape (Figs. 1.6.1 and 1.6.2).

Localized view (Fig. 1.6.3) of the percutaneous stereotactic biopsy depicts the linear tracts converging toward a central point in greater detail. Figure 1.6.4 confirms the location of the biopsy needle in relation to the lesion.

Case 7
■
Breast Cancer in Men

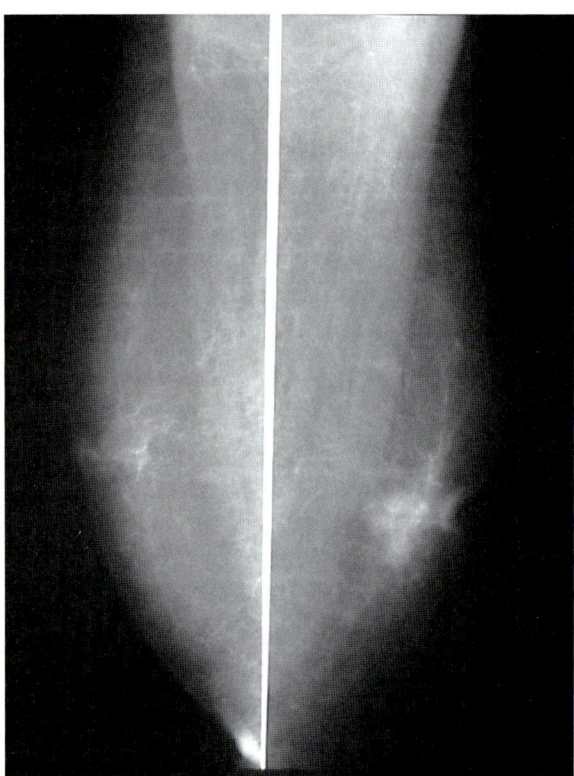

Fig. 1.7.1

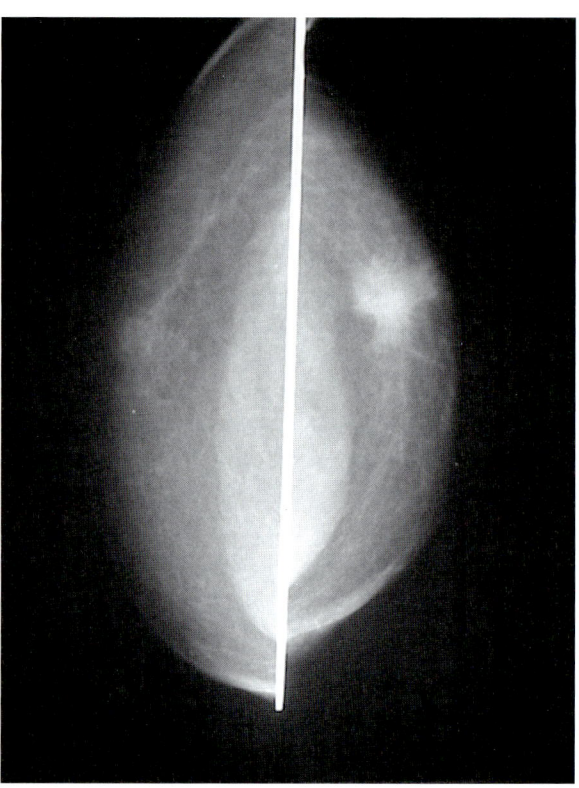

Fig. 1.7.2

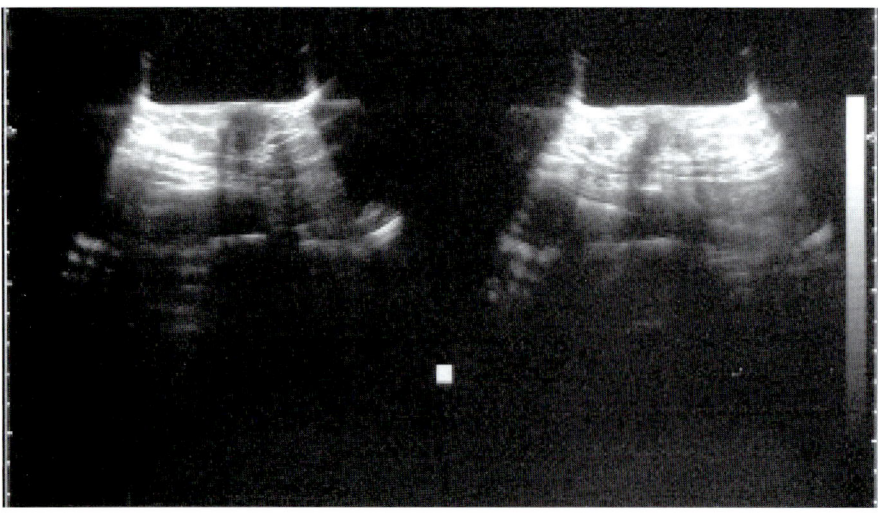

Fig. 1.7.3

A 58-year-old man, with no family or personal history of interest, presented with a mass in the left breast. The physical exam revealed the existence of a hard, fixed mass associated to nipple retraction.

Mammography and breast ultrasound confirmed the existence of a nodule highly suspicious for malignancy in the left breast.

Intraoperative biopsy followed by mastectomy and axillary emptying were carried out. Histopathologic study revealed infiltrating ductal carcinoma with axillary nodal extension.

Breast pathology in men constitutes less than 1% of all consultations in breast units.

Gynecomastia is clearly the most frequent breast pathology in men. It presents two peaks of incidence, one in puberty and another in the 6th or 7th decade of life. It is clinically characterized by a diffuse unilateral or bilateral increase in breast size or a retroareolar mass of soft consistency. Mammography shows an increase of breast tissue with a triangular morphology, central in relation to the nipple, without signs of malignancy.

After gynecomastia, breast carcinoma is the most frequent breast lesion in men. It constitutes less than 1% of breast carcinomas and less than 1% of malignant tumors in men. Clinically, it presents as a hard mass fixed to the surrounding tissues; it is eccentric to the nipple and may or may not be associated with other signs of malignancy. Mammographically, it is very similar to breast cancer in women but presents less varied forms. Given the smaller volume of male breast, extension to the nipple and the pectoral muscle is more frequent. Infiltration of the nipple favors lymphatic infiltration, and this has been considered one of the factors that worsens the prognosis of these patients.

Other breast lesions, such as cysts, abscesses, or lipomas, are less frequent in men.

Oblique (Fig. 1.7.1) and craniocaudal (Fig. 1.7.2) mammograms show a spiculated mass and nipple retraction, highly suspicious for malignancy (BI-RADS 5 category), in the left retroareolar region. The right breast shows fatty predominance with some isolated remains of fibroglandular tissue or rudimentary ducts in the retroareolar region.

Breast ultrasound confirms the existence of a solid and irregular nodule in this location.

Case 8
■
Breast Cancer and Simple Cyst

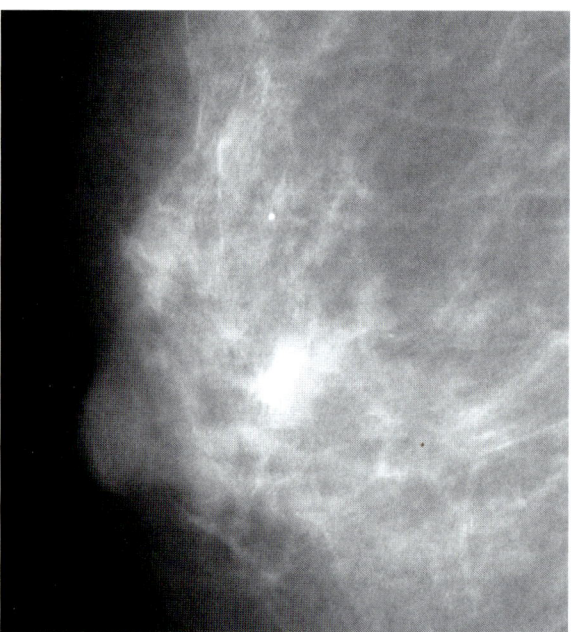

Fig. 1.8.1

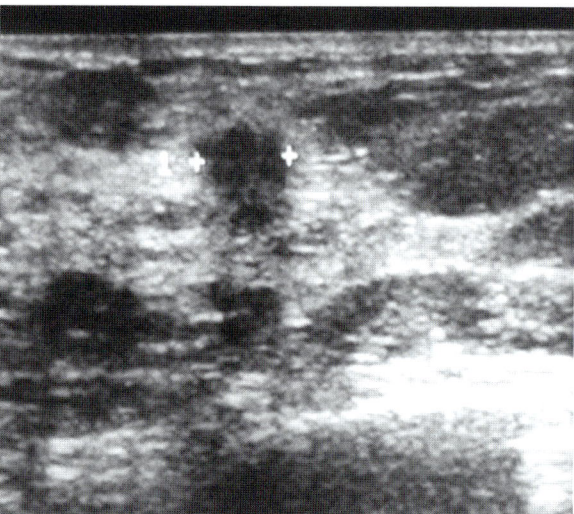

Fig. 1.8.2

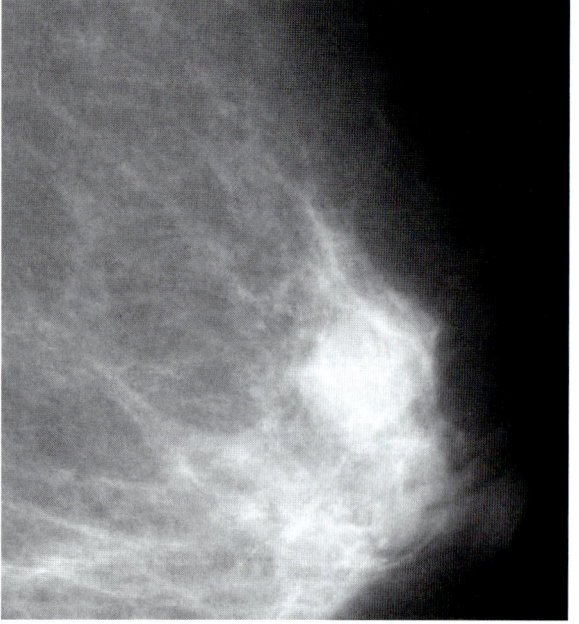

Fig. 1.8.3

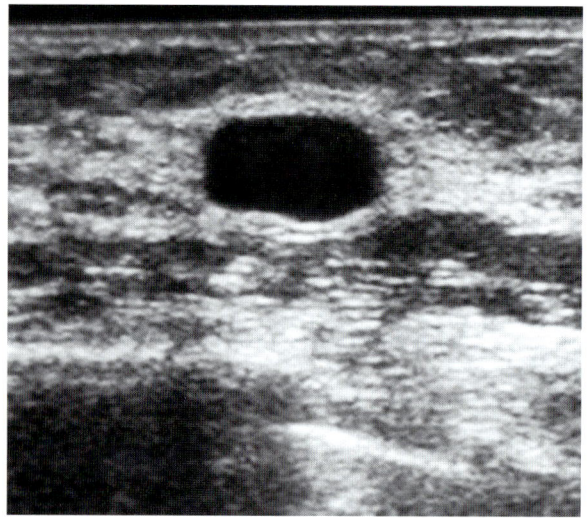

Fig. 1.8.4

A 64-year-old woman was referred from single-reader screening for a circumscribed retroareolar mass in the left breast.

Localized projections of both retroareolar regions and bilateral breast ultrasound showed an irregular solid mass in the right retroareolar region and a simple cyst in the left retroareolar region.

US-guided percutaneous breast biopsy confirmed the presence of an infiltrating ductal carcinoma in the right breast. The patient underwent mastectomy and axillary emptying, and the definitive classification was stage I (T1 N0 M0).

Mammography is the only accepted method for breast cancer screening and in recent years its use among healthy women has become more common through population-based screening programs. Population-based screening programs aim to reduce breast cancer mortality. These programs strive to obtain the maximum sensitivity (e.g., the highest detection rate) while keeping morbidity for participating women as low as possible. Some programs use double reading to improve their sensitivity.

The European guidelines recommend that a screening program should obtain a rate of participation of at least 70% of the target population and establish that the rate of detection should be higher than 3 in 1000 in women who participate for the first time and higher than 1.5 in 1000 in women who participate in successive rounds. The recall rate (i.e, the percentage of women sent for complementary tests) should also be kept within acceptable limits (lower than 7% in initial rounds and lower than 5% in successive rounds), since these practices cause anxiety and could affect the future involvement of women in the program.

The present case was referred to the breast unit by a single reader. The lesion that prompted the referral turned out to be a simple cyst. A carcinoma was detected in the other breast in the reference unit.

The localized mammographic views show an irregular-shaped mass with spiculated margins in the right retroareolar region (BI-RADS 5) (Fig. 1.8.1) and a well-circumscribed mass in left retroareolar region (BI-RADS 3) (Fig. 1.8.3).

Breast ultrasound confirmed the existence of a suspicious mass in right retroareolar region (Fig. 1.8.2).

The well-circumscribed mass in the left breast is anechoic with posterior acoustic enhancement; these findings are typical of a simple cyst, so the lesion that prompted referral is benign (BI-RADS 2) (Fig. 1.8.4).

Case 9
■
Breast Metastases

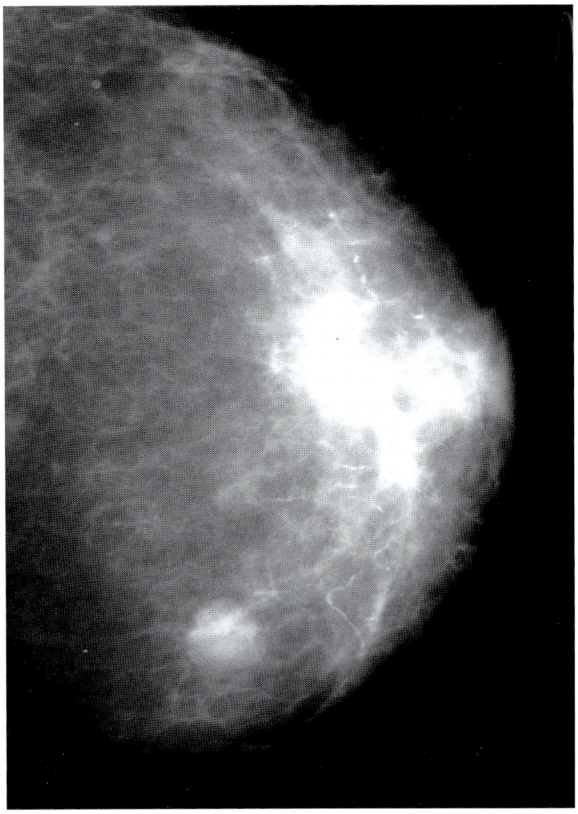

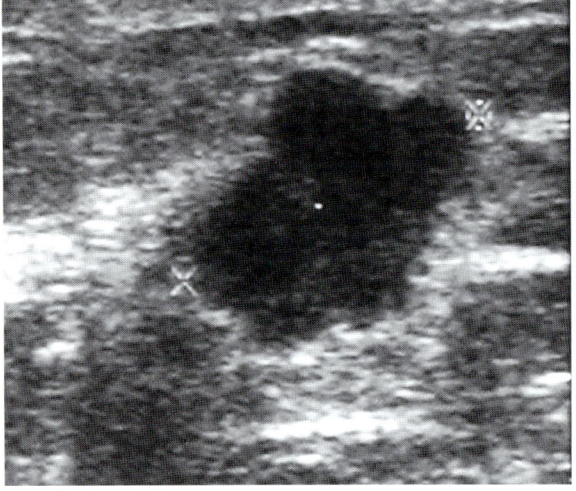

Fig. 1.9.1

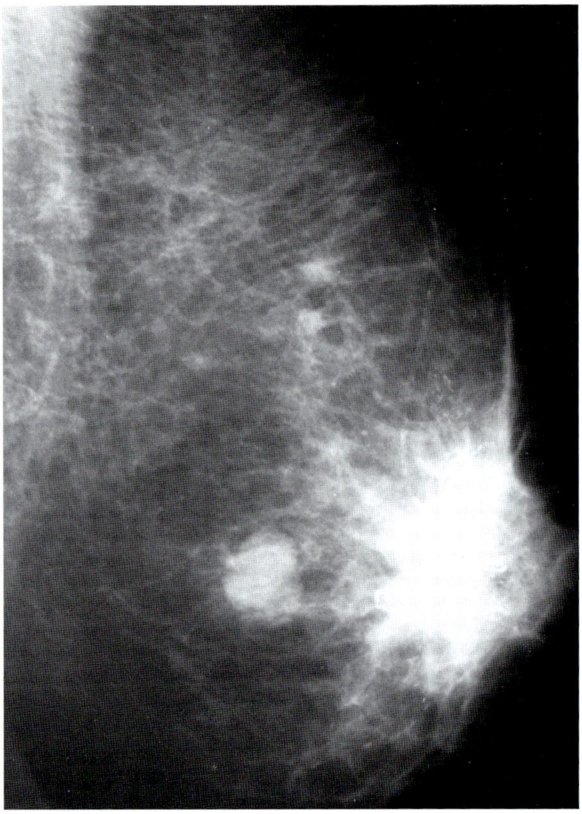

Fig. 1.9.2

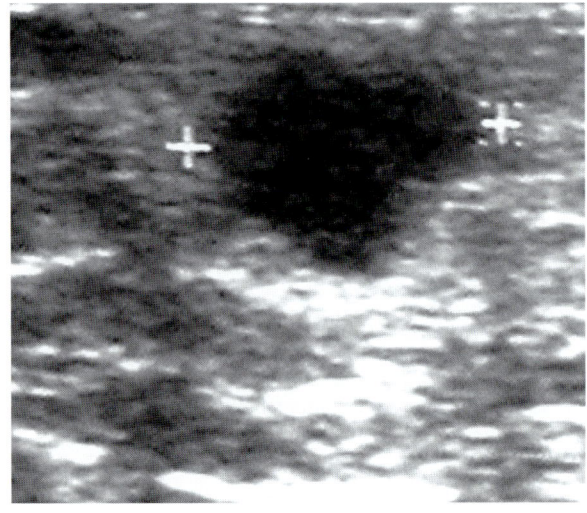

Fig. 1.9.3

Fig. 1.9.4

A 61-year-old woman, with no family history of interest, presented with an ipsilateral axillary node six years after the excision of a cutaneous melanoma. She underwent axillary emptying and nodal infiltration by melanoma was confirmed.

One year after axillary emptying, she presented with a right mammary nodule and an axillary node. Bilateral mammography confirmed the existence of a nodule in her right breast. Ultrasound demonstrated the solid nature of the nodule and revealed a right axillary node.

US-guided percutaneous biopsy of both the mammary nodule and the axillary node yielded melanoma metastases in both at histological examination. The patient underwent right tumorectomy and removal of the axillary node and was transferred to the oncology department to complete treatment.

Comments

The mammary gland is an infrequent site for metastasis. In 1903 the first case of mammary metastasis was reported and until 1991, only 300 cases of different metastatic tumors in the mammary gland had been published, the most frequent being leukemias, lymphomas, ovary neoplasms, and soft-tissue sarcomas.

The differential diagnosis between metastasis and primary neoplasms of the breast should be carried out due to the prognostic and therapeutic implications involved.

Mammographically, metastatic lesions tend to appear as single nodules, although they can also be multiple. They tend to be superficial and can be well- or ill-defined. Diagnostic ultrasound is used to confirm the solid nature of the lesions, to improve their characterization, and to guide biopsy.

Imaging Findings

In the oblique and craniocaudal mammographic projections, a well-delimited, high-density nodule is observed in the upper-outer quadrant of the right breast (Figs. 1.9.1 and 1.9.2).

Diagnostic ultrasound carried out in both breasts and axillae confirms the solid nature of the mammary nodule (Fig. 1.9.3). In addition, it revealed another right axillary node with the same characteristics (Fig. 1.9.4).

Case 10
■
Locorregional Staging

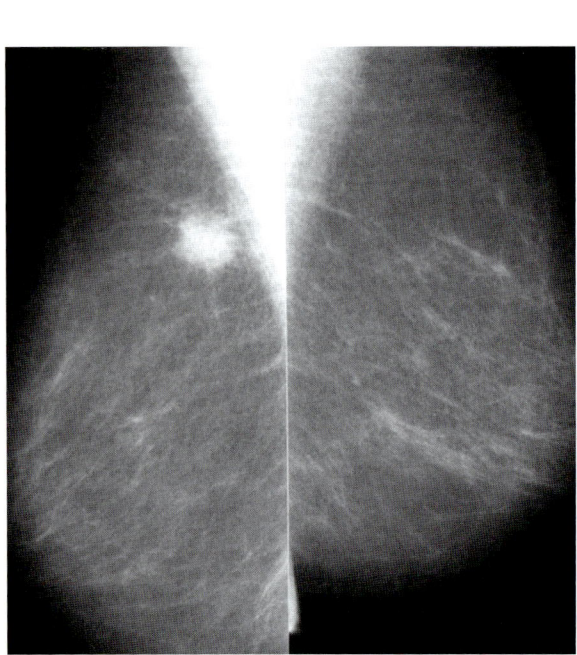

Fig. 1.10.1

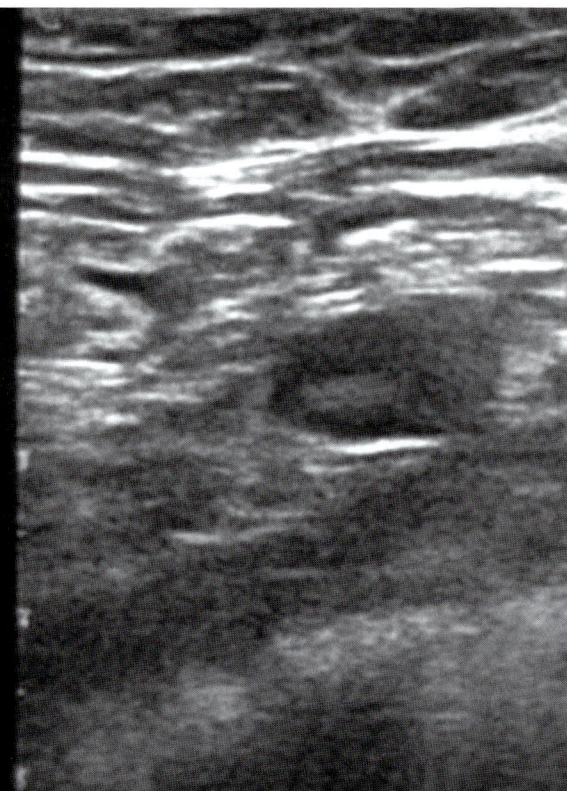

Fig. 1.10.3

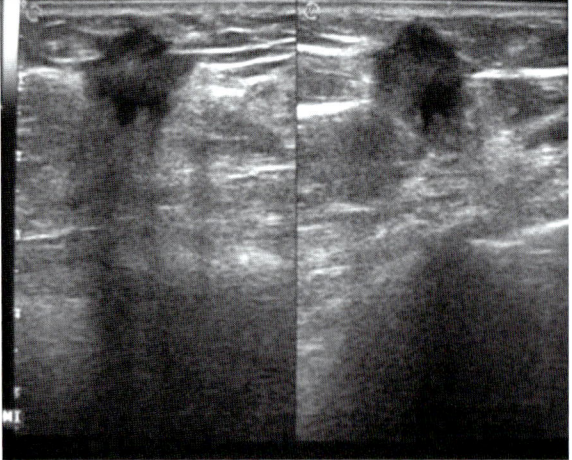

Fig. 1.10.2

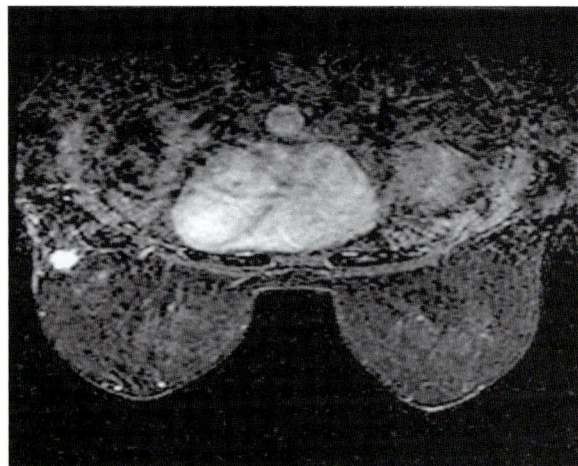

Fig. 1.10.4

56-year-old woman without prior history of interest presented with a nodule in her left breast after some months' evolution.

Bilateral mammography found a spiculated, hyperdense nodule in the upper-outer quadrant of the left breast, highly suspicious for malignancy (BI-RADS 5).

Diagnostic ultrasound confirmed its solid nature and revealed a suspicious node in the left axilla.

In the same diagnostic act, US-guided percutaneous mammary and axillary node core biopsy was carried out; infiltrating ductal carcinoma and axillary node infiltration were diagnosed at histology.

A dynamic breast MRI was performed to rule out other tumor foci in either breast. The patient underwent tumorectomy and axillary emptying, and the definitive classification was stage II (T1 N1 M0).

Comments

Nodules are one of the most frequent presentations of breast cancer. BIRADS recommends classifying them according to shape (round, oval-shaped, lobulated, or irregular), contour (circumscribed, ill-defined, microlobulated, darkened, or spiculated), and density (similar, equal or superior to the mammary parenchyma, or with fatty content).

Spiculated nodules have the highest probability of malignancy. Percutaneous biopsy enables histological study of lesions with less morbidity and lower costs than surgical biopsy and also allows women to participate in decisions about the therapeutic approach.

With the advent of selective sentinel node biopsy in the treatment of early stage breast cancer as an alternative to axillary dissection, sonographic assessment of the axilla with biopsy of suspicious adenopathies has gained great importance since it allows patients to be selected for the technique and helps to avoid false negatives. Loss of the oval-shaped morphology, loss of the fatty hilum, focal cortical enlargement, diffuse enlargement of the node cortex, and increased size are considered sonographic signs suspicious for neoplastic infiltration of a node.

Imaging Findings

Oblique mammographic projections (Fig. 1.10.1) show a round hyperdense nodule with spiculated contours in the upper-outer quadrant of the left breast. Diagnostic ultrasound confirms its solid nature and angular margins (Fig. 1.10.2).

A suspicious lymph node was identified on ultrasound. Although the node maintains its oval shape and fatty center, there is a focal enlargement of the lower pole cortex (Fig. 1.10.3).

Breast MRI (Fig. 1.10.4) confirms the existence of a contrast-enhanced nodule in the left breast. No other suspicious nodules were found.

Further Readings

Books

Americam College of Radiology. Breast Imaging Reporting and Data System. Reston VA; ACR, 2003

Breast Cancer – The Art and Science of Early Detection with Mammography. Tabar L, Tot T, Dean PB (2004). Thieme Medical Publishers. ISBN-13: 9781588902597

Breast Imaging. 3rd ed. Kopans DB (2006) Lippincott Williams & Wilkins. ISBN-13: 9780781747684

Breast Imaging Companion. Cardeñosa G (1997) Lippincott-Raven. ISBN-13: 9780397517787

Diagnostic Breast Imaging: Mammography, Sonography, Magnetic Resonance Imaging, and Interventional Procedures. 2nd ed. Heywang-Koebrunner S (2001) Thieme Medical Publishers. ISBN-13: 9781588900333

European guidelines for quality assurance in mammography screening. de Wolf CJ, Perry N (1996). European Communities / Union (EUR-OP/OOPEC/OPOCE). ISBN-13: 9789282774304

Practical Breast Pathology. Tot T, Tabar L, Dean PB (2002) Thieme Medical Publishers. ISBN-13: 9781588900913

Radiology: Diagnosis, Imaging, Intervention. Taveras JM, Ferrucci JT (2003) Lippincott Williams & Wilkins. ISBN-13: 9780015342449

The Practice of Breast Ultrasound: Techniques, Findings, Differential Diagnosis. Madjar H (2000) Thieme Medical Publishers. ISBN-13: 9781588904485

Diagnosis of Diseases of the Breast. 2nd ed. Bassett LW, Jackson V, Fu K, Fu Y (1997) Saunders Company. ISBN-13 9780721695631

Americam College of Radiology. Breast Imaging Reporting And Data System. Reston VA; ACR, 2003

Breast Imaging. Kopans DB 2001. Lippincott-Raven

Web-Links

http://acr.org/s_acr/sec.asp?CID=549&DID=14210
http://emedicine.com/radio/BREAST.htm
http://guideline.gov/Compare/comparison.aspx?file=BRSCREEN13.inc
http://imaginis.com/pro/teaching_files/
http://radiographics.rsnajnls.org/cgi/collection/breast_imaging
http://rad.washington.edu/breast/
http://radquiz.com/Breast%20Imaging.htm
http://rsna.org/education/archive/breast.cfm
http://sbi-online.org/sbi_home/education/fellowship_programs/breast_imaging__3
http://sprojects.mmi.mcgill.ca/mammography/cases.htm

Articles

Adepoju LJ, Chun J, El-Tamer M, Ditkoff BA, Schnabel F, Joseph KA. The value of clinical characteristics and breast-imaging studies in predicting a histopathologic diagnosis of cancer or high-risk lesion in patients with spontaneous nipple discharge. Am J Surg 2005; 190(4):644–646

Adrales G, Turk P, Wallace T, Bird R, Norton HJ, Greene F. Is surgical excision necessary for atypical ductal hyperplasia of the breast diagnosed by Mammotome? Am J Surg 2000; 180(4):313–315

Agoff SN, Lawton TJ. Papillary lesions of the breast with and without atypical ductal hyperplasia: can we accurately predict benign behavior from core needle biopsy? Am J Clin Pathol 2004; 122(3):440–443

Al Sarakbi W, Worku D, Escobar PF, Mokbel K. Breast papillomas: current management with a focus on a new diagnostic and therapeutic modality. Int Semin Surg Oncol 2006; 3:1

Alleva DQ, Smetherman DH, Farr GH, Cederbom GJ. Radial scar of the breast: Radiologic-pathologic correlation in 22 cases. Radiographics 1999; 19:S27–S35

Alonso-Bartolomé P, Vega-Bolívar A, Torres-Tabanera M, Ortega E, Acebal-Blanco M, Garijo-Ayensa F, Rodrigo I, Muñoz-Cacho P. Sonographically guided 11-G directional vacuum-assisted breast biopsy as an alternative to surgical excision: Utility and cost study in probably benign lesions. Acta Radiológica 2004; 4:390–396

Baker KS, Davey DD, Stelling CB. Ductal abnormalities detected with galactography: frequency of adequate excisional biopsy. AJR Am J Roentgenol 1994; 162(4):821–824

Baum F, Fischer U, Vosshenrich R, Grabbe E. Classification of hypervascularized lesions in CE MR imaging of the breast. Eur Radiol 2002; 12(5):1087–1092

Bedrosian I, Mick R, Orel SG et al. Changes in the surgical management of patients with breast carcinoma based on preoperative magnetic resonance imaging. Cancer 2003; 98:468–473

Berg WA. When is core breast biopsy or fine-needle aspiration not enough? Radiology 1996; 198:313–315

Berg WA, Arnoldus Ch L, Teferra E, Bhargavan M. Biopsy of amorphous breast calcifications: Pathologic outcome and yield at stereotactic biopsy. Radiology 2001; 221:495–503

Berube M, Curpen B, Ugolini P, Lalonde L, Ouimet-Olivia D. Level of suspicion of a mammographic lesion: use of features defined by BI-RADS lexicon and correlation with large-core breast biopsy. Can Assoc Radiol J 1998; 49(4):223–228

Brenner RJ. Strategies in the evaluation of breast asymmetries. Appl Radiol 1998; 27:15–20

Brenner RJ, Sickles EA. Surveillance mammography and stereotactic core breast biopsy for probably benign lesions: a cost comparison study. Acad Radiol 1997; 4:419–425

Ciatto S, Houssami N, Ambrogetti D, Bonardi R, Collini G, Del Turco MR. Minority report – false negative breast assessment in women recalled for suspicious screening mammography: imaging and pathological features, and associated delay in diagnosis. Breast Cancer Res Treat 2007; 105(1):37–43

Ciatto S, Morrone D, Catarzi S, Del Turco MR, Bianchi S, Ambrogetti D, Cariddi A. Radial scars of the breast: Review of 38 consecutive mammographic diagnoses. Radiology 1993; 187:757–760

Cohen MA, Sferlazza SJ. Role of sonography in evaluation of scars of the breast. AJR Am J Roentgenol 2000; 174:1075–1078

Costantini M, Belli P, Lombardi R, Franceschini G, Mule A, Bonomo L. Characterization of solid breast masses: use of the sonographic breast imaging reporting and data system lexicon. J Ultrasound Med 2006; 25(5):649–659

Dershaw DD, Morris EA, Liberman L, Abramson AF. Non-diagnostic stereotaxic core breast biopsy: Results of rebiopsy. Radiology 1996; 198:323–325

Diebold T, Hahn T, Solbach C, Rody A, Balzer JO, Hansmann ML, Marx A, Viana F, Peters J, Jacobi V, Kaufmann M, Vogl TJ. Evaluation of the stereotactic ^{8}G vacuum-assisted breast biopsy in the histologic evaluation of suspicious mammography findings (BI-RADS IV). Invest Radiol 2005; 40(7):465–471

Diebold T, Jacobi V, Krapfl E, von Minckwitz G, Solbach C, Ballenberger S, Hochmuth K, Balzer JO, Fellbaum M, Kaufmann M, Vogl TJ. The role of stereotactic 11G vacuum biopsy for clarification of BI-RADS IV findings in mammography. Rofo 2003; 175(4):489–494

Feig SA. Adverse effects of screening mammography. Radiol Clin N Am 2004; 42:807–819

Fine RE, Israel PZ, Walker LC, Corgan KR, Greenwald LV, Berenson JE, Boyd BA, Oliver MK, McClure T, Elberfeld J. A prospective study of the removal rate of imaged breast lesions by an 11-gauge vacuum-assisted biopsy probe system. Am J Surg 2001; 182(4):335–340

Frouge C, Tristant H, Guinebretiere JM, Meunier M, Conteso G, Paola R, Blery M. Mammographic lesions suggestive of radial scars: Microscopic findings in 40 cases. Radiology 1995; 195:623–625

Gill HK, Ioffe OB, Berg WA. When is a diagnosis of sclerosing adenosis acceptable at core biopsy? Radiology 2003; 228:50–57

Govindarajulu S, Narreddy SR, Shere MH, Ibrahim NB, Sahu AK, Cawthorn SJ. Sonographically guided mammotome excision of ducts in the diagnosis and management of single duct nipple discharge. Eur J Surg Oncol 2006; 32(7):725–728

Graf O, Helbich TH, Fuchsjaeger MH, Hopf G, Morgun M, Graf C, Mallek R, Sickles EA. Follow-up of palpable circumscribed noncalcified solid breast masses at mammography and US: Can biopsy be averted? Radiology 2004; 233:850–856

Guenin MA. Benign intraductal papilloma: Diagnosis and removal at stereotactic vacuum-assisted directional biopsy guided by galactography. Radiology 2001; 218:576–579

Gupta RK, Gaskell D, Dowle CS, Simpson JS, King BR, Naran S, Lallu S, Fauck R. The role of nipple discharge cytology in the diagnosis of breast disease: a study of 1948 nipple discharge smears from 1530 patients. Cytopathology 2004; 15(6):326–330

Harms SE. Breast magnetic resonance imaging. Semin Ultrasound CT MR 1998; 19:104–120

Harvey JA. Sonography of palpable breast masses. Semin Ultrasound CT MR 2006; 27(4):284–297

Helvie MA, Pennes DR, Rebner M, Adler DD. Mammographic follow-up of low suspicion lesions: Compliance rate and diagnostic yield. Radiology 1991; 178:155–158

Hendrick RE, smith RA, Rutlege JH, Smart CR. Benefit of screening mammography in women aged 40–49: a new meta-analysis of randomized controlled trials. Monogr natl Cancer Inst 1997; 22:87–92

Hou MF, Huang TJ, Liu GC. The diagnostic value of galactography in patients with nipple discharge. Clin Imaging. 2001; 25(2):75–81

Huber S, Wagner M, Medl M, Czembirek H. Benign breast lesions: minimally invasive vacuum-assisted biopsy with 11-gauge needles-Patient acceptance and effect on follow-up imaging findings. Radiology 2003; 226:783–790

Hunerbein M, Raubach M, Gebauer B, Schneider W, Schlag PM. Ductoscopy and intraductal vacuum assisted biopsy in women with pathologic nipple discharge. Breast Cancer Res Treat 2006; 99:301–307

Huynh PT, Jarolimek AM, Daye S. The false-negative mammogram. Radiographics 1998; 18:1137–1154

Jackman RJ, Nowelss KW, Rodriguez-Soto J, Marzoni FA, Finkelstein SL, Shepard MJ. Stereotactic, automated, Large-core needle biopsy of nonpalpable breast lesions: False-negative and histologic understimation rates after long-term follow-up. Radiology 1999; 210:799–805

Johnson AT, Henry-Tillman RS, Smith LF, et al. Percutaneous excisional breast biopsy. Am J Surg 2002; 184:550–554

Kerlikowske K, Grady D, Rubin SM, Sandrock C, Ernster VL. Efficacy of screening mammography: a meta-analysis. JAMA 1995; 273:149–154

Kerlikowske K, Smith-Bindman R, Abraham LA, Lehman CD, Yankaskas BC, Ballard-Barbash R, Barlow WE, Voeks JH, Geller BM, Carney PA, Sickles EA. Breast cancer yield for screening mammographic examinations with recommendation for short-interval follow-up. Radiology 2005; 234:684–692

Kettritz U, Morack G, Decker T. Stereotactic vacuum-assisted breast biopsies in 500 women with microcalcifications: radiological and pathological correlations. Eur J Radiol 2005; 5(2):270–276

King TA, Scharfenberg JC, Smetherman DH, Farkas EA, Bolton JS, Fuhrman GM. A better understanding of the term radial scar. Am J Surg 2000; 180:428–433

Kirwan SE, Denton ERE, Nash RM, Humphreys S, Michell MJ. Multiple ^{14}G Stereotactic core biopsies in the diagnosis of mammographically detected stellate lesions of the breast. Clin Radiol 2000; 55:763–766

Kuhl CK. MRI of breast tumor. Eur Radiol 2000; 10:46–58

Kuzmiak CM, Dancel R, Pisano E, Zeng D, Cole E, Koomen MA, McLelland R. Consensus review: A method of assessment of calcifications that appropriately undergo a six-month follow-up. Acad Radiol 2006; 13(5):621–629

Lacquement MA, Mitchell D, Hollingswotrth AB. Positive predictive value of the breast imaging reporting and data system. J Am Coll Surg 1999; 189(1):34–40

Lee Ch. Screening mammography: proven benefit, continued controversy. Radiol Clin North Am 2002; 40(3):395–407

Lee CH, Philpotts LE, Horvath LJ, Tocino I. Follow-up of breast lesions diagnosed as benign with stereotactic core-needle biopsy: Frequency of mammographic change and false-negative rate. Radiology 1999; 212:189–194

Lee JM, Orel SG, Czerniecki BJ, Solin LJ, Schnall MD. MRI before reexcision surgery in patients with breast cancer. AJR Am J Roentgenol 2004; 182:473–480

Liberman L. Clinical management issues in percutaneous core breast biopsy. Radiol Clin North Am 2000; 38(4):791–806

Liberman L, Dershaw DD, Morris EA, Abramson AF, Thornton CM, Rosen PP. Clip placement after sterotactic vacuum-assisted breast biopsy. Radiology 1997; 205:417–422

Liberman L, Abramson AF, Squires FB, Glassman JR, Morris EA, Dershaw DD. The Breast Imaging and Reporting Data System: Positive predictive value of mammographic features and final assessment categories. AJR Am J Roentgenol 1998; 171:35–40

Liberman L, Feng TL, Dershaw DD, Morris EA, Abramson AF. US-guided core breast biopsy: use and cost-effectiveness. Radiology 1998; 208(3):717–723

Liberman L, Bracero N, Vuolo MA, et al. Percutaneous large-core biopsy of papillary breast lesions. AJR Am J Roentgenol 1999; 172:331–337

Liberman L, Kaplan JB, Morris EA, Abramson AF, Menell JH, Dershaw DD. To excise or to sample the mammographic target: What is the goal of stereotactic 11-gauge vacuum-assisted breast biopsy? AJR Am J Roentgenol 2002; 179:679–683

Lindfors KK, O'Connor J, Acredolo CR, Liston SE. Short-interval follow-up mammography versus immediate core biopsy of benign breast lesions: Assessment of patient stress. AJR Am J Roentgenol 1998; 171:55–58

Litherland JC. Should fine needle aspiration cytology in breast assessment be abandoned? Clin Radiol 2002; 57:81–84

Lomoschitz FM, Helbich TH, Rudas M, Pfarl G, Linnau KF, Stadler A, Jackman RJ. Stereotactic 11-gauge vacuum-assisted breast biopsy: Influence of number of specimens on diagnostic accuracy. Radiology 2004; 232(3):897–903

Lorenzen J, Wedel AK, Lisboa BW, Loning T, Adam G. Diagnostic mammography and sonography: concordance of the breast imaging reporting assessments and final clinical outcome. Rofo 2005; 177(11):1545–1551

Mandelblatt JS, Wheat ME, Monane M, Moshief RD, Hollenberg JP, Tang J. Breast cancer screening for elderly women with and without comorbid conditions: a decision analysis model. Ann Intern Med 1992; 116:722–730

Mendelson EB, harris KM, Doshi N, Tobon H. Infiltrating lobular carcinoma: mammographic patterns with pathologic correlation. AJR Am J Roentgenol 1989; 153:265–271

Mendez A, Cabanillas F, Echenique M, Malekshamran K, Perez I, Ramos E. Mammographic features and correlation with biopsy findings using 11-gauge stereotactic vacuum-assisted breast biopsy (SVABB). Ann Oncol 2003; 14:450–454

Mercado CL, Hamele-Bena D, Singer C, Koenigsberg T, Pile-Spellman E, Higgins H, Smith SJ. Papillary Lesions of the Breast: Evaluation with stereotactic directional vacuum-assisted biopsy. Radiology 2001; 221:650–655

Morris EA. Breast cancer imaging with MRI. Radiol Clin North Am 2002; 40:443–466

Moy L, Slanetz PJ, Moore R, Satija S, Yeh FD, McCarthy KA, Hall D, Staffa M, Rafferty EA, Halpern E, Kopans DB. Specificity of mammography and US in the evaluation of a palpable abnormality: Retrospective review. Radiology 2002; 225:176–181

Orel SG. MR imaging of the breast. Radiol Clin North Am 2000; 38:899–913

Orel SG, Schnall MD. MR Imaging of the breast for the detection, diagnosis, and staging of breast cancer. Radiology 2001; 220:13–30

Parker SH, Burbank F, Jackman RJ, et al. Percutaneous large-core breast biopsy: A multi-institutional study. Radiology 1994; 193:359–364

Parker SH, Jobe WE, Dennis MA, et al. US-guided automated large-core breast biopsy. Radiology 1993; 187(2):507–511

Paterok EM, Rosenthal H, Sabel M. Nipple discharge and abnormal galactogram. Results of a long-term study (1964–1990). Eur J Obstet Gynecol Reprod Biol 1993; 50:227–234

Pearson LK, Sickles EA, Frankel SD, Leung J. Efficacy of step-oblique mammography for çconfirmation and localization of densities seen on only one standard mammographic view. AJR Am J Roentgenol 2000; 174:745–752

Philpotts LE, Shaheen NA, Jain KS, Carter D, Lee CCH. Uncommon high-risk lesions of the breast diagnosed at stereotactic core-needle biopsy: Clinical importance. Radiology 2000; 216:831–837

Pijnappel M, Peeters HM, Hendriks HC and Mali Th M. Reproducibility of mammographic classifications for non-palpable suspect lesions with microcalcifications. Br J Radiol 2004; 77:312–314

Puglisi F, Zuiani C, Bazzocchi M, Valent F, Aprile G, Pertoldi B, Minisini AM, Cedolini C, Londero V, Piga A, Di Loreto C. Role of mammography, ultrasound and large core biopsy in the diagnostic evaluation of papillary breast lesions. Oncology 2003; 65(4):311–315

Rahbar G, Sie AC, Hansen GC, et al. Benign versus malignant solid breast masses: US differentiation. Radiology 1999; 213:889–894

Rosen EL, Bentley RC, Baker JA, Soo MS. Imaging-guided core needle biopsy of papillary lesions of the breast. AJR Am J Roentgenol 2002; 179:1185–1192

Rosen EL, Blackwell KL, Baker JA, et al. Accuracy of MRI in the detection of residual breast cancer after neoadjuvant chemotherapy. AJR Am J Roentgenol 2003; 181:1275–1282

Samardar P, de Paredes SE, Grimes MM, Wilson JD. Focal asymmetric densities seen at mammography: US and pathologic correlation. Radiographics 2002; 22:19–33

Sardanelli F, Giusepetti G, Panizza P, et al. Sensitivity of MRI versus mammography for detecting foci of multifocal, multicentric breast cancer in fatty and dense breasts using the whole-breast pathologic examination as a gold standard. AJR Am J Roentgenol 2004; 183(4):1149–1157

Sauter ER, Schlatter L, Lininger J, Hewett JE. The association of bloody nipple discharge with breast pathology. Surgery 2004; 136(4):780–785

Shapiro S, Venet W, Strax P, Venet L, Rosser R. 10 to 14-year effect of screening on breast cancer mortality. J Natl cancer Inst 1982; 69:349–355

Shulman SG, March DE. Ultrasound-Guided Breast Interventions: Accuracy of biopsy techniques and applications in patient management. Sem Ultrasound CT MR 2006; 27(4):298–307

Sickles EA. Periodic mammographic follow-up of probably benign breast lesions: results in 3184 consecutive cases. Radiology 1991; 179:463–468

Sickles EA. Non-palpable circumscribed, non-calcified solid masses: Likelihood of malignancy based on lesion size and age of patient. Radiology 1994; 192:439–442

Sickles EA. Management of probably benign breast lesions. Radiol Clin North Am 1995; 33:1123–1130

Sickles EA. Probably benign breast lesions: When should follow-up be recommended and what is the optimal follow-up protocol? Radiology 1999; 213:11–14

Sickles EA, Parker SH. Appropriate role of core breast biopsy in the management of probably benign lesions. Radiology 1993; 188:315

Simon JR, Kalbhen CL, Cooper RA, Flisak ME. Accuracy and complication guided vacuum-assisted core breast biopsy: Initial results. Radiology 2000; 215: 694–697

Simsir A, Waisman J, Thorner K, Cangiarella J. Mammary lesions diagnosed as "papillary" by aspiration biopsy: 70 cases with follow-up. Cancer 2003; 99(3):156-165

Smith DN, Rosenfield Darling ML, Meyer JE, et al. The utility of ultrasonographically guided large-core needle biopsy: results from 500 consecutive breast biopsies. J Ultrasound Med 2001; 20(1):43–49

Smith RA, Duffy SW, MPhil RG, Tabar L, Yen A, Chen T. The randomized trials of breast cancer screening: What have we learned? Radiol Clin North Am 2004; 42:793–806

Smith-bindman R, Kerlikowske K, Gebretsadik T. Is screening mammography effective in elderly women? Am J Med 2000: 108:112–119

Spencer NJB, Evans AJ, Galea M, et al. Pathological-radiological correlations in benign lesions excised during a breast screening programme. Clin Radiol 1994; 49:853–856

Thurfjell MG, Lindgren A, Thurfjell E. Nonpalpable breast cancer: Mammographic appearance as predictor of histologic type. Radiology 2002; 222:165–170

Varas X, Leborgne F, Leborgne JH. Non-palpable, probably benign lesions: role of follow-up mammography. Radiology 1992, 184:409–414

Varas X, Leborgne JH, Leborgne F, Mezzera J, Jaumandreu S, Leborgne F. Revisiting the mammographic follow-up of BI-RADS category 3 lesions. AJR Am J Roentgenol 2002; 179(3):691–695

Vargas HI, Vargas MP, Eldrageely K, González KD, Burla MI, Venegas R, Khalkhali I. Outcomes of surgical and sonographic assessment of breast masses in women younger than 30. Am Surg 2005; 71(9):716–719

Vizcaíno I, Gadea L, Andreo L, Salas D, Ruiz-perales F, Cuevas D, Herranz C, Bueno F. Short-term Follow-up Results in 795 Nonpalpable probably benign lesions detected at screening mammography. Radiology 2001; 219:475–483

Yasmeen S, Romano PS, Pettinger M, Chlebowski RT, Robbins JA, Lane DS, Hendrix SL. Frequency and predictive value of a mammographic recommendation for short-interval follow-up. J Natl Cancer Inst 2003; 95:429–436

Cardiovascular Imaging

2

ELOISA FELIU, RAMON RIBES, and SERGIO MEJIA

Introduction**

Cardiovascular disease is the leading cause of death in developed countries and represents a serious social, economic, and health problem. In cardiology, clinical tasks were initially only supported by plain films and EKG. Later, interventional cardiology was introduced. Then, Doppler echocardiography and isotopic methods brought about a radical change, providing cardiologists with real noninvasive methods to document the diagnosis in practically all aspects of cardiac disease, except for the anatomy of coronary arteries. The development of new noninvasive imaging techniques for the diagnosis and follow-up of cardiovascular diseases has meant a great revolution in the last two decades.

Since cardiology departments have taken charge of cardiac catheterization as well as echocardiography, radiologists have played only a minor role in the diagnosis of cardiovascular diseases. However, recent technical developments in computed tomography (CT) and magnetic resonance imaging (MRI) have enabled us to perform not only studies of cardiac morphology and tissue characterization, but also qualitative, semiquantitative, and quantitative assessment of the parameters of cardiac function. This has definitely contributed to increased interest of radiologists in this field.

Echocardiography is still the first choice for the diagnosis and follow-up of multiple cardiac diseases and it is usually performed by cardiologists.

During the last decade MRI has developed into an important diagnostic clinical tool in cardiology. From a technical point of view, MRI offers some special advantages over other diagnostic imaging methods. First, it does not use ionizing radiation. Second, it provides additional diagnostic information about tissue characteristics. Finally, MRI provides three-dimensional (3D) images.

One of the main difficulties of imaging the heart is heart movement. However, this difficulty has been overcome with the development of new sequences synchronized with heart movement as well as with respiratory motion. At present, not only the anatomy of the heart but also its function, metabolism, perfusion, and, more recently, proximal coronary artery status can be assessed with cardiovascular MRI. Furthermore, the administration of intravenous contrast provides knowledge about myocardial viability in ischemic heart disease and about fibrosis in several other myocardiopathies. Hence, cardiac magnetic resonance (CMR) is emerging as one of the most promising techniques for the study of congenital and acquired cardiac pathology.

In general, CMR is considered a complementary study to echocardiography when the latter is inconclusive for a specific cardiac pathology or due to technical difficulties; however, it is considered the first choice technique for the study of certain cardiac pathologies. Since the introduction of CMR in regular clinical practice, the number of clinical situations in which CMR is indicated has continued to grow.

Multidetector CT (MDCT) coronary angiography is an indispensable tool that should be mastered by every department active in cardiac imaging. Close cooperation between radiologists and cardiologists is necessary to adequately exploit this powerful technique.

Case 1

■

Acute Myocardial Infarction

A 57-year-old obese male heavy smoker with history of an inferior myocardial infarction 2 years prior was admitted with angina of recent onset. Cardiac catheterization showed severe anterior descending and marginal branch coronary artery disease and total occlusion of the right coronary artery. A CMR viability study was performed to evaluate possible revascularization therapy.

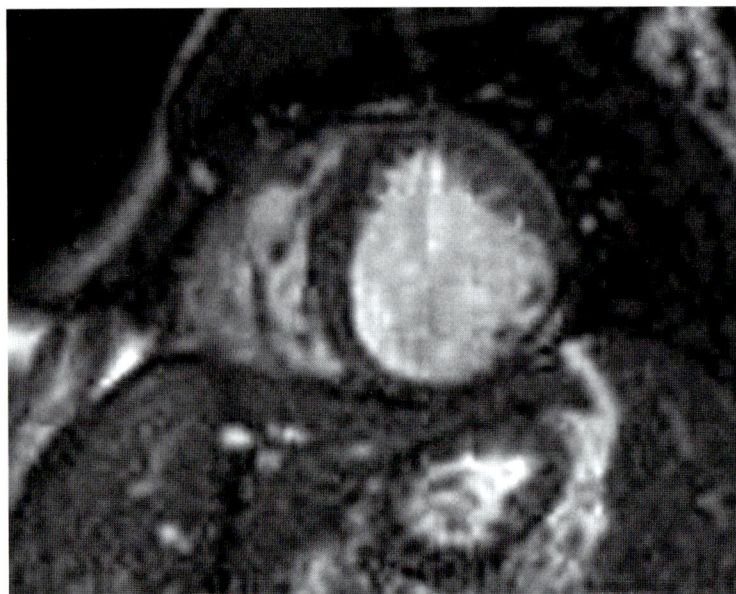

Fig. 2.1.1

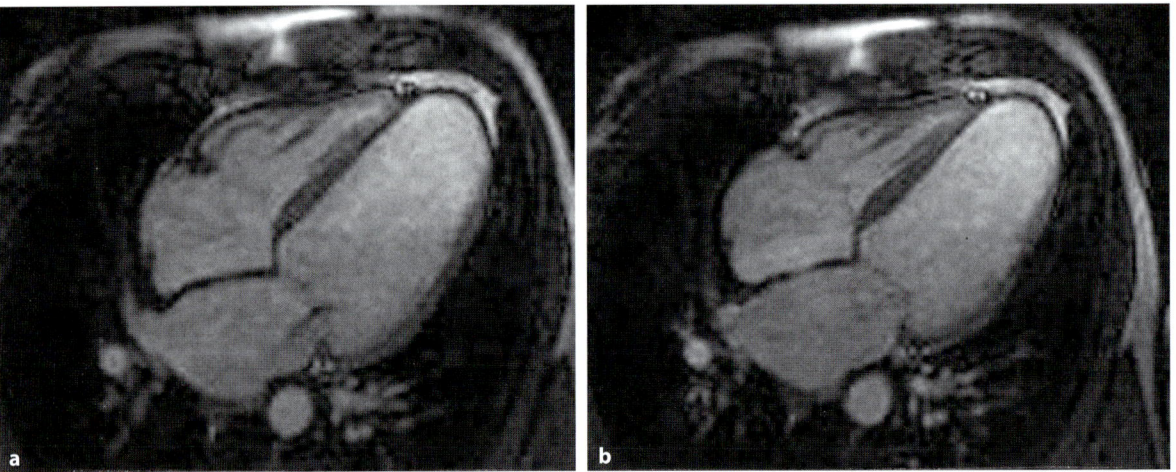

Fig. 2.1.2a,b

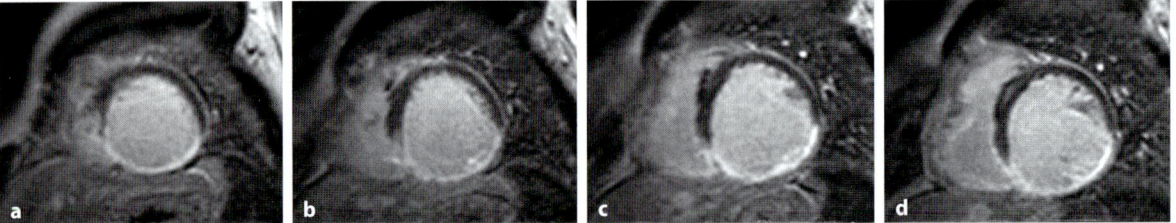

Fig. 2.1.3a–d

Acute myocardial infarction (AMI) results from a total thrombotic occlusion of an epicardial coronary artery. The absence of blood flow to the territory supplied by the occluded vessel causes cardiac tissue necrosis. Total occlusion of the vessel for more than 4–6 hours results in irreversible myocardial necrosis, but reperfusion within this period can salvage the myocardium and reduce morbidity and mortality.

AMI is classified as transmural when the full thickness of the muscle segment(s) is involved and nontransmural when the ischemic necrosis does not extend through the full thickness of myocardial wall segment(s). The endocardial and subendocardial zones of the myocardial wall are the least perfused regions of the heart and are most vulnerable to ischemia.

Classical symptoms of acute myocardial infarction include chest pain, dyspnea, nausea, vomiting, palpitations, sweating, and anxiety or a feeling of impending doom. Approximately one third of all myocardial infarctions are silent, without chest pain or other symptoms.

Coronary arteriography (CA) is the primary method of defining coronary anatomy in living patients. It provides not only an anatomic map of the coronary arteries, including the site, severity, and shape of stenotic lesions, but also information about the distal vessels. Furthermore, LV catheterization enables measurements of LV pressure and visual analysis of wall motion. Ventricular systolic and diastolic volume and ejection fraction can be calculated. Finally, apart from anatomic assessment of the coronary tree, CA also enables the culprit lesion(s) to be revascularized.

The accurate assessment of the extent and degree of myocardial injury is crucial in patients with acute or chronic myocardial infarction for individual risk stratification and therapy design. The differentiation of viable from nonviable myocardium helps to predict the success of revascularization (i.e., the recovery of regional function) and overall survival. The most common modalities used to this end are echocardiography, radionuclide angiography, and single photon emission computed tomography (SPECT). While all of these modalities have been used in clinical trials with good reproducibility, in clinical practice they are less precise. Cardiac magnetic resonance (CMR) has better sensitivity, reproducibility, and resolution. Cine-MR images allow assessment of cardiac morphology and function. Contrast-enhanced (CE) magnetic resonance imaging (MRI) can characterize acute myocardial infarction with two well-defined enhancement patterns: (1) First-pass images performed immediately after contrast injection often demonstrate areas of hypoenhancement in the endocardial core of the infarct, corresponding to microvascular obstruction. (2) Delayed images (10 to 20 minutes after contrast injection) demonstrate regional signal hyperenhancement, corresponding to myocardial necrosis.

Balanced fast field-echo cine MR images obtained in the cardiac short axis (Fig. 2.1.1) and at end-diastole (Fig. 2.1.2a) and end-systole vertical long axis (Fig. 2.1.2b): four chamber planes show dilatation of the left ventricle with thinning of the posteroinferior segments and the apex as well as akinesia of these segments. A jet of mitral regurgitation can be appreciated in Figure 2.1.2b.

Three-dimensional T1-weighted fast field-echo late-enhancement images (Fig. 2.1.3) obtained along the cardiac short-axis plane show marked hyperenhancement of the posteroinferior segments, indicating the absence of myocardial viability.

On the basis of these findings, with the absence of myocardial viability in the inferior wall, percutaneous angioplasty revascularization was performed instead of surgery.

Case 2
■
Hypertrophic Cardiomyopathy

A 45-year-old man who presented with syncope after exercising was admitted to our cardiology unit. An EKG revealed sinus bradycardia, LV hypertrophy, and negative T waves in derivations from the precordium and the extremities. Echocardiography revealed thickening of the myocardium with preserved LV systolic function (ejection fraction, 0.55). CMR was performed to assess cardiac morphology, LV outflow-tract obstruction, and the presence of myocardial fibrosis.

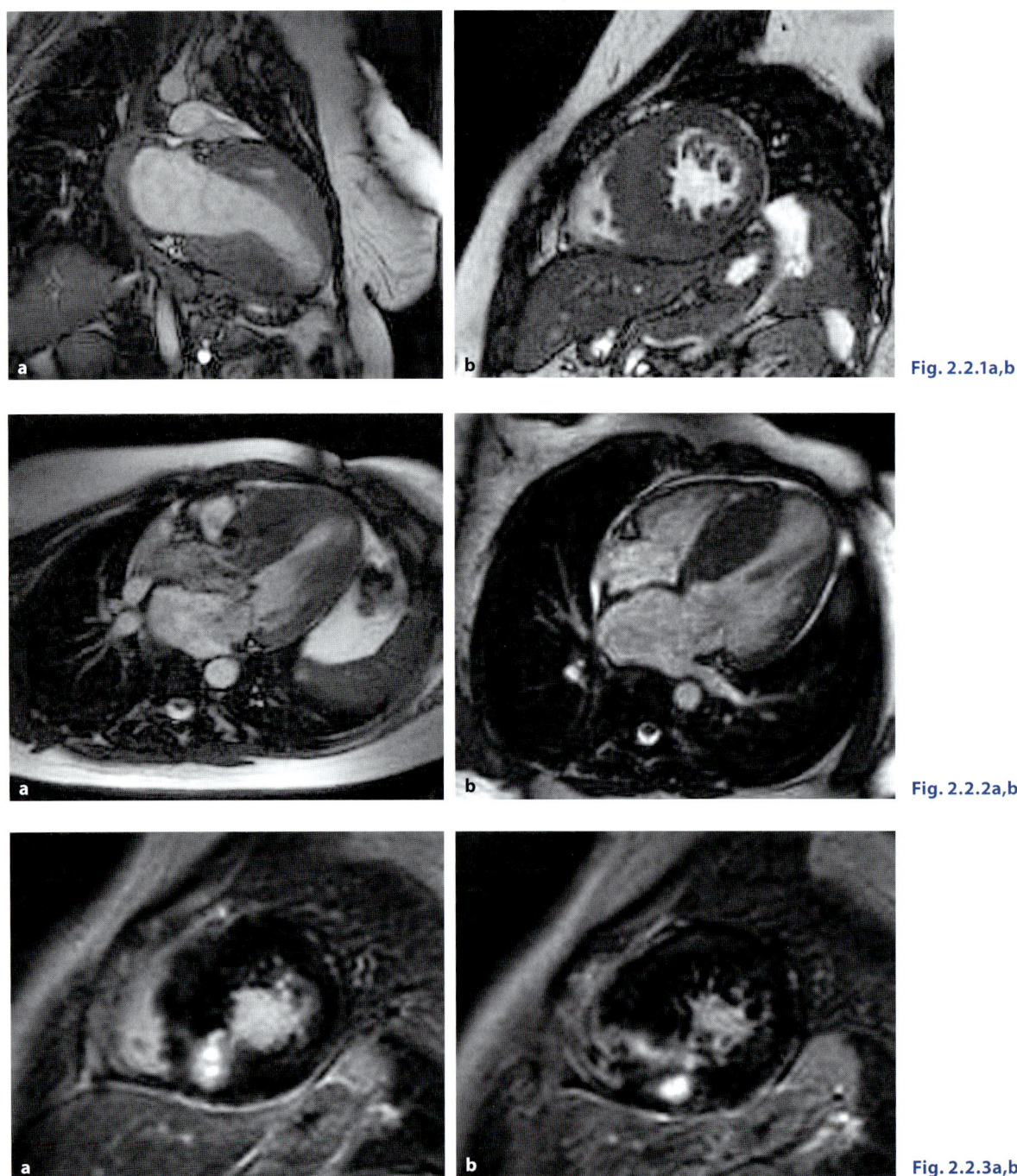

Fig. 2.2.1a,b

Fig. 2.2.2a,b

Fig. 2.2.3a,b

Hypertrophic cardiomyopathy (HCM) is a primary myocardial disease characterized by abnormal thickening of the left ventricular wall in the absence of dilatation. The prevalence of this entity is low, ranging from 0.02 to 0.2% in the general population, but HCM is the most frequent cause of sudden cardiac death in the young. In about 50% of cases this disorder is transmitted in an autosomal dominant pattern. Although the hypertrophy is most frequently confined to the basal anterior septum, it may be concentric or involve any other segments of the LV.

Histologically, HCM is characterized by the presence of extensive myocardial disarray (disruption of normal alignment of muscle cells) and various patterns of myocardial fibrosis. Furthermore, patients with HCM are prone to developing myocardial ischemia.

Pathophysiologically, HCM is characterized by outflow tract obstruction (obstructive hypertrophic cardiomyopathy), impaired regional myocardial performance, decreased myocardial compliance, decreased coronary flow reserve, and ventricular arrhythmias. Depending on the degree of obstruction of the outflow of blood from the LV, HCM can be defined as obstructive or non-obstructive. Dynamic outflow obstruction (when present in HCM) is usually due to systolic anterior motion of the anterior leaflet of the mitral valve, often aggravated by mid-septal bulging.

The clinical course of HCM is variable. Many patients are asymptomatic or mildly symptomatic. The symptoms of HCM include shortness of breath, chest pain, palpitations, lightheadedness, fatigue, syncope, and sudden cardiac death.

Echocardiography has been the standard method of assessing HCM. Thickening of 15 mm or more of the wall of the LV is usually identified in this disease. Echocardiograms will also show whether outflow tract obstruction is present (and to what degree) and whether there is mitral insufficiency. Nevertheless, echocardiography is limited by a variable acoustic window, inadequate LV wall visualization in more distant areas, and inaccurate evaluation of the LV mass in patients with asymmetric hypertrophy. In contrast, CMR can a) clearly define the areas of myocardial hypertrophy; b) assess regional and global LV function; c) depict outflow tract obstruction, mitral valve systolic anterior motion, and mitral regurgitation; d) calculate LV mass; and e) detect myocardial fibrosis using delayed enhancement techniques.

Comments

Balanced fast field-echo cine MR images obtained at end-diastole in the cardiac vertical long-axis (Fig. 2.2.1a) and short-axis (Fig. 2.2.1b) planes show asymmetric thickening of the myocardium with septal predominance.

Balanced fast field-echo cine MR image in the cardiac horizontal long-axis (Fig. 2.2.2a) reveals LV outflow-tract obstruction and mitral insufficiency. Four-chamber view (Fig. 2.2.2b) demonstrates predominant septal thickening and left atrial dilatation secondary to mitral insufficiency.

Three-dimensional T1-weighted fast field-echo late-enhancement images (Fig. 2.2.3) obtained along the cardiac short-axis plane display strong patchy enhancement at the junction of the interventricular septum (inferoseptal segment) and right ventricular free wall, indicating fibrous replacement of the myocardium.

CMR findings are consistent with the previous diagnosis of obstructive hypertrophic cardiomyopathy with septal predominance and multiple foci of myocardial fibrosis.

Imaging Findings

Case 3

■

**Arrhythmogenic Right
Ventricular Dysplasia**

A 45-year-old woman presented at our cardiology clinic for evaluation of dyspnea and palpitations. An EKG revealed nonsustained ventricular tachycardia, with left bundle branch block morphology. Echocardiography findings included moderate dilatation and increased trabeculation of the right ventricle. Coronary angiogram was normal. Cardiac MRI was performed to evaluate the right ventricular cardiomyopathy of uncertain origin.

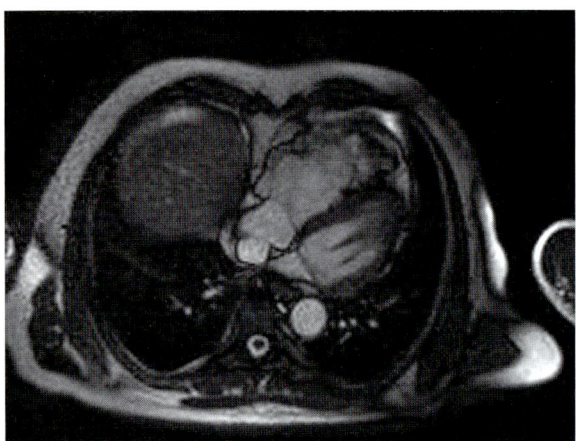

Fig. 2.3.1

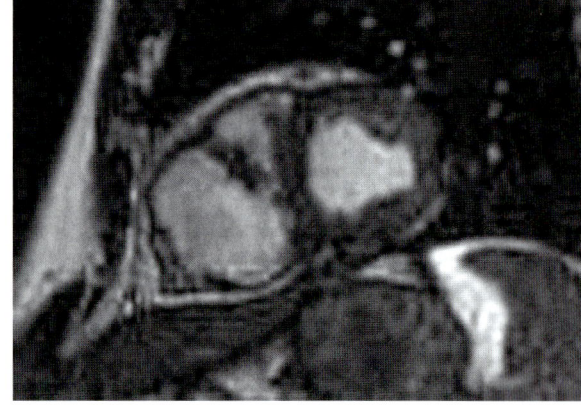

Fig. 2.3.2

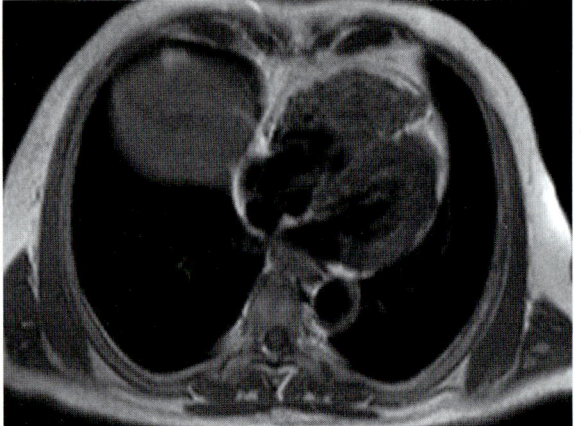

Fig. 2.3.3

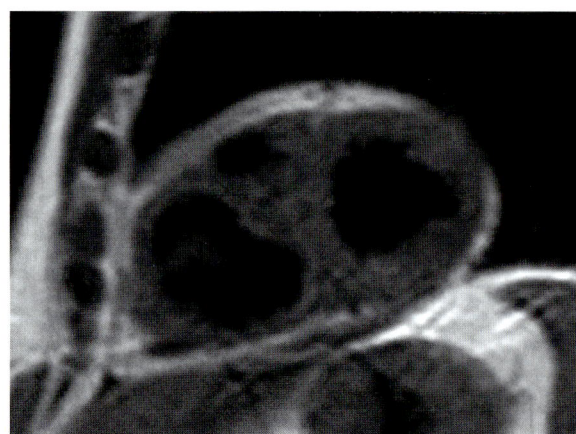

Fig. 2.3.4

Arrhythmogenic right ventricular dysplasia (ARVD) is a disorder characterized by progressive replacement of the right ventricular myocardium by fibrofatty tissue. Although this disorder usually involves the right ventricle, the left ventricle and septum also may be affected. This dysplasia can lead to extensive wall thinning, atypical arrangement of trabecular muscles, dilatations or aneurysms having paradoxical systolic motion, and, in rare cases, right-sided congestive heart failure.

Although the exact prevalence of ARVD is unknown, it has been estimated to occur in one in 5000 individuals from the general population. Several reports suggest that there is a familial occurrence of ARVD of about 30%–50%, with mainly autosomal dominant inheritance. It represents the second cause of sudden cardiac death in young persons, especially athletes, after hypertrophic heart disease.

Patients with ARVD are usually men younger than 35 years who complain of chest pain or tachycardia. In some cases, sudden cardiac death can be the first presentation.

The diagnosis of ARVD is based on the presence of major and minor criteria encompassing genetic, electrocardiographic, pathophysiologic, and histopathologic factors. Fifty to 90 percent of persons with ARVD will have characteristic findings on a resting electrocardiogram (ventricular tachycardia with LBBB, originating from the right ventricle). The imaging modalities used to evaluate right ventricular abnormalities include conventional angiography, echocardiography, radionuclide angiography, ultrafast computed tomography, and magnetic resonance (MR) imaging.

Right ventricular angiography has usually been regarded as the standard of reference for the diagnosis of ARVD, especially for discerning abnormalities such as akinetic or dyskinetic bulging in the infundibular, apical, and subtricuspid regions.

Echocardiography can detect regional or global changes in myocardial contractility, enlargement of the right ventricle, and right ventricular systolic dysfunction during a routine study. However, visibility of the apex and the right ventricular outflow tract is limited, areas of wall thinning may be very difficult to detect, and echocardiography lacks spatial resolution in depicting the typical fatty and fibrofatty changes in the right ventricular myocardium.

MR imaging allows visualization of ventricular cavities and walls with an excellent depiction of myocardial anatomy. Cine sequences detect regional motion changes such as global or local hypokinesia, localized early diastolic bulging, or circumscribed saccular outpouchings. T1-weighted sequences are able to detect intramyocardial fat in some cases. MR images obtained with the delayed-enhancement technique may reveal fibrous replacement of the right-ventricular free wall. Because MR imaging depicts both functional and structural abnormalities, positive MR imaging findings should be used as important additional criteria in the clinical diagnosis of ARVD. CMR appears to be the optimal technique for the detection and follow-up of clinically suspected ARVD.

Balanced fast field-echo cine MR images performed in the 4-chamber (Fig. 2.3.1) and short-axis (Fig. 2.3.2) projections show severe dilation of the right ventricle, along with wall thinning, increased trabeculation, multiple bulges with dyskinetic areas, and severe global dysfunction. The left ventricle is normal in size with mildly reduced global systolic function.

Black-blood T1-weighted MR images obtained in the 4-chamber (Fig. 2.3.3) and short-axis (Fig. 2.3.4) planes show the absence of areas of fatty replacement of the right ventricular wall.

On the basis of these findings, ARVD was diagnosed even though no fatty replacement of the RV wall was observed.

Comments

Imaging Findings

Case 4

■

Myocarditis

A 35-year-old woman with no relevant cardiovascular risk factors presented at the emergency department with a 5 hour history of oppressive central chest pain with typical characteristics and no other symptoms associated. She reported having gastroenteritis the week before and was afebrile. An EKG revealed ST elevation of 2 mm in

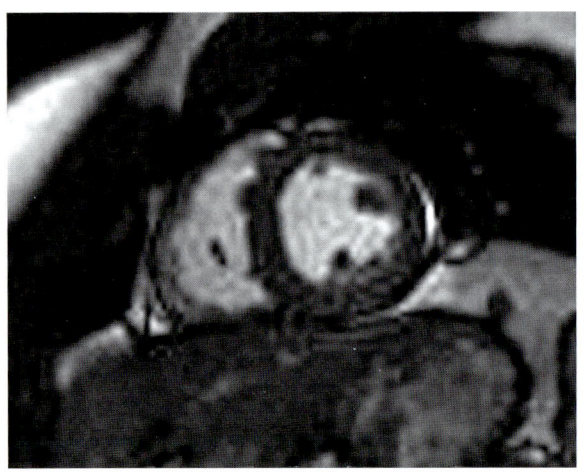

Fig. 2.4.1

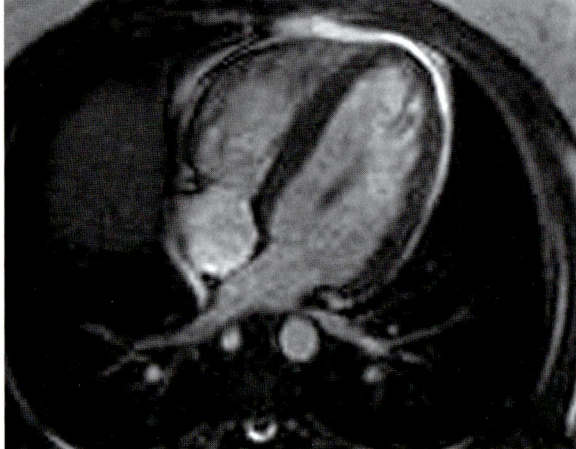

Fig. 2.4.2

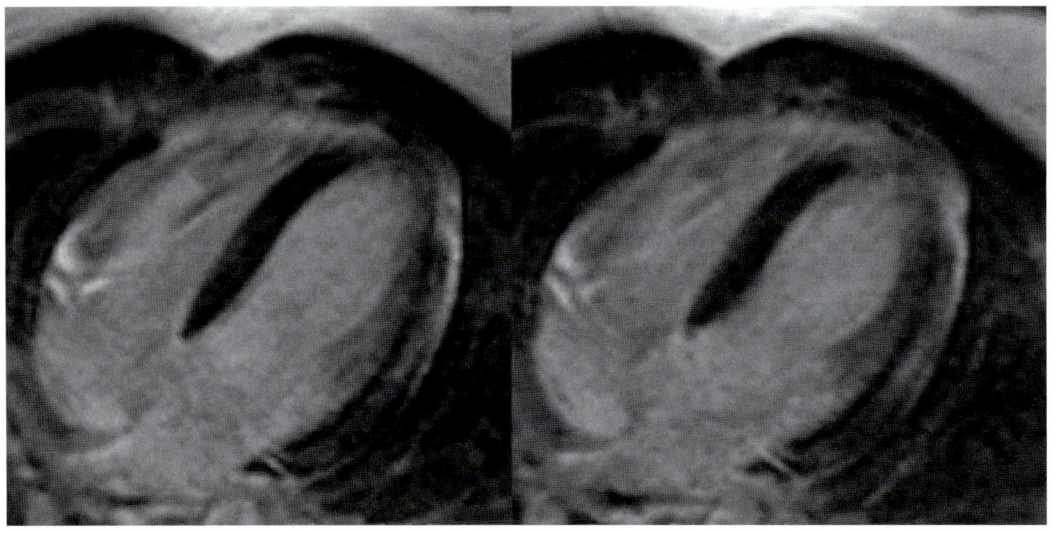

Fig. 2.4.3

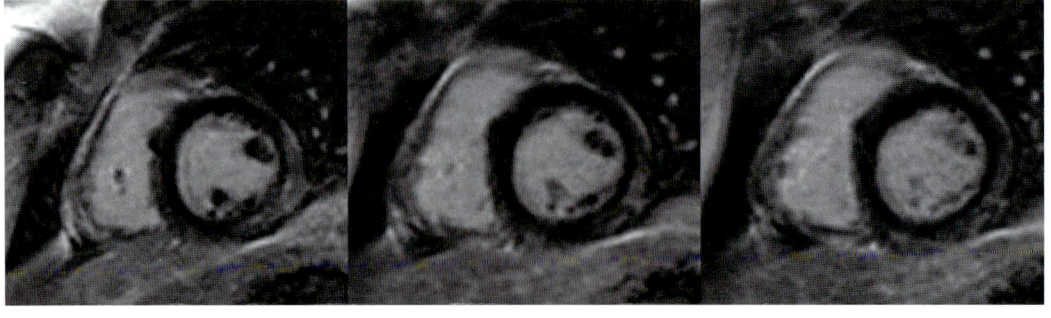

Fig. 2.4.4

the inferior, posterior, and lateral leads. Echocardiography performed in the emergency department showed mild hypokinesia of the inferolateral wall. There was no evidence of pericardial thickening or effusion. Initial cardiac enzyme tests revealed troponin I of 29.5 ng/mL (normal, < 0.4 ng/mL), CK of 2,585 U/L, and CK-MB of 389 ng/mL. The chest pain persisted despite sublingual and intravenous nitroglycerin administration, and she underwent urgent cardiac catheterization. Findings at coronary angiogram were normal and myocarditis was suspected. CMR was performed to assess cardiac morphology and function, as well as possible areas of inflammation.

Comments

Myocarditis is an acute inflammatory process that affects the myocardium in response to the action of various infectious (most frequently viruses), chemical, or physical agents.

In most patients, active myocarditis is clinically silent, with neither symptoms nor physical findings to suggest the diagnosis. The most obvious clue pointing to myocarditis is an antecedent viral syndrome. Sometimes clinical features are limited to minor signs such as fatigue, palpitations, and weakness in the days following an acute episode of fever and/or angina. However, in some cases acute myocarditis can mimic an acute coronary syndrome. Although the majority of patients recover fully, 5% to 10% may progress to chronic myocarditis and dilated cardiomyopathy, leading occasionally to sudden death due to disseminated myocarditis.

The diagnosis is often presumptive. Clinical and laboratory findings, EKG, echocardiography, and coronary angiography are of limited value except for eliminating acute coronary artery syndromes, and the final diagnosis is generally made after ruling out the most common causes of cardiac disease. Although endomyocardial biopsy is still considered the diagnostic gold standard (though it may lack sensitivity because the disease may be focal), the development of new imaging techniques such as CMR imaging have contributed greatly to the diagnosis of myocarditis. In addition to the evaluation of ventricular morphology and function, CMR studies can assess myocardial inflammation. In the delayed enhancement technique, contrast accumulates in the myocardium as a consequence of the breakdown of the myocyte membrane due to the inflammatory process. Contrast uptake usually occurs in a characteristic patchy pattern for about the first 2 weeks after the acute event, later becoming progressively more disseminated. This pattern of midwall enhancement with sparing of the subendocardial layer is easily distinguished from the subendocardial pattern of uptake seen in acute myocardial infarction. The association of changes in regional contractility in the areas of uptake considerably increases the degree of diagnostic accuracy. Moreover, CMR not only can define the site and extent of myocardial inflammation, but it can also serve to further evaluate the progression of the disease.

Imaging Findings

Balanced fast field-echo cine MR images performed in the short-axis plane (Fig. 2.4.1) and four-chamber (Fig. 2.4.2) projections show mild lateral hypokinesia.

Black-blood T1-weighted MR images obtained 10 min after injection of gadolinium in four-chamber view (Fig. 2.4.3) and in the short-axis (Fig. 2.4.4) planes show a large area of mid-myocardial delayed enhancement with sparing of the subendocardial tissue localized to the posterior and lateral regions.

These findings, taken together with the clinical and laboratory results, are highly suggestive of myocarditis.

Case 5
■
Aortic Coarctation

A 42-year-old man was referred for the study of treatment-refractory hypertension. Upon physical examination, his blood pressure was 175/95 mmHg in both superior extremities and 90/40 in both inferior extremities, with weak pulses in the latter. On auscultation, there was an extrasystolic sound in his back. The EKG sinus rhythm met the criteria for left ventricular hypertrophy. The echocardiogram confirmed severe left ventricular hypertrophy with normal ejection fraction, revealing a systolic gradient in the descending aorta. Suspected aortic coarctation was studied by CMR.

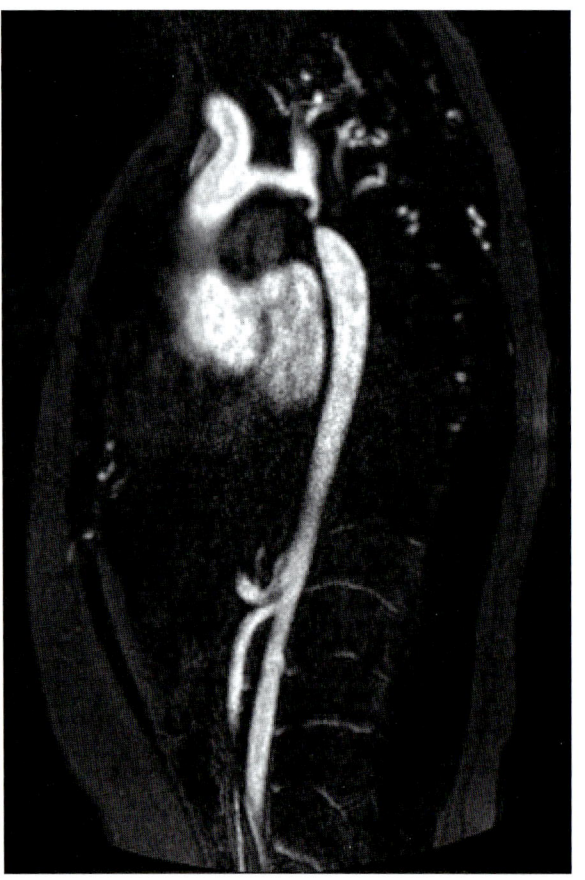

Fig. 2.5.1

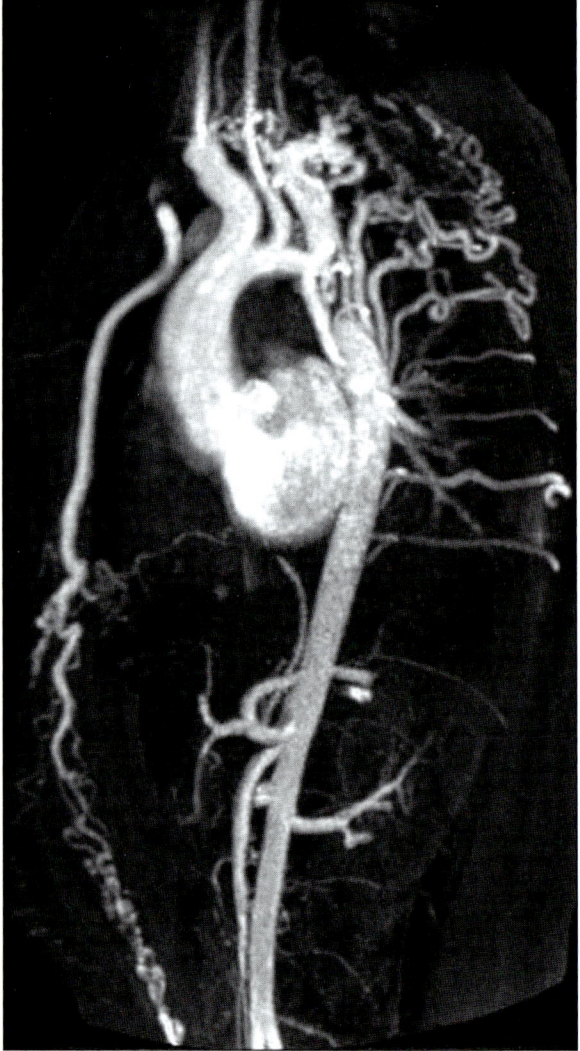

Fig. 2.5.2

Coarctation of the aorta represents a focal narrowing in the proximal descending thoracic aorta, most commonly found just distal to the origin of the left subclavian artery, usually in the region of the ductus arteriosus (juxtaductal). The gross morphology of the coarctation may vary from a discrete narrowing to a long-segment stenosis.

Coarctation of the aorta has a male preponderance and is relatively common, accounting for 5 percent to 10 percent of all congenital heart conditions. It often occurs together with other heart defects such as hypoplasia of the aortic arch and isthmus. Other associated conditions include bicuspid aortic valve (the most common associated anomaly, occurring in about half of the patients), patent ductus arteriosus, ventricular septal defect, tricuspid atresia, and mitral valve abnormalities. Noncardiac associations include berry aneurysms in the circle of Willis and Turner's syndrome.

In infants, the lesion lies either opposite the ductus or in a preductal location. In adolescents and adults, it is usually distal to the ligamentum arteriosum (postductal).

Patients with aortic coarctation may present with congestive heart failure as infants when a patent ductus arteriosus closes. Older children are for the most part asymptomatic, although a few will complain of mild fatigue, dyspnea, or symptoms of claudication in their legs when running. Adults usually present with hypertension and discrepant blood pressure measurements in the arms and legs.

Diagnosing coarctation early is important to prevent associated complications including aortic aneurysm, dissection, and bacterial endocarditis at the coarctation site or bicuspid aortic valve. The most specific chest radiograph findings in aortic coarctation are the aortic "Figure 2.5.3" sign and inferior rib notching due to pressure erosion from tortuous intercostal arteries acting as collaterals.

Transthoracic echocardiography is ideal for the initial assessment, since it provides comprehensive evaluation of valvular and ventricular function in addition to reliable assessment of the pressure gradient across the coarctation. Anatomic variations, such as isthmic or transverse arch hypoplasia, and the presence and severity of associated defects can also be evaluated.

CMR is now considered the standard noninvasive technique for the evaluation of aortic coarctation.

Cine phase-contrast techniques, including velocity-encoded cine MR, measure the peak velocity across the site of coarctation, thus enabling the pressure gradient across the coarctation to be estimated. Associated abnormalities, such as arch hypoplasia, bicuspid aortic valve, and ventricular septal defect, can also be assessed. Gadolinium-enhanced 3D MR angiography can readily demonstrate the presence of collateral circulation. It also provides excellent anatomic images of the extent of the coarctation and allows reconstruction of 3D data into multiple planes. CMR is also well suited for assessing re-stenosis after surgical repair and complications such as postoperative pseudoaneurysms.

Oblique sagittal partition (Fig. 2.5.1) and maximum intensity projection (Fig. 2.5.2) images from breath-hold gadolinium-enhanced three-dimensional MR angiogram show severe postductal aortic coarctation with extensive collateral circulation, as well as mild hypoplasia of the aortic arch.

Comments

Imaging Findings

Case 6
■ Constrictive Pericarditis

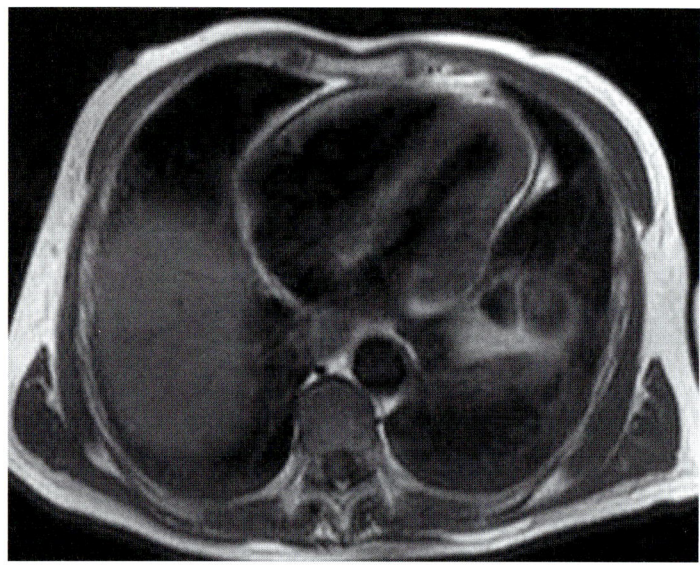

Fig. 2.6.1

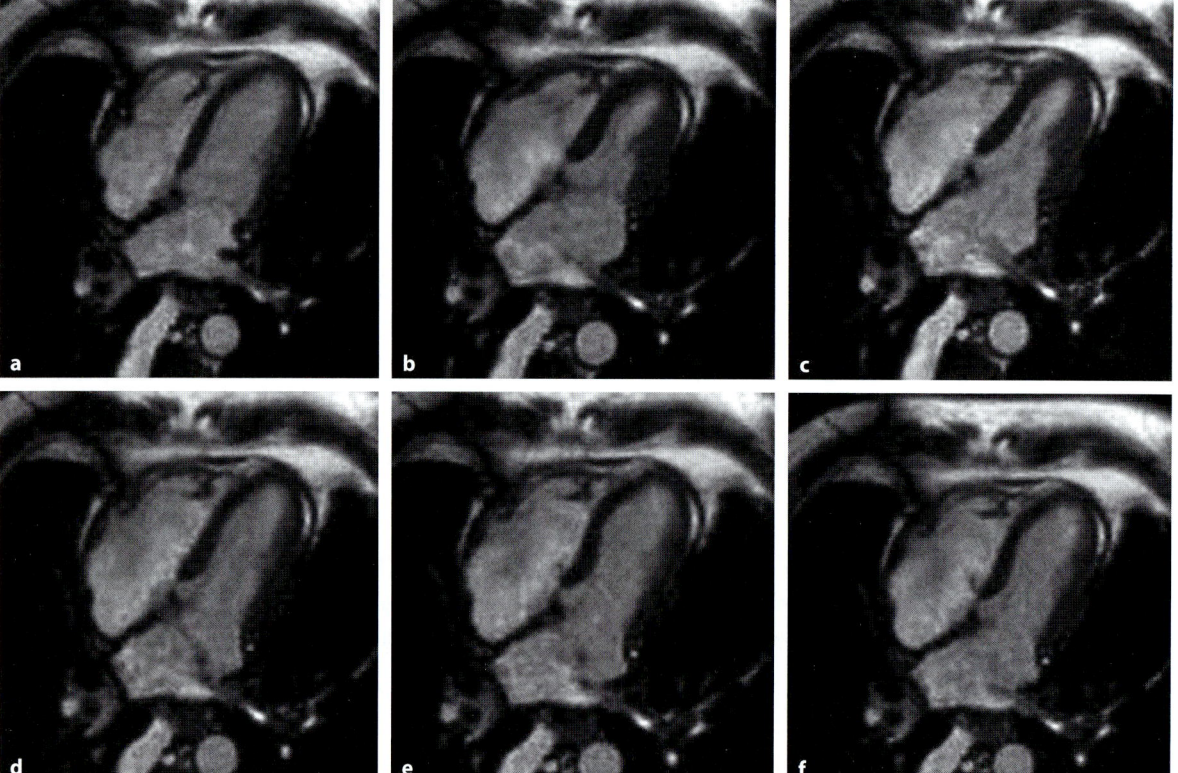

Fig. 2.6.2a–f

A 62-year-old male active smoker with history of tuberculosis in his youth consulted his cardiologist for dyspnea on exertion, coughing, and orthopnea associated to increased abdominal perimeter. At physical examination, elevated venous pressure and hepatomegaly were observed. On auscultation there were tele-inspiratory crepitus. Chest X-ray showed subtle pericardial calcifications. The EKG revealed auricular fibrillation and the echocardiogram suggested possible pericardial thickening along with dilatation of the inferior vena cava. CMR was requested to study the pericardium.

Comments

Constrictive pericarditis (CP) is a disorder caused by inflammation and subsequent thickening, scarring, and contracture of the pericardium. The most common presentation is an initial episode of acute pericarditis, which may go undetected clinically. This then slowly progresses to a subacute stage of organization and resorption of effusion, followed by a chronic stage consisting of fibrous scarring and thickening of the pericardium resulting in diastolic dysfunction of both ventricles. In this stage, calcium deposition may contribute to stiffening of the pericardium.

Almost half the cases of CP are idiopathic. However, there is a small but definite incidence of CP complicating operations on the heart and pericardium. At present, the most frequent known causes are cardiac surgery and radiation therapy. Other causes include infection (viral or tuberculous), connective-tissue disease, uremia, or neoplasm.

Patients with CP frequently present with symptoms of heart failure, such as dyspnea, orthopnea, and fatigability, and occasionally may present with liver enlargement and ascites.

Diseases that reduce myocardial compliance, such as restrictive cardiomyopathy (RCM), however, are also characterized by impaired ventricular filling, and the clinical manifestation of these diseases can be very similar to that of CP. Distinguishing between the two entities is crucial, because CP can be successfully treated with early pericardiectomy, whereas medical treatment is recommended for RCM.

Transthoracic echocardiography is not highly accurate in the depiction of pericardial thickening. Transesophageal imaging allows better visualization of the pericardium; however, it is limited by a narrow field of view and is relatively invasive. CT and MR imaging provide an excellent depiction of the pericardium. A pericardial thickness of 4 mm or more accompanied by clinical findings of heart failure is highly suggestive of CP. CT presents the additional advantage of its high sensitivity in depicting pericardial calcification. MR studies allow perfect depiction of increased ventricular interdependence, a phenomenon whereby the function of one ventricle is altered by changes in the filling of the other ventricle. Because the pericardial sac has a fixed volume in CP, the position of the ventricular septum during diastole will depend on the filling characteristics of both ventricles. The rapid change in ventricular pressure that takes place in CP can lead to abrupt changes in septal position, with septal flattening or eventually septal inversion (i.e., paradoxical motion).

Black-blood axial T1-weighted image (Fig. 2.6.1) shows thickening of the pericardium.

Imaging Findings

Balanced fast field-echo cine MR images (Fig. 2.6.2) performed in the 4 chamber projection also show a thickened pericardium, as well as paradoxical movement of the septum.

Case 7
■
Restrictive Cardiomyopathy

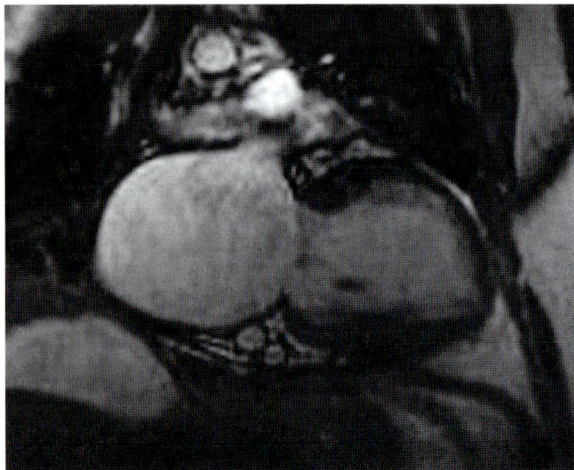

Fig. 2.7.1

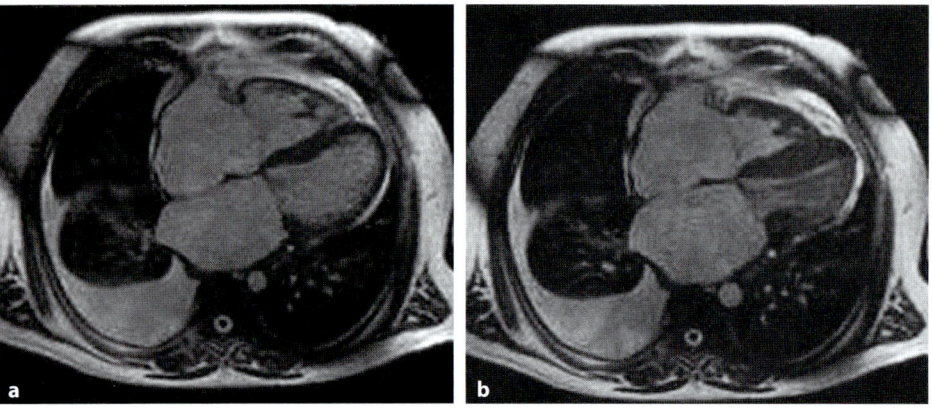

a   b   Fig. 2.7.2a,b

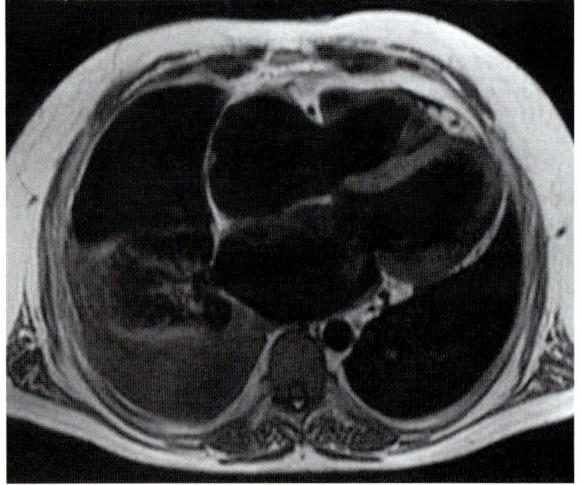

Fig. 2.7.3

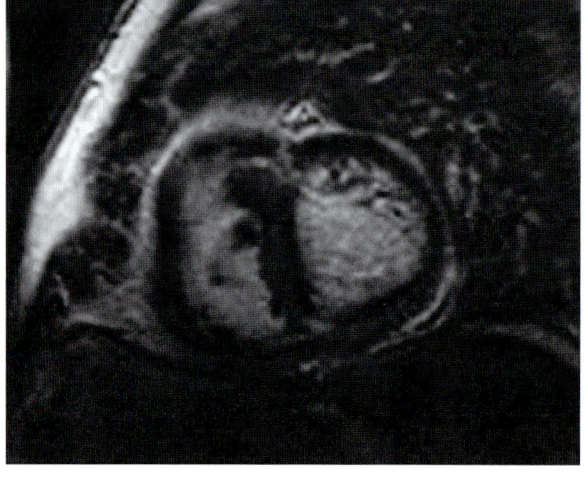

Fig. 2.7.4

An obese 65-year-old woman with history of light congestive heart failure consulted for worsening of her status during the previous month, with dyspnea on slight exertion, weakness, and severe edema in the lower extremities. At physical examination elevated central venous pressure and severe hepatomegaly were noteworthy findings. The EKG showed decreased voltage of the QRS complex in all leads. An echocardiogram revealed moderate thickening of both ventricles with severe dilatation of both atria, as well as mitral and tricuspid insufficiency.

Comments

Restrictive cardiomyopathy (RCM) is the least common form of cardiomyopathy. RCM is defined as heart-muscle disease consisting of an increased stiffness of the myocardium that results in impaired ventricular filling, with normal or decreased diastolic volume of either or both ventricles. Systolic function usually remains normal, at least early in the disease, and wall thickness may be normal or increased, depending on the underlying cause.

RCM may be idiopathic or secondary to infiltrative diseases such as amyloidosis, hemochromatosis, hypereosinophilic syndrome and Löffler endocarditis, sarcoidosis, radiation toxicity, glycogen storage diseases, and Gaucher disease. It also frequently occurs after a heart transplant.

The initial symptoms at presentation may be those of congestive heart failure (dyspnea, peripheral edema, and ascites) and arrhythmias. Up to a third of patients may present with an embolic complication. In advanced cases, all the signs of heart failure are present except cardiomegaly. The findings are similar to those seen in severe constrictive pericarditis.

The diagnosis is based largely on the findings at physical examination, electrocardiography (EKG), and echocardiography. EKG abnormalities are not specific enough for a diagnosis. Echocardiography may show biatrial enlargement, normal-to-symmetrically-thickened ventricular walls, rapid early-diastolic filling, slow late-diastolic filling, and normal or slightly reduced ventricular volume and systolic function

CMR can provide additional information about the structure of the heart. With the delayed-enhancement technique, areas of hyperenhancement suggest myocardial fibrosis in patients with RCM. A precise diagnosis usually requires cardiac catheterization to measure pressures in the heart chambers and take biopsy samples.

The diagnosis of restrictive cardiomyopathy should therefore be considered in a patient presenting with heart failure but no evidence of cardiomegaly or systolic dysfunction. Although therapy is generally unsatisfactory, the importance of an accurate diagnosis lies in distinguishing restrictive cardiomyopathy from constrictive pericarditis, which can also present with "restrictive physiology" but which is often cured surgically.

Imaging Findings

Vertical long-axis (two-chamber) view cine-MR image (Fig. 2.7.1) shows marked dilatation of the left auricle.

Balanced fast field-echo cine MR (Fig. 2.7.2) and black-blood T1-weighted (Fig. 2.7.3) images performed in the 4 chamber projection show marked dilatation of both atria, as well as impaired diastolic filling. No pericardial thickening or effusion is observed.

Black-blood T1-weighted MR image obtained 10 min after injection of gadolinium in the short-axis (Fig. 2.7.4) plane shows a large area of mid-myocardial delayed enhancement localized to the septum, consistent with fibrosis.

Case 8

■

**Congenital Anomalies of
Coronary Arteries**

An obese 71-year-old woman with history of hypertension, insulin-dependent diabetes mellitus, and atypical chest pain episodes was admitted to the emergency department for long-lasting chest pain with dubious changes at EKG. Cardiac enzyme tests were negative. The exercise test was inconclusive, so cardiac catheter-

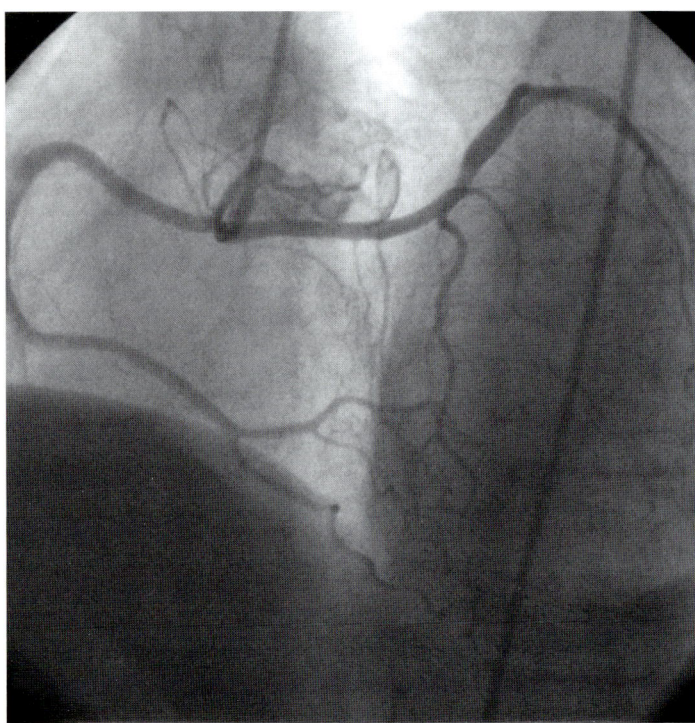

Fig. 2.8.1

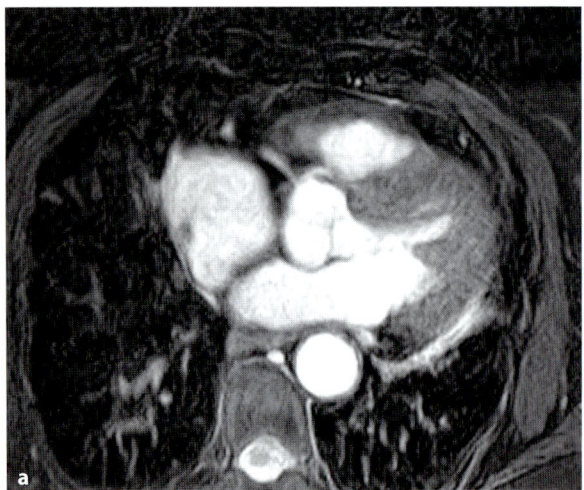
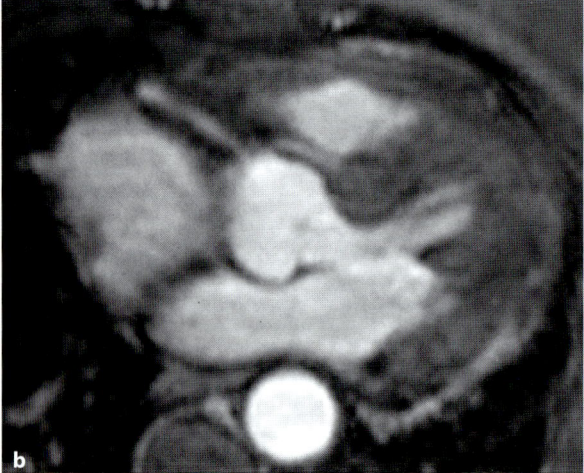

Fig. 2.8.2a,b

ization was requested. In the angiogram, an abnormal origin of the left coronary artery arising from the right coronary sinus along with the right coronary artery was observed. Given the diagnostic and therapeutic implications of this finding, CMR was performed to determine the course of the abnormal left coronary vessel and its relation with the great vessels.

The term coronary artery anomaly (CAA) refers to a wide range of congenital abnormalities involving the origin, course, and structure of epicardial coronary arteries. CAAs are found in approximately 1% of all patients undergoing coronary angiography and in approximately 0.3% of patients undergoing autopsy. Although coronary anomalies can be an incidental autopsy finding, they are found relatively more frequently in young persons who die during exercise. Coronary artery anomalies are frequently found in association with other major congenital cardiac defects.

These anomalies may show a wide range of potential pathologic alterations that is matched by the variability in their clinical presentations. In their mildest form, they can be asymptomatic with no clinical consequences. Symptoms are reported in less than 30% of patients before a diagnosis of coronary anomaly is made. These generally include palpitation, dyspnea on exertion, angina, syncope, fatigue, or fever. These symptoms rarely raise clinical suspicion of coronary artery anomalies. However, other CAAs are more frequently fatal, usually in the absence of warning symptoms. In particular, the pattern with proximal coronary artery segments crossing between the aorta and the pulmonary trunk has been reported to be potentially lethal.

The current diagnostic method of choice for detecting CAAs is conventional X-ray coronary angiography. However, X-ray angiography provides only a two-dimensional view of a vessel's complex three-dimensional path, so the anatomic course of the anomalous vessel with respect to the aorta and pulmonary artery may be difficult to discern. In addition, the anomalous vessel may be erroneously overlooked or assumed to be occluded if not selectively engaged.

Transesophageal echocardiography can also detect coronary anomalies, but this method is not totally noninvasive and is too costly for screening large populations. CT has also been recommended. It offers excellent spatial resolution and identifies most anomalies in the course of the coronary arteries, but it uses ionizing radiation and potentially nephrotoxic or allergenic contrast agents.

MR coronary angiography is a novel noninvasive technique that has proved accurate in the imaging of proximal coronary anatomy in patients. The free choice of the imaging plane is an advantage over the limited possibilities of angulations in conventional coronary angiography. Also, MRA is a tomographic technique that is potentially better in elucidating three-dimensional anatomy than a projection technique.

Its greatest limitation is in determining the distal coronary course.

Left anterior oblique coronary angiogram projection (Fig. 2.8.1) showing both right and left coronary arteries arising from the right coronary sinus.

3D coronary MRA images (Fig. 2.8.2) show the left coronary artery (LCA) arising from the right anterior sinus along with the right coronary artery (RCA). The anomalous course of the LCA between the aorta and pulmonary arteries can also be observed.

Case 9
■
Coronary Artery S Stenoses

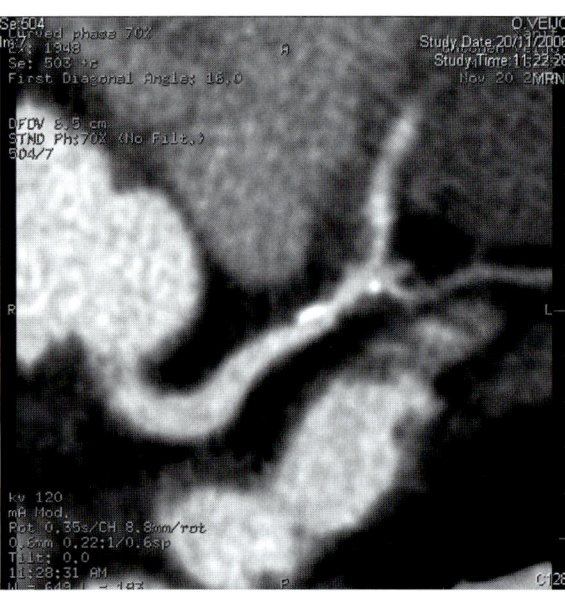

Fig. 2.9.1

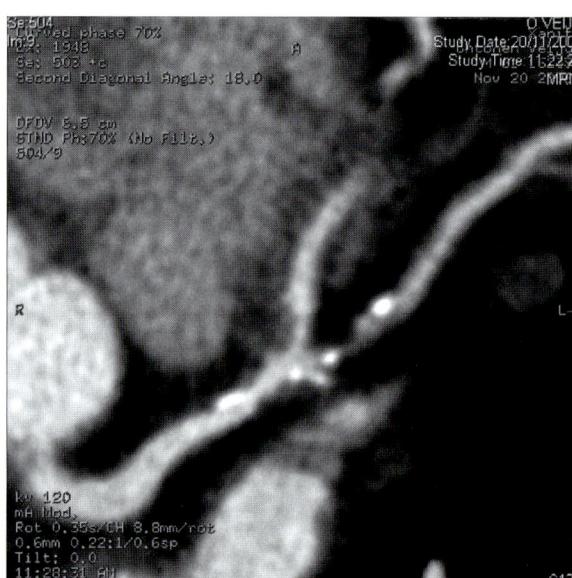

Fig. 2.9.2

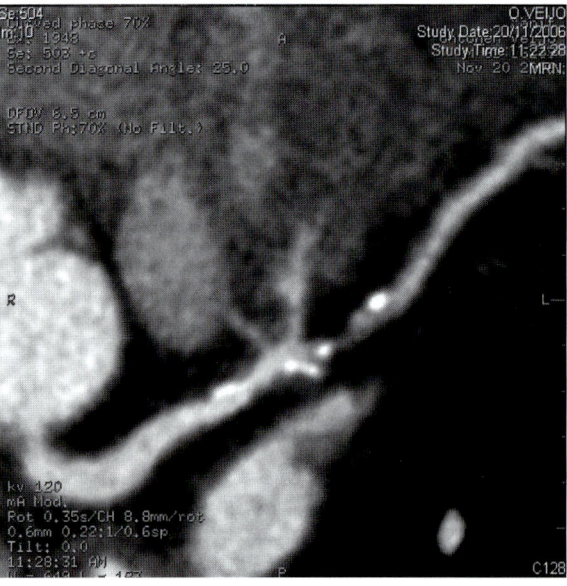

Fig. 2.9.3

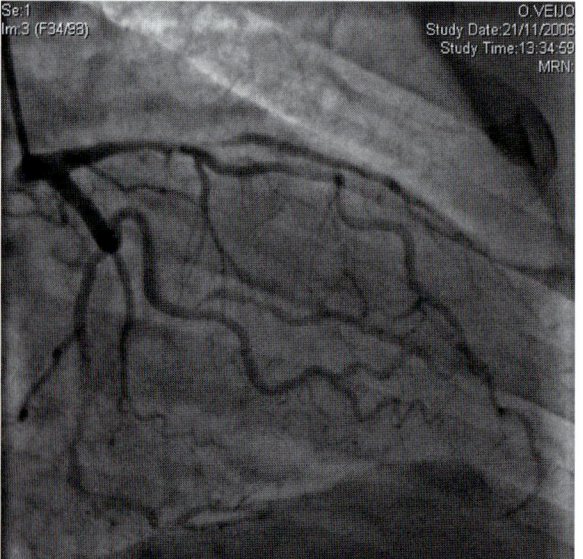

Fig. 2.9.4

A 61-year-old man with a history of systemic hypertension, dyslipemia, heavy smoking ceased 24 years prior, and a family history of ischemic heart disease was referred for chest discomfort that was sometimes related to exercise and sometimes occurred at rest.

No other symptoms were reported.

Physical examination revealed blood pressure of 160/100 mmHg with no other abnormal cardiovascular findings.

EKG showed a sinus rhythm with left axis deviation and high T-waves in precordial leads with up-sloping of the J point.

Two-dimensional echocardiography showed normal dimensions for the cardiac chambers and severe hypokinesia of the lateral wall of the LV, with preserved global systolic function (ejection fraction EF: 50%). The heart valves had a normal anatomic appearance and no functional disturbances.

Comments

Diagnostic accuracy of MDCT for the detection and assesment of lesions on native coronary arteries is high in proximal and middle segments of the vessels. Both sensitivity and specificity decrease when distal segments or secondary branches are studied due to their reduced diameter and contrast opacification.

The left main (LM) and left anterior descending (LAD) arteries are the most readily visualized ones being the accuracy of MDCT in right coronary artery (RAC) and left circumflex artery (LCx) lower than in the case of both LM and LAD.

Imaging Findings

The CT coronary scan revealed a significant ostial stenosis of the main diagonal branch of the left anterior descending (LAD) artery along with a non-calcified 50% stenosis in the mid-portion of the LAD. The right coronary artery and left circumflex artery were free of lesions.

A cardiac catheterization with angioplasty procedure was successfully performed. Two days after the revascularization procedure, the patient started complaining of atypical chest pain but no myocardial damage was found on the EKG. Blood work findings were normal. The patient was discharged on antiplatelet medication and in good health.

Case 10

Aortocoronary Bypass

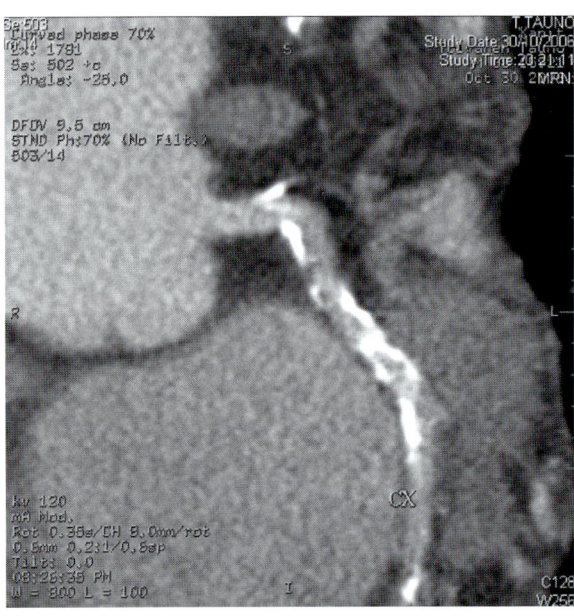

Fig. 2.10.1

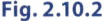

Fig. 2.10.2

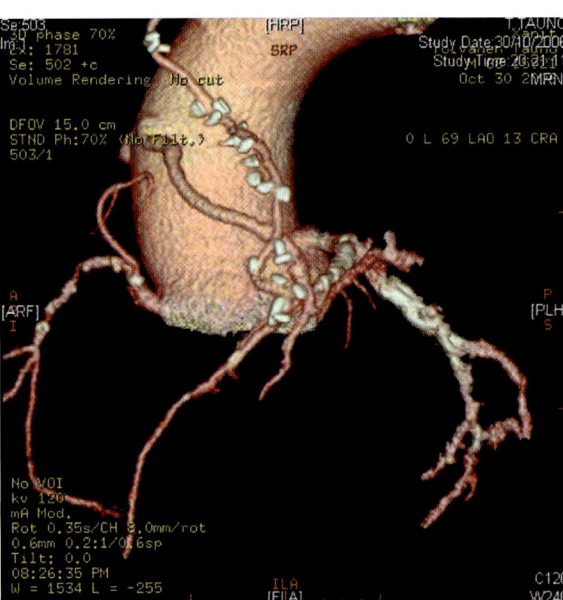

Fig. 2.10.3

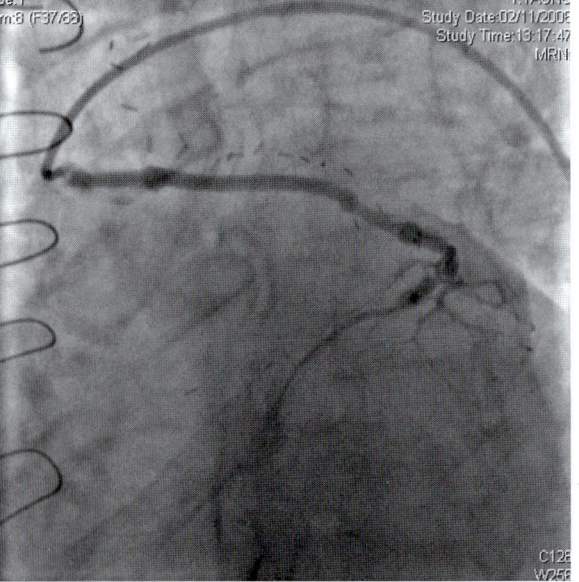

Fig. 2.10.4

A 70-year-old man with a past history of aortocoronary bypass surgery in 1992 after acute myocardial infarction and a one-week history of severe chest pain (clearly related to physical exertion and emotional stress but also present at rest) was referred for cardiological evaluation.

Physical examination was within normal limits.

The EKG showed normal sinus rhythm, with a horizontal electrical axis, QS in leads V1 and V2, with ST elevation and T-wave inversion.

Two-dimensional echocardiography showed a dilated LV with akynesia of the anterior segment, inferior hypokinesia, and depressed systolic function (ejection fraction: 30%). Valve examination showed low grade mitral regurgitation and low-grade tricuspid regurgitation. The pulmonary artery systolic pressure was 43 mmHg.

The patient was admitted to the ICU. No enzyme movement was recorded and the patient remained free of angina.

Comments

Coronary artery bypass grafts (CABG) are more amenable to multidetector computed tomography (MDCT) imaging than native arteries due to their larger diameter and lower pulsatile movements along the cardiac cycle.

Although metallic clips in mammary arteries and radial artery grafts can interfere with the visualization of lesions, reports on diagnostic accuracy of MDCT in CABG have shown values of sensitivity and specificity over 95% for the presence of stenoses in these vessels.

Imaging Findings

A CT scan showed severe RCA lesions, occlusion of the saphenous graft to the left marginal branch, patency of the LIMA graft to the LAD artery, and patency of the saphenous graft to a diagonal branch.

Coronary angiography was performed to confirm these findings and evaluate the possibility of percutaneous revascularization. The angiographic appearance of the RCA was not good enough to warrant an angioplasty procedure and the patient was discharged on antianginal and antiplatelet drugs.

Further Readings

Books

Atlas of Non-Invasive Coronary Angiography by Multidetector Computed Tomography. Pons-Lladó G, Leta-Petracca R (2006) Springer-Verlag, Berlin. ISBN-13: 9780387330440

Atlas of Practical Applications of Cardiovascular Magnetic Resonance (Developments in Cardiovascular Medicine). Pons-Lladó G, Carreras F (2005) Springer-Verlag, Berlin. ISBN-13: 9780387236322

Cardiac CT Imaging: Diagnosis of Cardiovascular Disease. Budoff MJ, Shinbane JS (2006) Springer, London. ISBN-13: 9781846280283

Cardiac CT Made Easy: An Introduction to Cardiovascular Multi-Detector Computed Tomography. Schoenhagen P, Stillman AE, White RD (2005) Informa Healthcare. ISBN-13: 9781841846187

Cardiovascular Magnetic Resonance. Manning WJ, Pennell DJ (2002) Churchill Livingstone, Philadelphia. ISBN-13: 9780443075193

Cardiovascular Magnetic Resonance: Established and Emerging Applications. Lardo AC, Fayad ZA, Chronos NAF, Fuster V (2003) Informa Healthcare. ISBN-13: 1841842028

Computed Tomography of the Coronary Arteries. de Feyter PJ, Krestin GP (2005) Informa Healthcare. ISBN-13: 9781841844398

CT of the Heart: Principles and Applications (Contemporary Cardiology). Schoepf UJ. Humana Press, New Jersey. ISBN-13: 9781588293039

MRI and CT of the Cardiovascular System. 2nd ed. Higgins CB, de Roos A (2005) Lippincott Williams & Wilkins. ISBN-13: 9780781762717

Pocket Atlas of Cardiac MRI (Radiology Pocket Atlas Series). 2nd ed. Woodard PK, Brown JJ, Higgins CB (2004) Lippincott Williams & Wilkins. ISBN-13: 9780781748704

Weblinks

http://diagnosticimaging.com/cardiovascular/
http://emedicine.com/radio/CARDIAC.htm
http://gehealthcare.com/euen/ct/products/products_technologies/products/lsvct_index.html
http://mayoclinic.com/health/heart-disease/HB99999
http://medstudents.com.br/cardio
http://med.yale.edu/intmed/cardio/imaging/
http://radiographics.rsnajnls.org/cgi/collection/cardiac_radiology
http://scmr.org/
http://search.medscape.com/all-search?queryText=Coronary%20CT%20scan
http://theheart.org/search.do?searchString=Coronary+CT&x=29&y=5

Articles

CMR

Abdel-Aty H, Boye P, Zagrosek A, Wassmuth R, Kumar A, Messroghli D, Bock P, Dietz R, Friedrich MG, Schulz-Menger J. Diagnostic performance of cardiovascular magnetic resonance in patients with suspected acute myocarditis: comparison of different approaches. J Am Coll Cardiol 2005; 45(11):1815–1822

Bogaert J, Kuzo R, Dymarkowski S, Janssen L, Celis I, Budts W, Gewillig M. Follow-up of patients with previous treatment for coarctation of the thoracic aorta: comparison between contrast-enhanced MR angiography and fast spin-echo MR imaging. Eur Radiol 2000; 10(12):1847–1854

Bogaert J, Goldstein M, Tannouri F, Golzarian J, Dymarkowski S. Late myocardial enhancement in hypertrophic cardiomyopathy with contrast-enhanced MR imaging. AJR Am J Roentgenol 2003; 180(4):981–985

Bucciarelli-Ducci C, Locca D, Barbeau G, Prasad SK. Value of cardiovascular magnetic resonance for determining cardiac involvement in systemic amyloidosis. Eur Heart J 2006; 28:1186. Epub 2006 Nov 22

Bunce NH, Pennell DJ. Magnetic resonance of coronary arteries. Eur Radiol 2001; 11(5):721–731

Cheng AS, Banning AP, Mitchell AR, Neubauer S, Selvanayagam JB. Cardiac changes in systemic amyloidosis: visualisation by magnetic resonance imaging. Int J Cardiol 2006; 113(1):E21–23

Cheong B, Huber S, Muthupillai R, Flamm SD. Evaluation of myocardial iron overload by T2* cardiovascular magnetic resonance imaging. Tex Heart Inst J 2005; 32(3):448–449

Chinnaiyan KM, Leff CB, Marsalese DL. Constrictive pericarditis versus restrictive cardiomyopathy: challenges in diagnosis and management. Cardiol Rev 2004; 12(6):314–320

Constantine G, Shan K, Flamm SD, Sivananthan MU. Role of MRI in clinical cardiology. Lancet 2004; 363(9427):2162–2171

Dall'armellina E, Hamilton CA, Hundley WG. Assessment of blood flow and valvular heart disease using phase-contrast cardiovascular magnetic resonance. Echocardiography 2007; 24(2):207–216

Debl K, Djavidani B, Buchner S, Lipke C, Nitz W, Feuerbach S, Riegger G, Luchner A. Delayed hyperenhancement in magnetic resonance imaging of left ventricular hypertrophy caused by aortic stenosis and hypertrophic cardiomyopathy: visualisation of focal fibrosis. Heart 2006; 92(10):1447–1451. Epub 2006 Apr 10

Desai MY, Lima JA, Bluemke DA. Cardiovascular magnetic resonance imaging: current applications and future directions. Methods Enzymol 2004; 386:122–148

Didier D, Saint-Martin C, Lapierre C, Trindade PT, Lahlaidi N, Vallee JP, Kalangos A, Friedli B, Beghetti M. Coarctation of the aorta: pre and postoperative evaluation with MRI and MR angiography; correlation with echocardiography and surgery. Int J Cardiovasc Imaging 2006; 22(3–4):457–475

Dodd JD, Ferencik M, Liberthson RR, Cury RC, Hoffmann U, Brady TJ, Abbara S. Congenital anomalies of coronary artery origin in adults: 64-MDCT appearance. AJR Am J Roentgenol 2007; 188(2):W138–W146

Dumont CA, Monserrat L, Soler R, Rodriguez E, Fernandez X, Peteiro J, Bouzas B, Pinon P, Castro-Beiras A. Clinical significance of late gadolinium enhancement on cardiovascular magnetic resonance in patients with hypertrophic cardiomyopathy. Rev Esp Cardiol 2007; 60(1):15–23

Finsterer J, Stollberger C. Cardiac involvement in primary myopathies. Cardiology 2000; 94(1):1–11

Francone M, Dymarkowski S, Kalantzi M, Bogaert J. Magnetic resonance imaging in the evaluation of the pericardium. A pictorial essay. Radiol Med (Torino) 2005; 109(1–2):64–74; quiz 75–76

Giorgi B, Mollet NR, Dymarkowski S, Rademakers FE, Bogaert J. Clinically suspected constrictive pericarditis: MR imaging assessment of ventricular septal motion and configuration in patients and healthy subjects. Radiology 2003; 228(2):417–424

Hancock EW. Differential diagnosis of restrictive cardiomyopathy and constrictive pericarditis. Heart 2001; 86(3):343–349

Hunold P, Schlosser T, Vogt FM, Eggebrecht H, Schmermund A, Bruder O, Schuler WO, Barkhausen J. Myocardial late enhancement in contrast-enhanced cardiac MRI: distinction between infarction scar and non-infarction-related disease. AJR Am J Roentgenol 2005; 184(5):1420–1426

Ichikawa Y, Sakuma H, Suzawa N, Kitagawa K, Makino K, Hirano T, Takeda K. Late gadolinium-enhanced magnetic resonance imaging in acute and chronic myocardial infarction. Improved prediction of regional myocardial contraction in the chronic state by measuring thickness of nonenhanced myocardium. J Am Coll Cardiol 2005; 45(6):901–909

Ingkanisorn WP, Rhoads KL, Aletras AH, Kellman P, Arai AE. Gadolinium delayed enhancement cardiovascular magnetic resonance correlates with clinical measures of myocardial infarction. J Am Coll Cardiol 2004; 43(12):2253–2259

Isbell DC, Kramer CM. The evolving role of cardiovascular magnetic resonance imaging in nonischemic cardiomyopathy. Semin Ultrasound CT MR 2006; 27(1):20–31

Keenan NG, Pennell DJ. CMR of Ventricular Function. Echocardiography 2007; 24(2):185–193

Kim SY, Seo JB, Do KH, Heo JN, Lee JS, Song JW, Choe YH, Kim TH, Yong HS, Choi SI, Song KS, Lim TH. Coronary artery anomalies: classification and ECG-gated multidetector row CT findings with angiographic correlation. Radiographics 2006; 26(2):317–333

Klessen C, Post F, Meyer J, Thelen M, Kreitner KF. Depiction of anomalous coronary vessels and their relation to the great arteries by magnetic resonance angiography. Eur Radiol 2000; 10(12):1855–1857

Krinsky GA, Rofsky NM, DeCorato DR, Weinreb JC, Earls JP, Flyer MA, Galloway AC, Colvin SB. Thoracic aorta: comparison of gadolinium-enhanced three-dimensional MR angiography with conventional MR imaging. Radiology 1997; 202(1):183–193

Kuijpers D. Diagnosis of coronary artery disease with dobutamine-stress MRI. Eur Radiol 2005; 15 Suppl 2:B48–51

Kwong RY, Falk RH. Cardiovascular magnetic resonance in cardiac amyloidosis. Circulation 2005; 111(2):122–124

Laissy JP, Hyafil F, Feldman LJ, Juliard JM, Schouman-Claeys E, Steg PG, Faraggi M. Differentiating acute myocardial infarction from myocarditis: diagnostic value of early-

and delayed-perfusion cardiac MR imaging. Radiology 2005; 237(1):75–82

Liu PP, Yan AT. Cardiovascular magnetic resonance for the diagnosis of acute myocarditis: prospects for detecting myocardial inflammation. J Am Coll Cardiol 2005; 45(11):1823–1825

Lund GK, Stork A, Saeed M, Bansmann MP, Gerken JH, Muller V, Mester J, Higgins CB, Adam G, Meinertz T. Acute myocardial infarction: evaluation with first-pass enhancement and delayed enhancement MR imaging compared with ^{201}Tl SPECT imaging. Radiology 2004; 232(1):49–57

Luo AK, Wu KC. Imaging microvascular obstruction and its clinical significance following acute myocardial infarction. Heart Fail Rev 2006; 11(4):305–312

Mahrholdt H, Wagner A, Judd RM, Sechtem U. Assessment of myocardial viability by cardiovascular magnetic resonance imaging. Eur Heart J 2002; 23(8):602–619

Mahrholdt H, Wagner A, Deluigi CC, Kispert E, Hager S, Meinhardt G, Vogelsberg H, Fritz P, Dippon J, Bock CT, Klingel K, Kandolf R, Sechtem U. Presentation, patterns of myocardial damage, and clinical course of viral myocarditis. Circulation 2006; 114(15):1581–1590

Marcu CB, Nijveldt R, Beek AM, Van Rossum AC. Delayed contrast enhancement magnetic resonance imaging for the assessment of cardiac disease. Heart Lung Circ 2007; 16(2):70–78. Epub 2007 Feb 21

Masui T, Finck S, Higgins CB. Constrictive pericarditis and restrictive cardiomyopathy: evaluation with MR imaging. Radiology 1992; 182(2):369–373

Matsunaka T, Hamada M, Matsumoto Y, Higaki J. First-pass myocardial perfusion defect and delayed contrast enhancement in hypertrophic cardiomyopathy assessed with MRI. Magn Reson Med Sci 2003; 2(2):61–69

McConnell MV, Ganz P, Selwyn AP, Li W, Edelman RR, Manning WJ. Identification of anomalous coronary arteries and their anatomic course by magnetic resonance coronary angiography. Circulation 1995; 92(11):3158–3162

Mollet NR, Dymarkowski S, Volders W, Wathiong J, Herbots L, Rademakers FE, Bogaert J. Visualization of ventricular thrombi with contrast-enhanced magnetic resonance imaging in patients with ischemic heart disease. Circulation 2002; 106(23):2873–2876

Moon JC, Prasad SK. Cardiovascular magnetic resonance and the evaluation of heart failure. Curr Cardiol Rep. 2005; 7(1):39–44

Moon JC, McKenna WJ, McCrohon JA, Elliott PM, Smith GC, Pennell DJ. Toward clinical risk assessment in hypertrophic cardiomyopathy with gadolinium cardiovascular magnetic resonance. J Am Coll Cardiol 2003; 41(9):1561–1567

Moon JC, Mogensen J, Elliott PM, Smith GC, Elkington AG, Prasad SK, Pennell DJ, McKenna WJ. Myocardial late gadolinium enhancement cardiovascular magnetic resonance in hypertrophic cardiomyopathy caused by mutations in troponin I. Heart 2005; 91(8):1036–1040

Mulder BJ, van der Wall EE. Optimal imaging protocol for evaluation of aortic coarctation; time for a reappraisal. Int J Cardiovasc Imaging 2006; 22(5):695–697

Nishimura RA. Constrictive pericarditis in the modern era: a diagnostic dilemma. Heart 2001; 86(6):619–623

Oyama N, Oyama N, Komuro K, Nambu T, Manning WJ, Miyasaka K. Computed tomography and magnetic resonance imaging of the pericardium: anatomy and pathology. Magn Reson Med Sci 2004; 3(3):145–152

Paelinck BP, Lamb HJ, Bax JJ, Van der Wall EE, de Roos A. Assessment of diastolic function by cardiovascular magnetic resonance. Am Heart J 2002; 144(2):198–205

Pons-Llado G. Assessment of cardiac function by CMR. Eur Radiol 2005; 15 Suppl 2:B23–32

Post JC, van Rossum AC, Bronzwaer JG, de Cock CC, Hofman MB, Valk J, Visser CA. Magnetic resonance angiography of anomalous coronary arteries. A new gold standard for delineating the proximal course? Circulation 1995; 92(11):3163–3171

Rerkpattanapipat P, Gregory Hundley W. Dobutamine stress magnetic resonance imaging. Echocardiography 2007; 24(3):309–315

Rochitte CE, Tassi EM, Shiozaki AA The emerging role of MRI in the diagnosis and management of cardiomyopathies. Curr Cardiol Rep 2006; 8(1):44–52

Saeed M, Weber O, Lee R, Do L, Martin A, Saloner D, Ursell P, Robert P, Corot C, Higgins CB. Discrimination of myocardial acute and chronic (scar) infarctions on delayed contrast enhanced magnetic resonance imaging with intravascular magnetic resonance contrast media. J Am Coll Cardiol 2006; 48(10):1961–1968

Sipola P, Lauerma K, Jaaskelainen P, Laakso M, Peuhkurinen K, Manninen H, Aronen HJ, Kuusisto J. Cine MR imaging of myocardial contractile impairment in patients with hypertrophic cardiomyopathy attributable to Asp[175]Asn mutation in the alpha-tropomyosin gene. Radiology 2005; 236(3):815–824

Soler R, Rodriguez E, Remuinan C, Bello MJ, Diaz A. Magnetic resonance imaging of primary cardiomyopathies. J Comput Assist Tomogr 2003; 27(5):724–734

Soler R, Rodriguez E, Monserrat L, Mendez C, Martinez C. Magnetic resonance imaging of delayed enhancement in hypertrophic cardiomyopathy: relationship with left ventricular perfusion and contractile function. J Comput Assist Tomogr 2006; 30(3):412–420

Stern HC, Locher D, Wallnofer K, Weber F, Scheid KF, Emmrich P, Buhlmeyer K. Noninvasive assessment of coarctation of the aorta: comparative measurements by two-dimensional echocardiography, magnetic resonance, and angiography. Pediatr Cardiol 1991; 12(1):1–5

Syed MA, Carlson K, Murphy M, Ingkanisorn WP, Rhoads KL, Arai AE. Long-term safety of cardiac magnetic resonance imaging performed in the first few days after bare-metal stent implantation. J Magn Reson Imag 2006; 24(5):1056–1061

Tarantini G, Razzolini R, Cacciavillani L, Bilato C, Sarais C, Corbetti F, Marra MP, Napodano M, Ramondo A, Iliceto S. Influence of transmurality, infarct size, and severe microvascular obstruction on left ventricular remodeling and function after primary coronary angioplasty. Am J Cardiol 2006; 98(8):1033–1040

Taylor AJ, Al-Saadi N, Abdel-Aty H, Schulz-Menger J, Messroghli DR, Friedrich MG. Detection of acutely impaired microvascular reperfusion after infarct angioplasty with magnetic resonance imaging. Circulation 2004; 109(17):2080–2085. Epub 2004 Apr 26

Vliegen HW, Doornbos J, de Roos A, Jukema JW, Bekedam MA, van der Wall EE. Value of fast gradient echo magnetic resonance angiography as an adjunct to coronary arteriography in detecting and confirming the course of clinically significant coronary artery anomalies. Am J Cardiol 1997; 79(6):773–776

Vogel-Claussen J, Rochitte CE, Wu KC, Kamel IR, Foo TK, Lima JA, Bluemke DA. Delayed enhancement MR imaging: utility in myocardial assessment. Radiographics 2006; 26(3):795–810

Wang ZJ, Reddy GP, Gotway MB, Yeh BM, Hetts SW, Higgins CB. CT and MR imaging of pericardial disease. Radiographics 2003; 23 Spec No:S167–S180

Waxman S, Eustace S, Hartnell GG. Myocardial involvement in primary hemochromatosis demonstrated by magnetic resonance imaging. Am Heart J 1994; 128(5):1047–1049

Wilson JM, Villareal RP, Hariharan R, Massumi A, Muthupillai R, Flamm SD. Magnetic resonance imaging of myocardial fibrosis in hypertrophic cardiomyopathy. Tex Heart Inst J 2002; 29(3):176–180

Yan AT, Gibson CM, Larose E, Anavekar NS, Tsang S, Solomon SD, Reynolds G, Kwong RY. Characterization of microvascular dysfunction after acute myocardial infarction by cardiovascular magnetic resonance first-pass perfusion and late gadolinium enhancement imaging. J Cardiovasc Magn Reson 2006; 8(6):831–837

MDCT

Beck T, Burgstahler C, Reimann A, Kuettner A, Heuschmid M, Kopp AF, Schroeder S. Technology insight: possible applications of multislice computed tomography in clinical cardiology. Nat Clin Pract Cardiovasc Med 2005; 2(7):361–368

Cademartiri F, Aldrovandi A, Palumbo A, Maffei E, Fusaro M, Tresoldi S, Messalli G, Rossi A, Rengo M, Pugliese F, Salamousas BV, Reverberi C, Meijboom WB, Mollet NR, Ardissino D, De Feyter PJ. Multislice computed tomography coronary angiography: clinical applications. Minerva Cardioangiol 2007; 55(5):647–658

Cademartiri F, Palumbo A, Maffei E, Casolo G, Mollet NR, Meijboom BW, Ligthart JM. Follow-up of internal mammary artery stent with 64-slice CT. Int J Cardiovasc Imaging 2007; 23(4):537–539

Cademartiri F, Schuijf JD, Pugliese F, Mollet NR, Jukema JW, Maffei E, Kroft LJ, Palumbo A, Ardissino D, Serruys PW, Krestin GP, Van der Wall EE, de Feyter PJ, Bax JJ. Usefulness of 64-slice multislice computed tomography coronary angiography to assess in-stent restenosis. J Am Coll Cardiol 2007; 49(22):2204–2210

de Feyter PJ, Mollet NR, Cademartiri F, Nieman K, Pattynama P. MS-CT coronary imaging. J Interv Cardiol 2003; 16(6):465–468

de Feyter PJ, Meijboom WB, Weustink A, Van Mieghem C, Mollet NR, Vourvouri E, Nieman K, Cademartiri F. Spiral multislice computed tomography coronary angiography: a current status report. Clin Cardiol 2007; 30(9):437–442

Dewey M, Rutsch W, Schnapauff D, Teige F, Hamm B. Coronary artery stenosis quantification using multislice computed tomography. Invest Radiol 2007; 42(2):78–84

Ehara M, Surmely JF, Kawai M, Katoh O, Matsubara T, Terashima M, Tsuchikane E, Kinoshita Y, Suzuki T, Ito T, Takeda Y, Nasu K, Tanaka N, Murata A, Suzuki Y, Sato K, Suzuki T. Diagnostic accuracy of 64-slice computed tomography for detecting angiographically significant coronary artery stenosis in an unselected consecutive patient population: comparison with conventional invasive angiography. Circ J 2006; 70(5):564–571

Gilard M, Cornily JC, Pennec PY, Joret C, Le Gal G, Mansourati J, Blanc JJ, Boschat J. Accuracy of multislice computed tomography in the preoperative assessment of coronary disease in patients with aortic valve stenosis. J Am Coll Cardiol 2006; 47(10):2020–2024

Goldstein JA, Gallagher MJ, O'Neill WW, Ross MA, O'Neil BJ, Raff GL. A randomized controlled trial of multi-slice coronary computed tomography for evaluation of acute chest pain. J Am Coll Cardiol 2007; 49(8):863–871

Haberl R, Tittus J, Bohme E, Czernik A, Richartz BM, Buck J, Steinbigler P. Multislice spiral computed tomographic angiography of coronary arteries in patients with suspected coronary artery disease: an effective filter before catheter angiography? Am Heart J 2005; 149(6):1112–1119

Hoffmann MH, Shi H, Schmitz BL, Schmid FT, Lieberknecht M, Schulze R, Ludwig B, Kroschel U, Jahnke N, Haerer W, Brambs HJ, Aschoff AJ. Noninvasive coronary angiography with multislice computed tomography. JAMA 2005; 293(20):2471–2478. Erratum in: JAMA 2005; 294(10):1208

Mather R. Multislice CT: 64 slices and beyond. Radiol Manage 2005; 27(3):46–48, 50–52

Meijboom WB, van Mieghem CA, Mollet NR, Pugliese F, Weustink AC, van Pelt N, Cademartiri F, Nieman K, Boersma E, de Jaegere P, Krestin GP, de Feyter PJ. 64-slice computed tomography coronary angiography in patients with high, intermediate, or low pretest probability of significant coronary artery disease. J Am Coll Cardiol 2007; 50(15):1469–1475

Meijboom WB, van Pelt N, de Feyter P. Use of High-resolution Spiral CT for the Diagnosis of Coronary Artery Disease. Curr Treat Options Cardiovasc Med 2007; 9(1):29–36

Mollet NR, Cademartiri F, van Mieghem CA, Runza G, McFadden EP, Baks T, Serruys PW, Krestin GP, de Feyter PJ. High-resolution spiral computed tomography coronary angiography in patients referred for diagnostic conventional coronary angiography. Circulation 2005; 112(15):2318–2323

Motoyama S, Kondo T, Sarai M, Sugiura A, Harigaya H, Sato T, Inoue K, Okumura M, Ishii J, Anno H, Virmani R, Ozaki Y, Hishida H, Narula J. Multislice computed tomographic characteristics of coronary lesions in acute coronary syndromes. J Am Coll Cardiol 2007; 50(4):319–326

Nicol ED, Underwood SR. X-ray computed tomography coronary angiography-defining the role of a new technique. Int J Cardiovasc Imaging 2007; 23(5):615–616

Nikolaou K, Knez A, Rist C, Wintersperger BJ, Leber A, Johnson T, Reiser MF, Becker CR. Accuracy of 64-MDCT in the diagnosis of ischemic heart disease. AJR Am J Roentgenol 2006; 187(1):111–117

Pontone G, Andreini D, Quaglia C, Ballerini G, Nobili E, Pepi M. Accuracy of multidetector spiral computed tomography in detecting significant coronary stenosis in patient populations with differing pre-test probabilities of disease. Clin Radiol 2007; 62(10):978–985

Pundziute G, Schuijf JD, Jukema JW, de Roos A, van der Wall EE, Bax JJ. Advances in the noninvasive evaluation of coronary artery disease with multislice computed tomography. Expert Rev Med Devices 2006; 3(4):441–451

Raff GL, Gallagher MJ, O'Neill WW, Goldstein JA. Diagnostic accuracy of noninvasive coronary angiography using 64-slice spiral computed tomography. J Am Coll Cardiol 2005; 46(3):552–557

Ropers D. Multislice computer tomography for detection of coronary artery disease. J Interv Cardiol 2006; 19(6):574–582

Schuijf JD, Pundziute G, Jukema JW, Lamb HJ, van der Hoeven BL, de Roos A, van der Wall EE, Bax JJ. Diagnostic accuracy of 64-slice multislice computed tomography in the noninvasive evaluation of significant coronary artery disease. Am J Cardiol 2006; 98(2):145–148

Schussler JM, Grayburn PA. Non-invasive coronary angiography using multislice computed tomography. Heart 2007; 93(3):290–297

Shrivastava V, Vundavalli S, Mitchell L, Dunning J. Is cardiac computed tomography a reliable alternative to percutaneous coronary angiography for patients awaiting valve surgery? Interact Cardiovasc Thorac Surg 2007; 6(1):105–109

Soon KH, Kelly AM, Cox N, Chaitowitz I, Bell KW, Lim YL. Non-invasive multislice computed tomography coronary angiography for imaging coronary arteries, stents and bypass grafts. Intern Med J 2006; 36(1):43–50

Sun Z, Jiang W. Diagnostic value of multislice computed tomography angiography in coronary artery disease: a meta-analysis. Eur J Radiol 2006; 60(2):279–286

Van Mieghem CA, Cademartiri F, Mollet NR, Malagutti P, Valgimigli M, Meijboom WB, Pugliese F, McFadden EP, Ligthart J, Runza G, Bruining N, Smits PC, Regar E, van der Giessen WJ, Sianos G, van Domburg R, de Jaegere P, Krestin GP, Serruys PW, de Feyter PJ. Multislice spiral computed tomography for the evaluation of stent patency after left main coronary artery stenting: a comparison with conventional coronary angiography and intravascular ultrasound. Circulation 2006; 114(7):645–653

Vembar M, Walker MJ, Johnson PC. Cardiac imaging using multislice computed tomography scanners: technical considerations. Coron Artery Dis 2006; 17(2):115–123

Thoracic Radiology

3

Santiago E. Rossi and Joaquina Lopez Mora

Introduction

Chest radiology plays an essential role in the detection and characterization of conditions involving the thorax. Knowledge of a patient's clinical history is particularly important in thoracic radiology, since the radiological findings may suggest a myriad of possible interpretations in any given case. A wide range of imaging techniques is useful in the study of the thorax. The different imaging procedures in thoracic radiology can be summarized as:

- Chest X-rays are usually the first-line imaging modality in thoracic pathology and give a detailed overview of the lungs, heart, and chest wall.
- Computed Tomography (CT) is generally performed to characterize a chest X-ray finding. High resolution CT (HRCT) has a significant contribution in the evaluation of diffuse lung diseases.
- Magnetic Resonance (MR) has a limited use in thoracic imaging; it is especially useful in the evaluation of mediastinal and pleural masses. It has the advantage of not using ionizing radiation.
- Ventilation-perfusion scan (V/Q) is a type of diagnostic scintigraphy used to study the distributions of pulmonary blood flow and alveolar ventilation.
- PET-CT has all the advantages of the two methods that make up this dual imaging modality, computed tomography and positron emission tomography, and combines both anatomical and metabolic findings. It is especially used in oncology, including the evaluation of solitary pulmonary nodules, lung cancer staging and re-staging, and the response to therapy.

With the increasing number of diagnostic modalities, thoracic radiologists must master a wide spectrum of different technologies and determine the most appropriate diagnostic test for each clinical situation. Chest radiology includes the evaluation of different systems: the lung and airways, heart and great vessels, chest wall, diaphragm, and mediastinum. The evaluation of the heart and great vessels is a growing area of interest for thoracic radiologists, and the development of cardiovascular applications of both MR and multislice CT has expanded the role of the thoracic radiologist in the study diseases affecting the heart and great vessels. The recent introduction of multislice CT and PET-CT has also had a great impact on patient management.

Although, this chapter focuses on pulmonary imaging cases, interventional radiology plays a vital role in daily clinical practice. Among other invasive diagnostic and therapeutic techniques, thoracic radiologists biopsy pulmonary nodules and treat lung tumors using radiofrequency ablation.

In conclusion, thoracic radiology is in constant evolution and includes much more than reading chest X-rays. In our opinion, its versatility makes thoracic radiology one of the most attractive radiology subspecialties.

Case 1
■ Usual Interstitial Pneumonia (UIP)

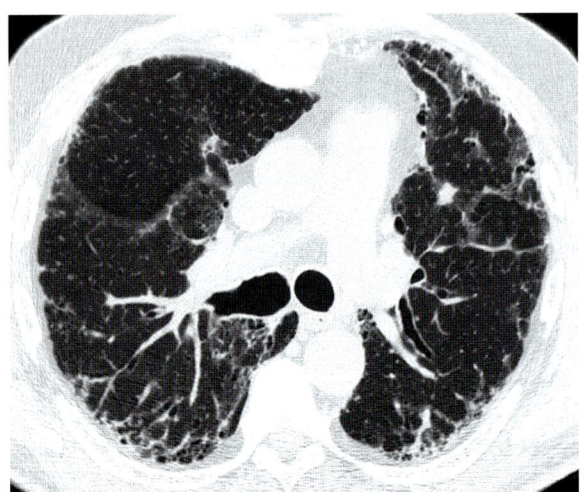

Fig. 3.1.1

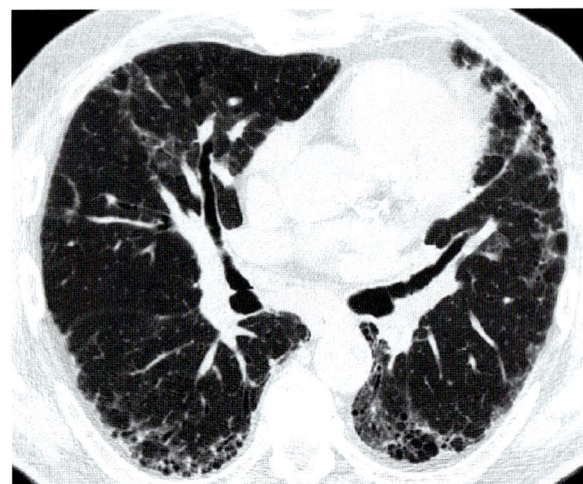

Fig. 3.1.2

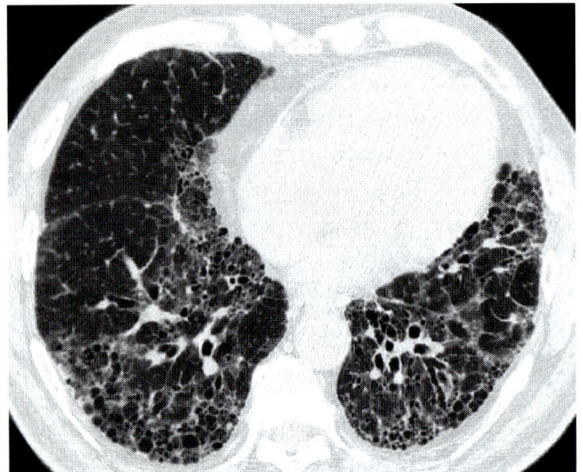

Fig. 3.1.3

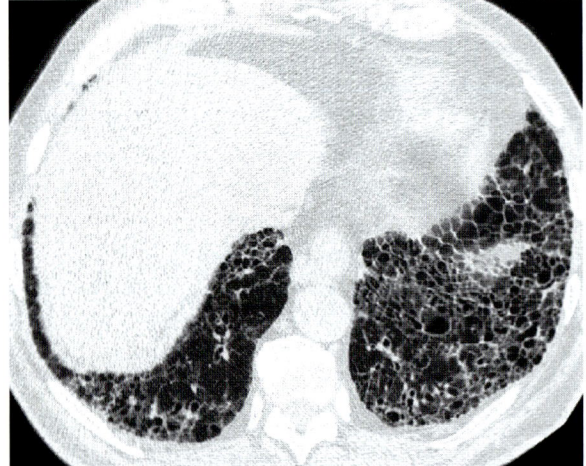

Fig. 3.1.4

A 54-year-old man presented with progressive dyspnea and non-productive cough. Drug toxicity, environmental exposure, and collagen vascular disease were ruled out. Bibasilar velcro-type end-inspiratory crackles were detected on auscultation. Lung function tests revealed a moderate restrictive defect, decreased PAO2, and decreased diffusing capacity of the lung for carbon monoxide (DLCO).

Idiopathic pulmonary fibrosis (IPF) is the clinical syndrome associated with an interstitial pneumonia of unknown cause. Histopathological findings show a pattern of usual interstitial pneumonia.

Surgical lung biopsy is the most definitive method for establishing the diagnosis. Pathologic changes have a predilection for the subpleural and paraseptal parenchyma. Fibrotic zones with associated honeycombing alternate with areas of relatively unaffected lung tissue. Areas of chronic lung injury contrast with regions of acute injury with foci of actively proliferating fibroblasts and myofibroblasts. Interstitial inflammation is mild and generally associated with fibrosis. Spatial and temporal heterogeneity are characteristic.

Patients with IPF have an increased incidence of lung carcinoma. The disease follows a progressive course with a mean survival time of 3 years. Treatment options include corticosteroids, azathioprine, and lung transplantation.

Differential diagnoses:
- Nonspecific interstitial pneumonia (ground-glass pattern predominance, usually no honeycombing)
- Asbestosis (subpleural lines and parenchymal bands)
- Drug toxicity (ground glass and consolidations)

Chest radiograph demonstrates:
- Bilateral reticular opacities
- Lower lobes, peripheral predominance
- Cystic dilatation of the distal air spaces "honeycombing"
- Traction bronchiectasis

High resolution computed tomography (HRCT) increases spatial resolution, facilitating visualization of parenchymal detail to the level of the secondary pulmonary lobule.

HRCT (UIP) demonstrates:
- Interlobular septal thickening
- Ground-glass attenuation pattern
- Traction bronchiectasis and bronchiolectasis
- Architectural distortion
- Honeycomb pattern
- Basal and peripheral predominance

Case 2
■
Lymphangitic Carcinomatosis

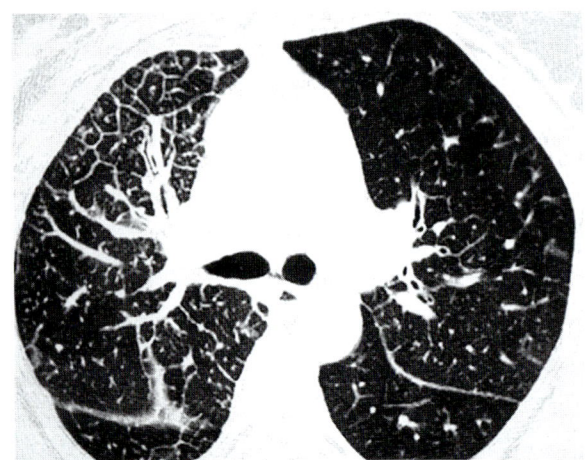

Fig. 3.2.1

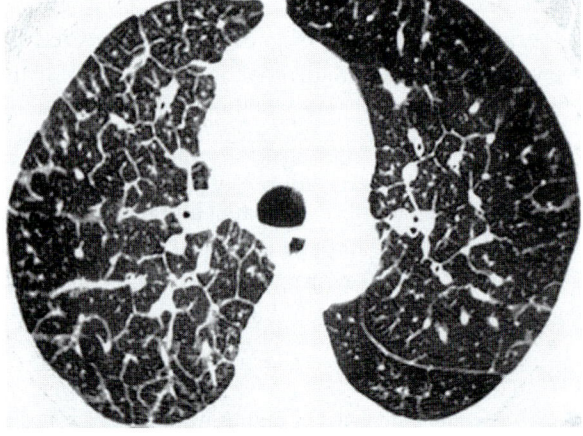

Fig. 3.2.2

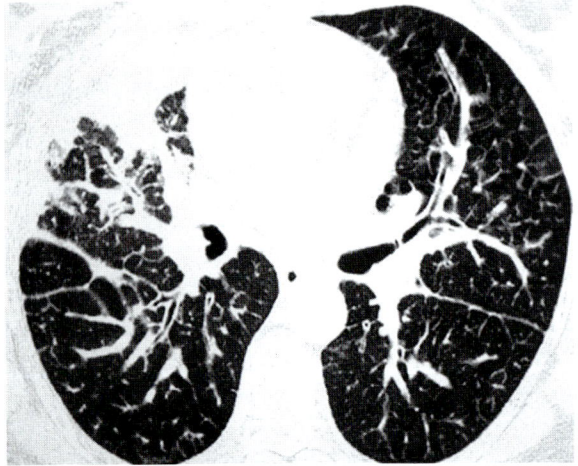

Fig. 3.2.3

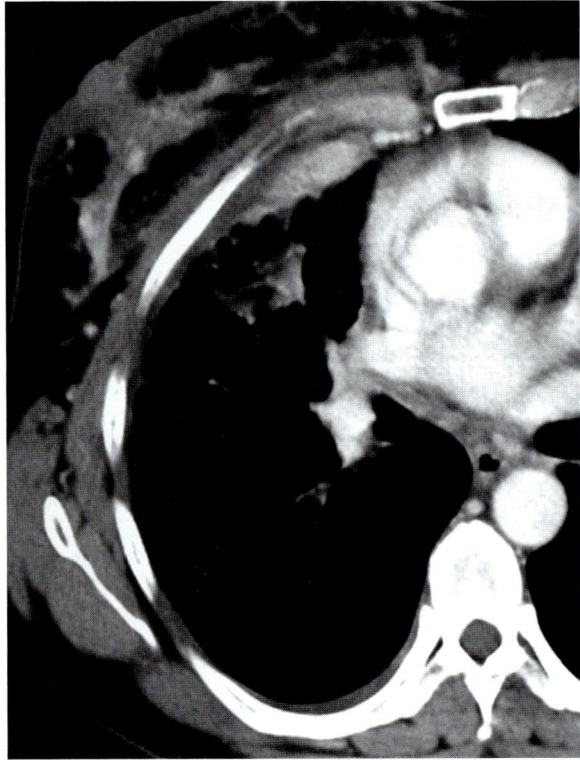

Fig. 3.2.4

A 59-year-old woman with a 30 pack/year history of smoking presented with shortness of breath, nonproductive cough, fatigue, and weakness. Physical examination revealed tachypnea; tachycardia, and cyanosis. Auscultation revealed diffuse fine rales in the basal regions and a restrictive ventilatory defect. Past medical included a history of breast carcinoma 10 years prior. Bronchoalveolar lavage detected neoplastic cells and an increased number of lymphocytes.

Lymphangitic carcinomatosis represents intrapulmonary spread of metastatic neoplasm via lymphatics and adjacent connective tissue. It is a frequent pattern of neoplastic spread to the lungs (35–55%). The most common primary malignancies producing lymphangitic spread include adenocarcinomas of the breast, lung, stomach, pancreas, cervix, and colon. Most cases of lymphangitic spread occur as a result of tumor microembolization. Other potential mechanisms include retrograde spread from involved lymph nodes, local extension from a primary pulmonary tumor, and transdiaphragmatic spread. Pulmonary architecture is preserved, although the lymphatic vessels appear distended by neoplastic cells and a perilymphatic fibrotic reaction is usual. In the presence of an unknown primary tumor, the diagnosis is based on histopathologic specimens.

Differential Diagnosis:
- Pulmonary edema (interlobular septal thickening, nodules are absent, ground-glass, and consolidation)
- Sarcoidosis (bilateral, peribronchovascular, upper lobes predominance, distortion of pulmonary architecture)
- Silicosis (upper lobes, associated with masses and parenchymal distortion)
- Pneumoconiosis
- Hypersensitivity pneumonitis
- Lymphoma and Kaposi's Sarcoma

Chest radiograph shows:
- Normal findings, usually (25% sensitivity)
- Reticulonodular pattern, more frequent in the lower lobes
- Kerley B lines (Kerley B lines in the absence of congestive heart failure is very suggestive of lymphangitic carcinomatosis)
- Pleural effusion
- Hilar and mediastinal adenopathy

High resolution computed tomography (HRCT) shows:
- Nodular, irregular or smooth reticular pattern (beaded appearance)
- Peribronchovascular, centrilobular, septal, and subpleural distribution
- Unilateral, bilateral, or patchy distribution
- Pulmonary architecture is preserved
- Normal lung volume
- Pleural effusion
- Hilar or mediastinal adenopathy

Case 3
■
**Thrombotic
Pulmonary Embolism**

A 70-year-old-woman presented with pleuritic chest pain irradiated to the right shoulder, hemoptysis, and sudden shortness of breath. She had a history of 20-pack/year smoking habit, hypertension, and obesity. She had been immobilized after hip replacement surgery for 20 days and left hospital three days prior. On admission the patient was tachypneic; oxygen saturations on air were 80%, and decreased air entry to her right lung base was noted with pleural rub.

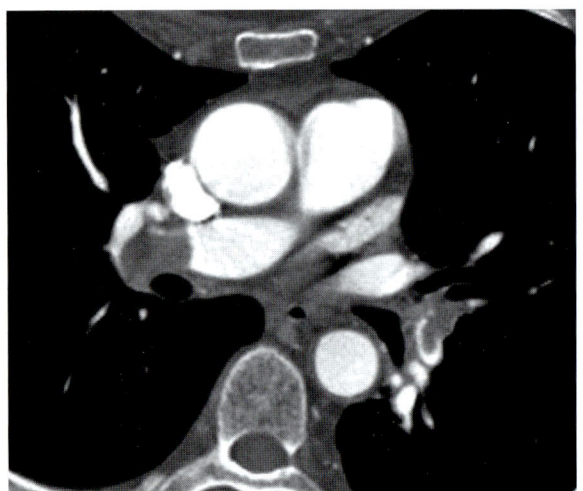

Fig. 3.3.1

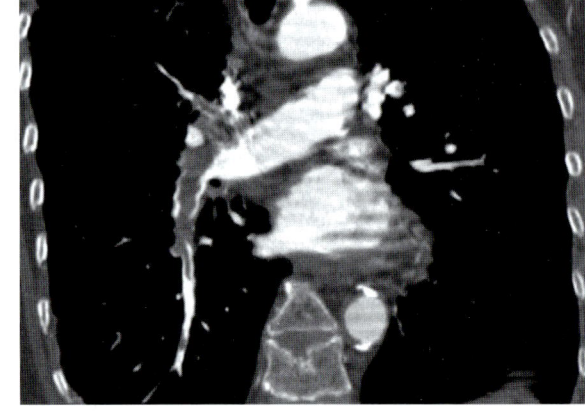

Fig. 3.3.2

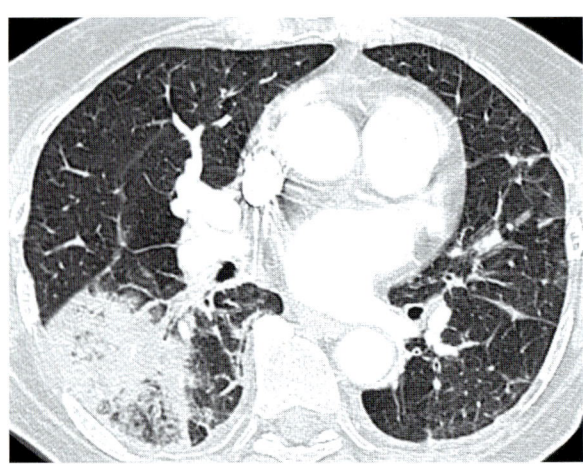

Fig. 3.3.3

Thrombotic pulmonary embolism is a major cause of death in hospitalized patients. Predisposing factors include hypercoagulable state, orthopedic surgery, malignancy, and pregnancy. Most emboli arise from the deep veins of the legs and lodge within the branches of the pulmonary arteries, and a few straddle the bifurcation of the main pulmonary artery. The effects of emboli are due to vascular obstruction. Pulmonary arterial obstruction and release of vasoactive agents elevate pulmonary vascular resistance, increasing alveolar dead space and causing redistribution of blood flow. Reflex bronchoconstriction augments airway resistance, lung edema decreases pulmonary compliance, and right ventricular afterload increases. Embolic infarction is unusual (15%) and occurs only when the combined bronchial and pulmonary arterial circulation is inadequate (peripheral arterial tree or heart failure). The main cause of death in pulmonary embolism is circulatory collapse secondary to right-sided heart failure.

Differential Diagnosis:
- Chronic pulmonary embolism: eccentric defect at an obtuse angle with the arterial wall, nodular arterial wall, abrupt narrowing of the arterial diameter, recanalization of thrombosed vessel
- Septic pulmonary embolism
- Hydatid embolism
- Fat embolism
- Amniotic fluid embolism
- Tumor embolism
- Air embolism

Chest radiographs are usually used only to exclude other causes since they have low sensitivity and specificity. Main signs include:
- Enlargement of the central pulmonary artery (Fleischner sign)
- Oligemia of the lung beyond the occluded vessel (Westermark sign)
- Pleura-based areas of consolidation (Hampton hump sign)
- Pleural effusion
- Hemidiaphragm elevation
- Linear atelectasis

Contrast-enhanced CT detects intraluminal filling defects in the main, lobar, segmental, and subsegmental arteries.
- Total filling defect occluding the entire lumen of an artery, which might be enlarged
- Partial filling defect ("polo mint" sign on images acquired perpendicular to the long axis of a vessel and "railway track" sign on longitudinal images of the vessel)
- Peripheral intraluminal filling defect that forms acute angles with the arterial wall
- Infarcts (peripheral wedge-shaped areas of hyperattenuation)
- Linear bands
- Right ventricular dilatation or deviation of the interventricular septum

Ventilation-perfusion scan (V/Q) is a type of diagnostic scintigraphy used to study the distributions of pulmonary blood flow and alveolar ventilation. In pulmonary embolism, pulmonary perfusion is abnormal while the lung parenchyma remains intact and ventilation remains normal ("mismatched perfusion defect"). If embolism results in infarction, a ventilation defect corresponding to the perfusion defect appears.

Case 4
■
Metastases

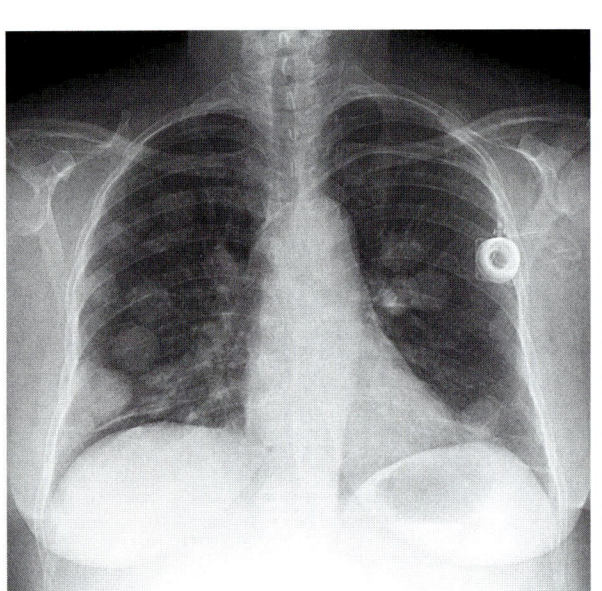

Fig. 3.4.1

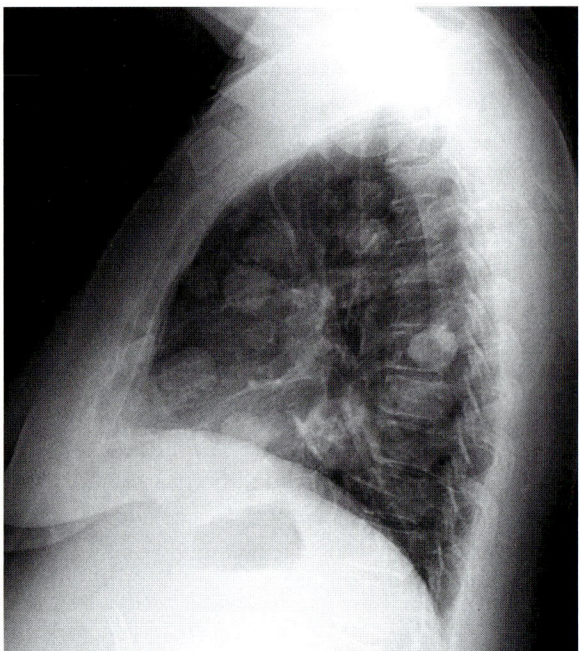

Fig. 3.4.2

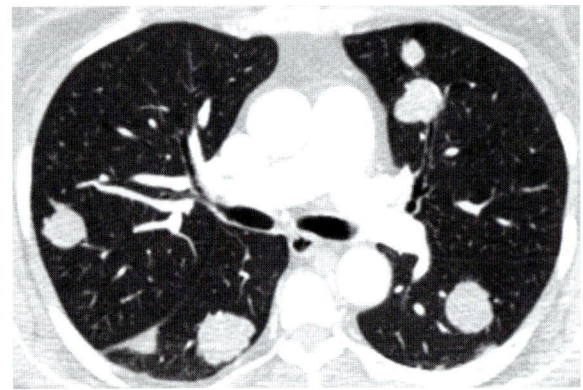

Fig. 3.4.3

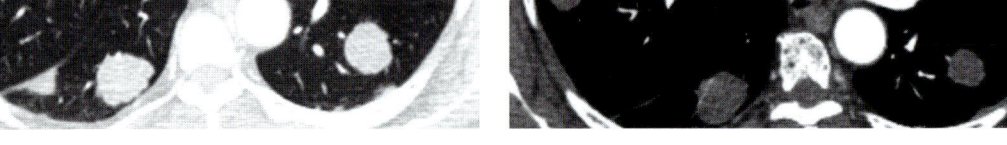

Fig. 3.4.4

A 63-year-old-woman with a past history of colon carcinoma.

In autopsy series, pulmonary metastases are found in 20–50% of patients with colon cancer. The most common sources of metastases include colon, breast, kidney, prostate, head, and neck carcinoma. Tumors with a high incidence of pulmonary metastases are choriocarcinoma, osteosarcoma, melanoma, and thyroid carcinoma. Early diagnosis of pulmonary metastases may be critical in planning and evaluating the accuracy of therapy. The most frequent mechanisms of dissemination to the lungs are: hematogenous (nodules), lymphangitic (interstitial disease), and endobronchial spread, and tumor embolization.

Chest radiograph shows:
- Spherical nodules
- Solitary or multiple
- Variable in size
- Bilateral
- Peripheral (outer third of the lungs or subpleural)
- IMiddle or lower zones of the lungs

CT shows:
- Oval or spherical discrete nodules
- Solitary or multiple
- Well-defined, smooth or irregular outlines
- Soft-tissue density
- Pulmonary vessels leading to metastases ("afferent vessel sign")

Atypical radiologic findings:
- Cavitation: cervix, colon, or head and neck metastases
- Calcification: osteosarcoma, chondrosarcoma, breast, ovarian, colon, thyroid, or treated metastases
- Miliary dissemination: thyroid, renal metastases
- Spontaneous pneumothorax: sarcoma metastases
- Ground-glass attenuation around mass ("halo sign"): choriocarcinoma or angiosarcoma metastases
- Solitary mass: melanoma, sarcoma, colon, testicle, breast, or kidney metastases

Case 5
■
Thoracic Neurofibroma

A 34-year-old man with neurofibromatosis type I presented with radicular thoracic pain involving the left hemithorax from spine to sternum.

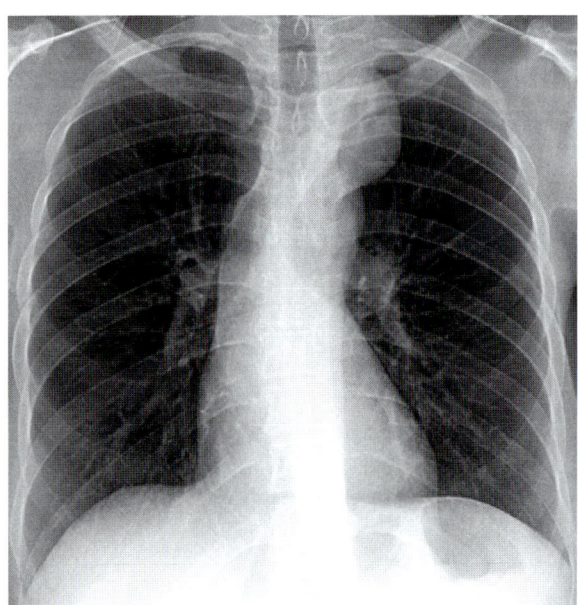

Fig. 3.5.1

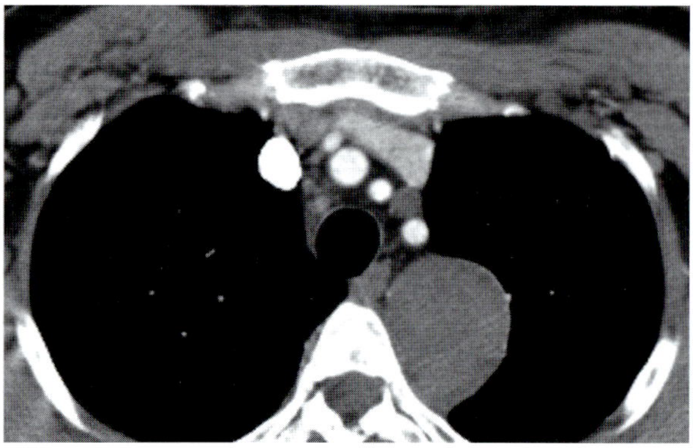

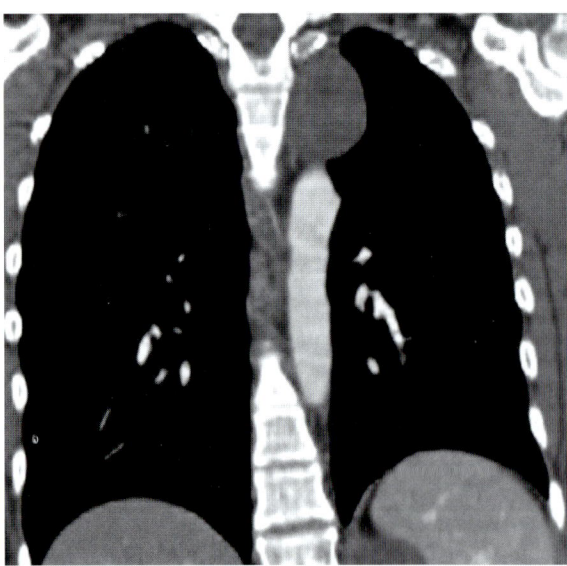

Fig. 3.5.3

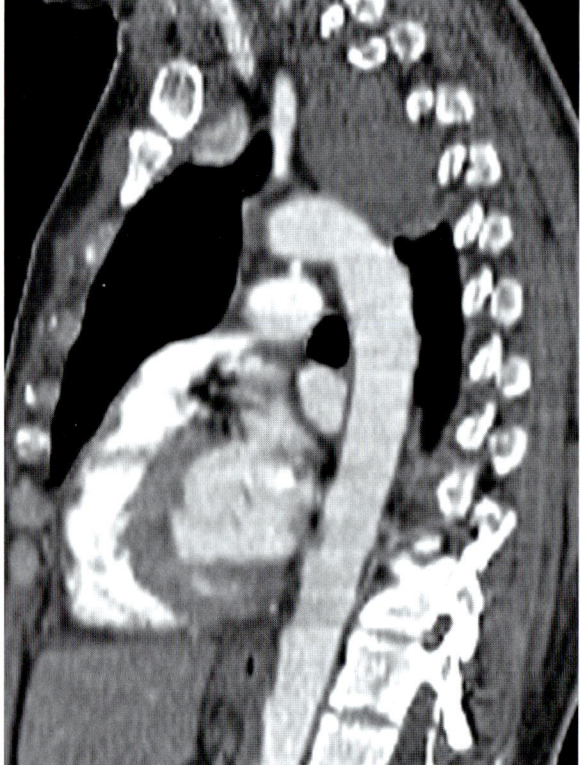

Fig. 3.5.2

Fig. 3.5.4

Neurogenic tumors account for about 9% of primary mediastinal masses in adults and 30% of mediastinal tumors in children. Neurofibromas are slow-growing neoplasms that originate from the nerve sheath and are derived from Schwann cells. They are seen most commonly in patients between 20 and 30 years of age. Most are benign, although malignant degeneration occasionally occurs (up to 25%). Almost all arise from intercostal or sympathetic nerves, adjacent to the spine. They are usually not encapsulated. Neurofibromas demonstrate proliferation of nerve sheath cells interspersed with thick collagen bundles and may show variable degrees of myxoid degeneration and calcifications.

Differential Diagnosis:
● Other neurogenic tumors including schwannoma, neuroblastoma, ganglioneuroma
● Adenopathies (lymphoma, tuberculosis, sarcoid, or metastases)
● Extramedullary hematopoiesis
● Neurenteric cysts
● Pancoast tumor

Radiographs of the spine may show:
● Widening of neural foramina
● Focal scoliosis
● Rib abnormalities

Chest radiographs may show:
● Well-defined mass
● Smooth or lobulated contours
● Round or oval
● Variable size
● Situated in the posterior mediastinum or grow along intercostal nerves

CT may show:
● Homogeneous mass
● Soft-tissue density and may have low attenuation zones
● Calcification (not usual): finely stippled
● Heterogeneous enhancement after intravenous administration of contrast material
● Bone erosions of ribs and vertebrae: the cortex is preserved and thickened
● Malignant degeneration: heterogeneous density, local invasion, bone destruction, and metastasis to the pleura or lungs

MR may show:
● Intermediate signal intensity on T1-weighted images
● Heterogeneous signal intensity on T2-weighted images: areas of collagen and fibrous tissue (low-signal) and areas of myxoid tissue or cystic degeneration (high-signal)
● "Target pattern": central portion shows higher intensity on T1, and the periphery shows higher intensity on T2 (due to highly cellular central zone and abundant stromal material in the peripheral zone)
● MR shows intraspinal extension best
● Plexiform neurofibroma: extensive fusiform or infiltrating mass that tends to surround mediastinal vessels with loss of fat planes

Comments

Imaging Findings

Case 6
Hodgkin Lymphoma

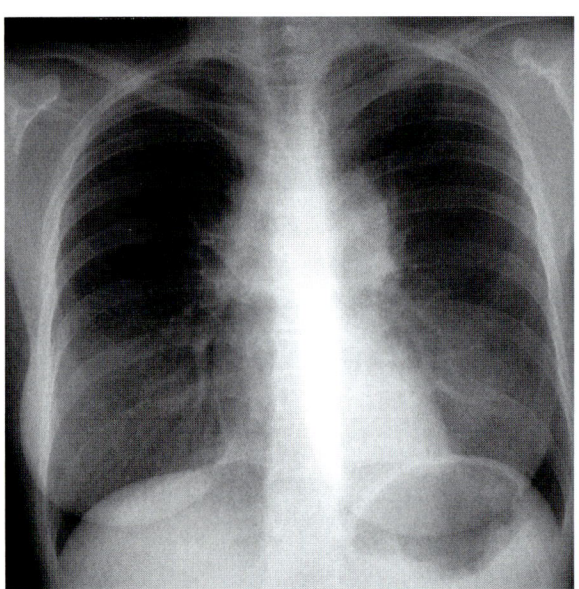

Fig. 3.6.1

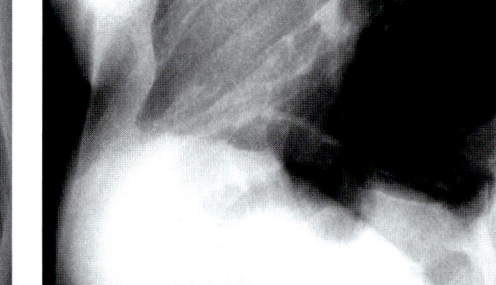

Fig. 3.6.2

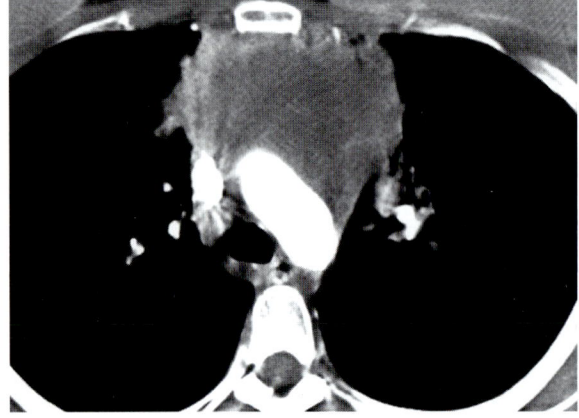

Fig. 3.6.3

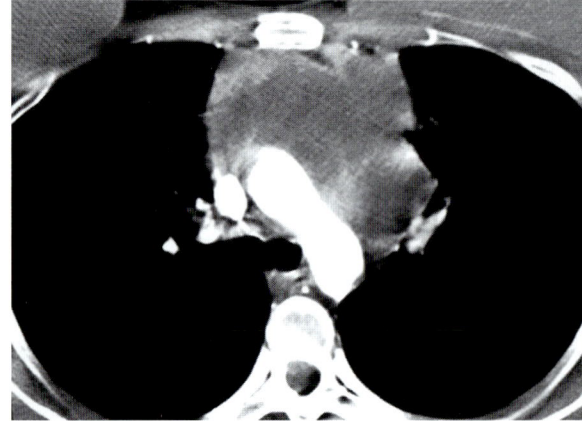

Fig. 3.6.4

A 30-year-old-woman presented with a one-month history of swollen neck lymph nodes, weight loss, fever, and night sweats. Her past medical history was unremarkable.

Lymphomas are divided into Hodgkin disease (HD) and non-Hodgkin lymphoma. Hodgkin disease is a lymphoid neoplasm of B lymphocyte lineage, characterized by the presence of Reed-Sternberg cells. Nodular sclerosis HD is the most common lymphoma of the anterior mediastinum, and patients are usually women between 20 and 50 years old. It most frequently involves the anterior mediastinal and paratracheal regions. Usually several nodal groups are involved at the moment of the diagnosis. It characteristically spreads by means of contiguous lymph node groups. Isolated hilar involvement should suggest other diagnoses. Staging of HD takes into account the extent of nodal disease, presence of extranodal disease, and clinical symptoms.

Differential diagnoses:
- Seminoma: heterogeneous, younger patients
- Thymoma: calcifications are usually seen
- Metastases: history of head and neck carcinoma
- Goiter: higher attenuation, extension to the neck (thyroid gland)
- Sarcoidosis: symmetrical hilar and paratracheal adenopathy
- Tuberculosis: lymph nodes with annular enhancement

Chest Radiograph shows:
- Rounded or lobulated mass
- Sharply marginated borders
- Widening of the mediastinum or hilum
- Increased opacity of the retrosternal area on the lateral view
- Calcifications after treatment
- Unilateral pleural effusions (15%)
- Lung involvement (10%)

CT appearance:
- Nodal enlargement: short axis > 1 cm
- Soft-tissue attenuation mass or adenopathy
- Slight-to-moderate enhancement after intravenous contrast material
- Necrotic nodes (central low attenuation) 20–45%
- Calcification after therapy: irregular, eggshell or diffuse pattern
- Pulmonary involvement: nodules, consolidations, or interstitial infiltration

MR appearance:
- Intermediate signal intensity on T1-weighted images
- High-signal intensity on T2-weighted images
- Demonstrates vascular invasion or compression

Case 7
■
Lung Cancer

A 50-year-old-man presented with upper back pain and progressive dyspnea; he had a history of smoking 30 packs/year. At physical examination, he showed signs of weight loss and expiratory wheezing at auscultation.

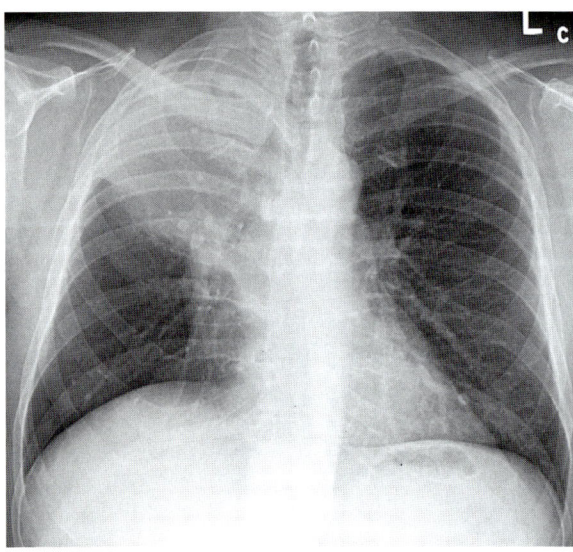

Fig. 3.7.1

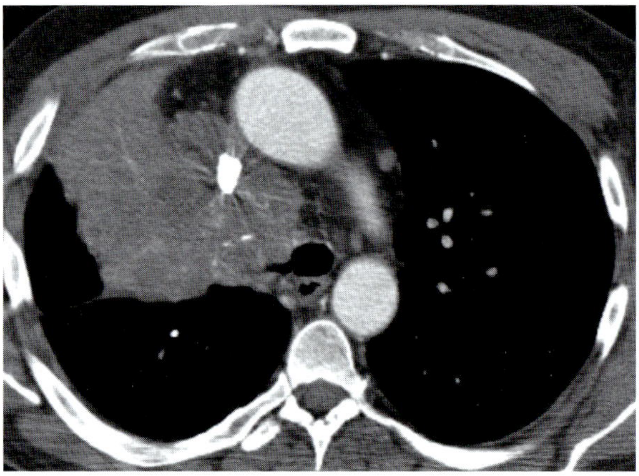

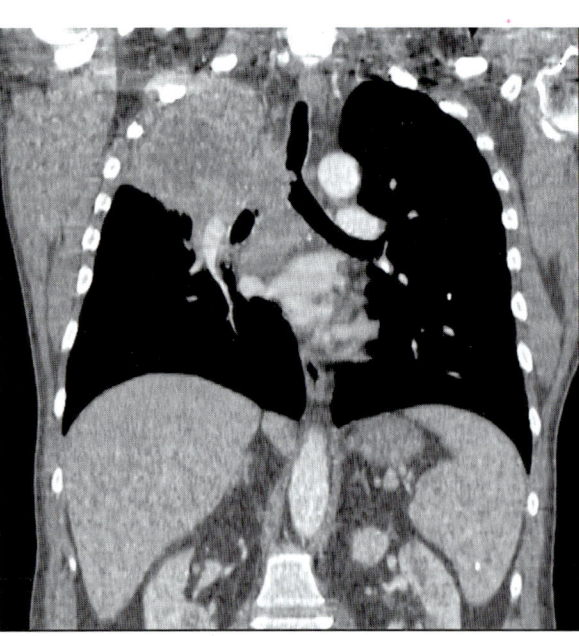

Fig. 3.7.3

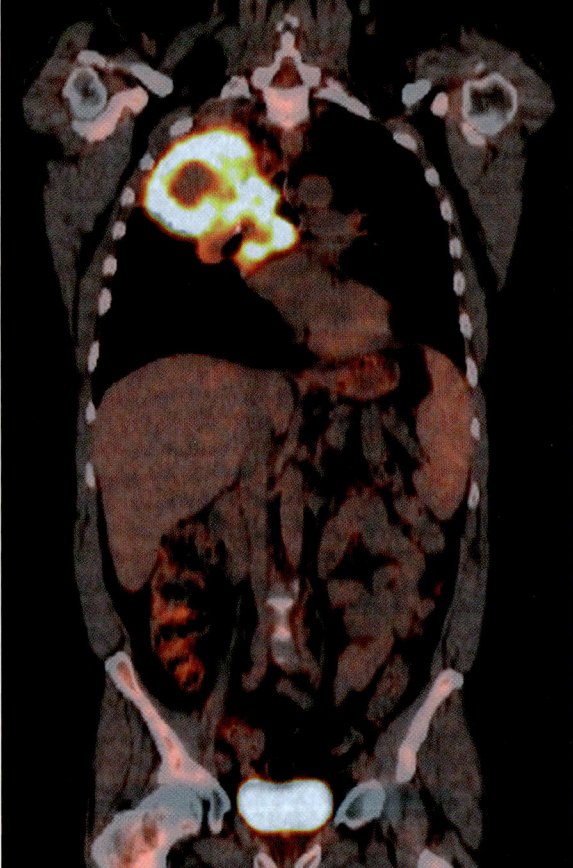

Fig. 3.7.2

Fig. 3.7.4

Bronchogenic carcinoma is the most common cause of cancer-related death in both men and women. It is divided into four main histologic subtypes: adenocarcinoma (the most common), squamous cell carcinoma, small cell carcinoma, and large cell carcinoma.

Adenocarcinoma:
- Symptoms include dyspnea or cough, pleuritic pain depending on extension
- Upper lobe, peripheral, or subpleural predominance
- Adrenal, brain, bone, or liver metastases
- Radiographic finding of a solitary pulmonary node or mass with well-marginated, lobulated, irregular, or poorly defined borders

Squamous cell carcinoma:
- Symptoms include cough and hemoptysis
- Central location with endobronchial component
- Direct extension to the local lymph nodes
- Slowest growth rate
- Radiographic finding of a hilar mass with or without obstructive pneumonitis or atelectasis
- Central necrosis is common in large tumors and central cavitation in 15%
- Can manifest as a Pancoast tumor (superior sulcus tumor): with invasion of the pleura and rib producing shoulder pain and involvement of the brachial plexus causing arm pain and paresthesia.

Differential Diagnosis:
- Bronchial carcinoid tumor: calcification, enhances with IV contrast, widening of the approaching bronchus
- Solitary metastases
- Primary pulmonary sarcoma
- SPN benign causes including hamartoma (fat/calcium), granuloma, and arteriovenous malformation.

Chest radiograph shows:
- Nodule or mass
- Hilar or mediastinal adenopathy or mass
- Pleural effusion
- Obstructive findings: atelectasis, pneumonia, mucoid impaction

CT shows:
- Nodule or mass
- Morphology: spherical or oval, lobulated or spiculated
- Density: soft-tissue density, amorphous calcification, cavitation with thick walls
- Contrast enhancement related to angiogenesis
- Evaluate growth rate
- Presence of associated collapse and/or consolidation
- Hilar and mediastinal adenopathies
- IMediastinal and chest wall invasion

PET-CT Noninvasive diagnostic metabolic and anatomic technique. PET-CT can aid in diagnosis, staging, assessing recurrence, and monitoring response to therapy.

Comments

Imaging Findings

Case 8
■
Bronchiectasis

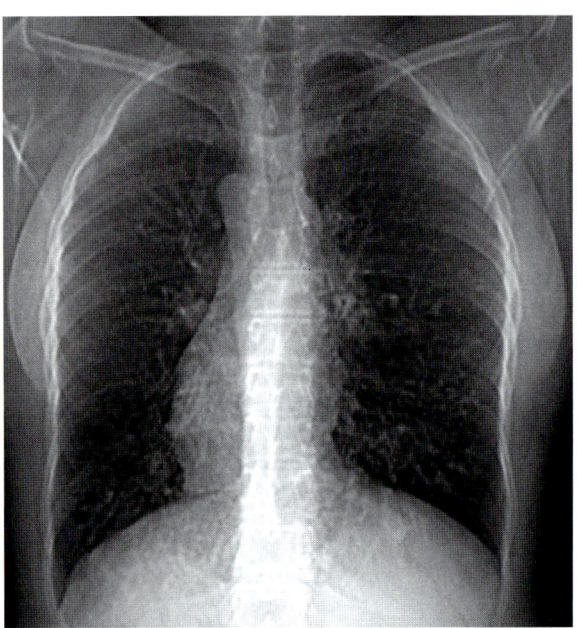

Fig. 3.8.1

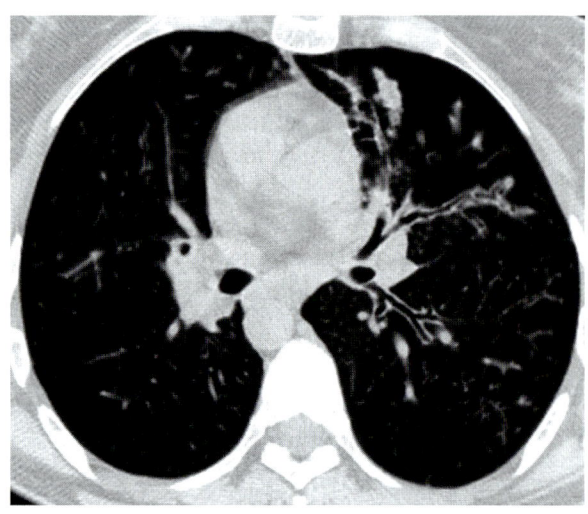

Fig. 3.8.2

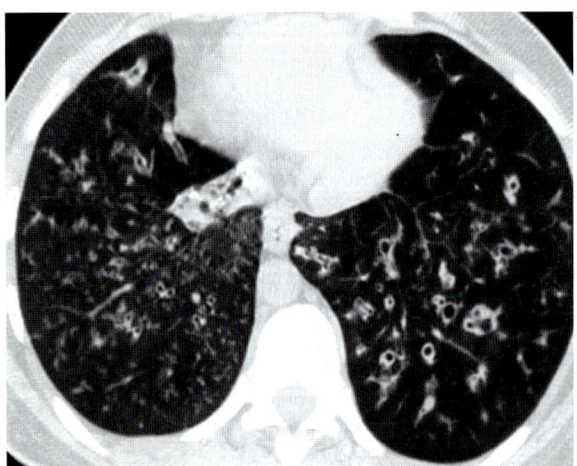

Fig. 3.8.3

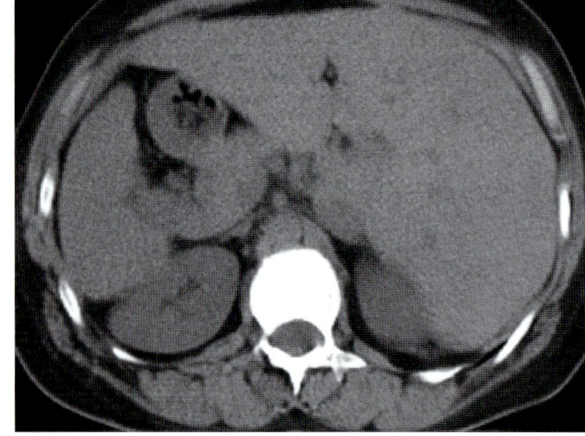

Fig. 3.8.4

A 15-year-old girl with chronic sinusitis and bronchitis presented with a productive cough without fever. Diffuse rhonchi were detected at physical examination.

Bronchiectasis is characterized by the permanent dilation of bronchi with destruction of the elastic and muscular components of bronchial walls. It is usually caused by acute or chronic infection. The main symptoms of bronchiectasis include chronic cough and sputum production. Recurrent bacterial colonization and infection lead to progressive airway injury.

Inflammatory mediators produce inflammation and destruction of the elastic and muscular components of bronchial walls, while the contractile force of the surrounding lung tissue exerts traction, expanding the diameter of involved airways.

Bronchiectasis is also associated with increased bronchial arterial proliferation and arteriovenous malformations, predisposing to recurrent hemoptysis in some patients. Bronchiectasis may have a focal or diffuse distribution.

Kartagener's syndrome refers to the triad of situs inversus, bronchiectasis, and recurrent sinusitis, occurring in half of patients with primary ciliary dyskinesia. This is an autosomal-recessive disorder associated with defective ciliary structure and function.

Differential Diagnosis:
- Cystic fibrosis
- Allergic bronchopulmonary aspergillosis (ABPA)
- Mycobacterium avium complex infection
- Pulmonary fibrosis
- Bronchial obstruction

Chest radiograph shows:
- Dilated and thickened airways (ring-like shadows of airways that are seen on end, or tram lines of airways that are perpendicular to the X-ray beam)
- Focal pneumonitis
- Scattered irregular opacities
- Plate-like atelectasis

High resolution CT (HRCT) shows:
- Bronchial wall thickening
- Bronchial dilatation
- Bronchus is larger than the adjacent pulmonary artery (signet ring sign)
- Bronchi are visible within 1 cm of pleura
- Cylindrical bronchiectasis (smooth bronchial dilatation)
- Varicose bronchiectasis (beaded bronchial dilatation)
- Cystic bronchiectasis (air-fluid levels in dilated airways)
- Mucoid impaction (tree-in-bud pattern)
- Atelectasis distal to mucoid plug
- Focal air-trapping distal to mucoid plug

Case 9
Malignant Mesothelioma

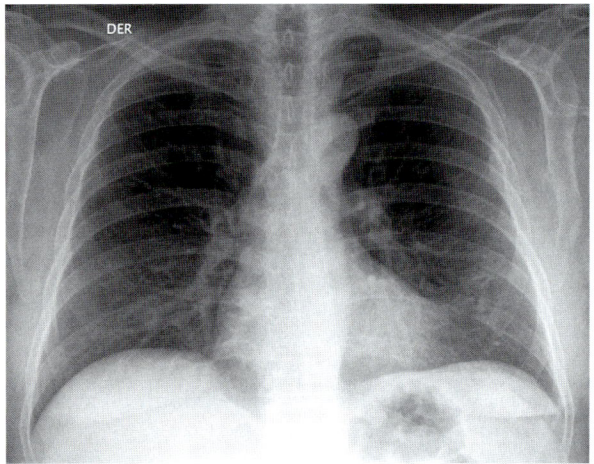

Fig. 3.9.1

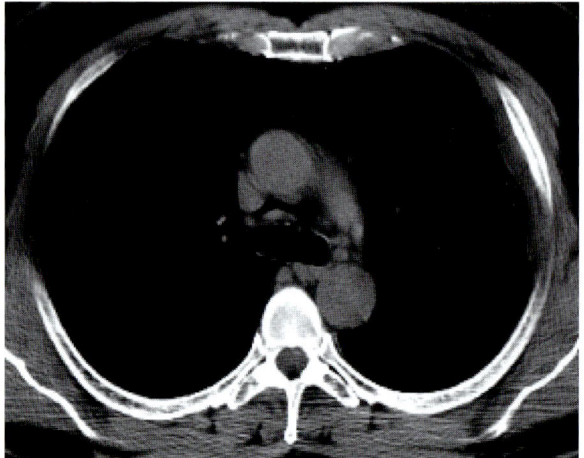

Fig. 3.9.2

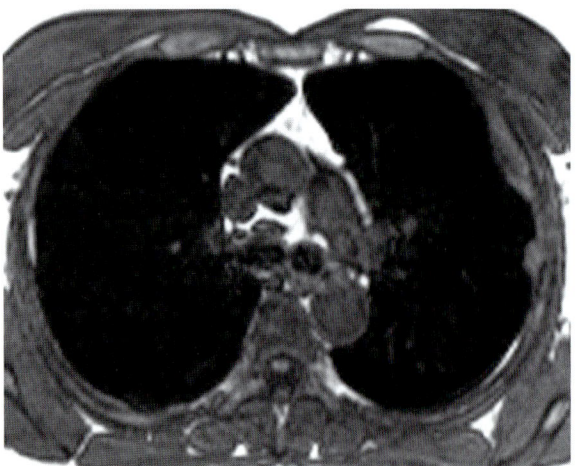

Fig. 3.9.3

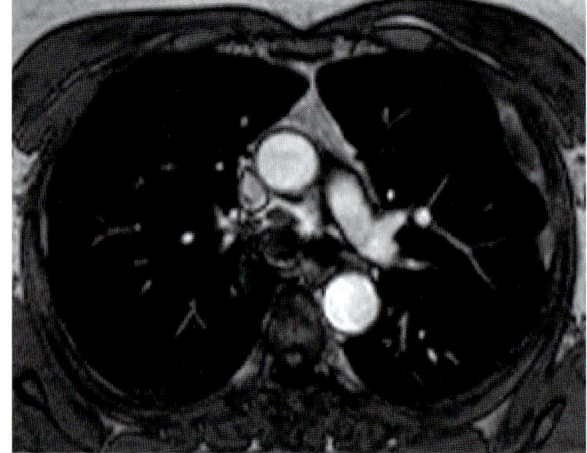

Fig. 3.9.4

A 64-year-old man presented with shortness of breath, pleuritic pain, and weight loss. The patient referred pleural effusions drained two years prior and had worked in an electric wiring factory for 20 years. He had no history of smoking.

Malignant mesothelioma is the most common primary neoplasm of the pleura. It has a strong association with asbestos exposure, with a latency of 35–40 years. Median survival time after diagnosis is between 12–15 months. The main histologic subtypes are epithelial, sarcomatous, and mixed. It is locally aggressive, with frequent invasion of the chest wall, mediastinum, and diaphragm. Metastases to the hilar and mediastinal lymph nodes are usual at the moment of diagnosis. The most frequent hematogenous metastases are to the lungs, liver, kidneys, and adrenal glands.

Differential diagnoses:
- Adenocarcinoma
- Lymphoma
- Thymoma (drop metastases)
- Asbestos-related benign pleural disease
- Infections

Chest radiograph shows:
- Pleural effusion
- Circumferential pleural thickening
- Lung nodules or masses

CT shows:
- Unilateral pleural effusion
- Sheetlike or lobulated pleural thickening
- Interlobar fissure thickening
- Tumor encasement of the lung with a rindlike appearance
- Contraction of the affected hemithorax with associated ipsilateral mediastinal shift, narrowed intercostal spaces, and elevation of the ipsilateral hemidiaphragm
- Chest wall invasion: obliteration of fat planes, invasion of intercostal muscles, infiltration or separation of ribs, bone destruction
- Invasion into the mediastinum: obliteration of fat planes or direct tumor invasion to the heart, great vessels, esophagus, and trachea

MR imaging provides excellent soft-tissue contrast, showing:
- Isointense to muscle or slightly hyperintense on T1-weighted images
- Hyperintense on T2-weighted images
- Enhances after contrast administration

PET-CT shows:
- More extensive disease involvement
- Most appropriate biopsy site for obtaining positive results
- Occult distant metastases

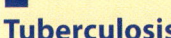

Case 10
■
Tuberculosis

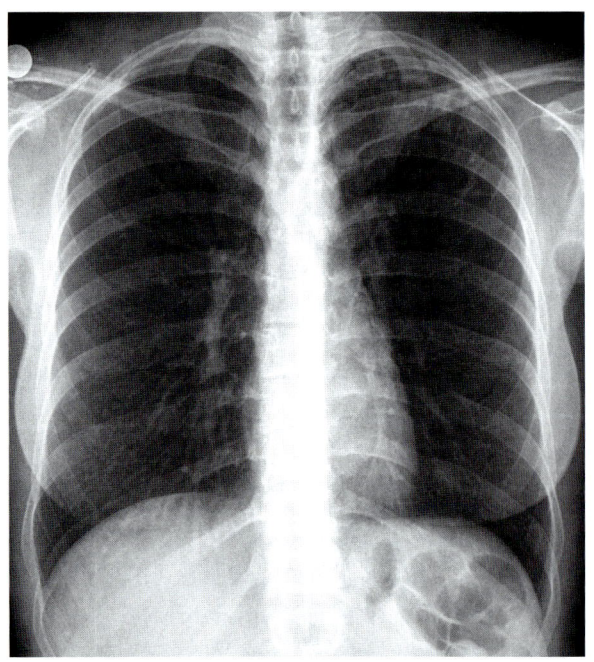

Fig. 3.10.1

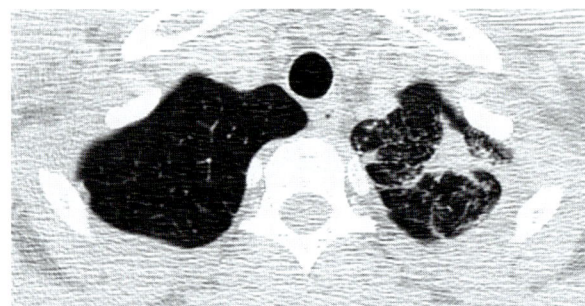

Fig. 3.10.2

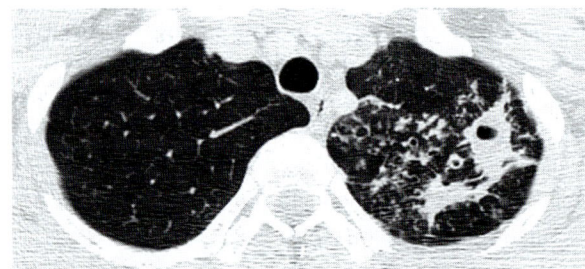

Fig. 3.10.3

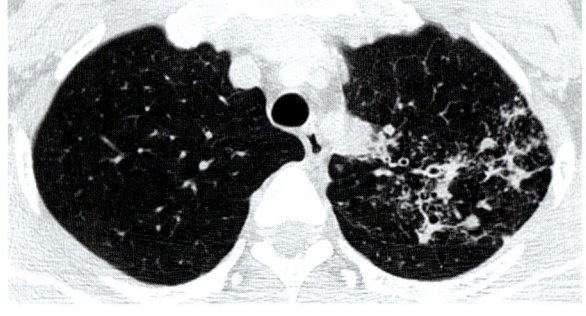

Fig. 3.10.4

A 35-year-old woman presented with a three-month history of non-productive cough, low-grade fever, anorexia, night sweats, and weight loss. Laboratory tests revealed raised peripheral blood leukocyte count and anemia and the absence of HIV antibodies.

Comments

Pulmonary tuberculosis is caused by inhalation of droplets laden with Mycobacterium tuberculosis bacilli. The most common site of implantation is the middle and lower lung lobes. The course of the disease depends on the interaction between the host response and organism's virulence. Primary tuberculosis typically appears as air-space consolidation in the lower lobes, hilar and mediastinal lymphadenopathy, and pleural effusion. Postprimary tuberculosis occurs in persons with a degree of acquired immunity from prior infection and usually appears as nodular and linear areas of increased opacity or attenuation in the lung apex. Active and inactive disease can only be reliably differentiated radiographically on the basis of temporal evolution (no change over a 4–6 month interval).

Imaging Findings

Primary disease:
- Lymphadenopathy: right paratracheal and hilar stations most frequently involved.
- Central areas of low attenuation with peripheral rim enhancement (most frequently HIV)
- Parenchymal consolidation: homogeneous, patchy, linear or nodular; segmental or lobar distribution
- Obstructive atelectasis, usually right-sided
- Unilateral pleural effusion
- Radiographs are normal (15%)

Post primary disease:
- Parenchymal disease with cavitation: heterogeneous opacities in the apical and posterior segments of the upper lobes and the superior segment of the lower lobes
- Cavitation: usually multiple, with thin and smooth or thick and irregular walls. May have air-fluid levels
- Tuberculoma: solitary round sharply marginated mass with calcification
- Bronchogenic spread: 4 mm centrilobular nodules and sharply marginated linear branching opacities ("tree-in-bud" appearance)
- Pleural effusion
- Fibroproliferative disease: upper lobe volume loss with cicatricial atelectasis, architectural distortion, and traction bronchiectasis

Complications:
- Mycetomas: mobile intracavitary masses, air crescent sign
- Traction bronchiectasis
- Residual cavities
- Rasmussen aneurysm: pseudoaneurysm of a pulmonary artery
- Broncholithiasis: calcified peribronchial nodes

Further Readings

Books

Chest Radiology: Plain Film Patterns and Differential Diagnosis, 5th ed. Reed JC (2003) Philadelphia, Pa: Elsevier Science. ISBN-13: 9780323026178

CT and MR Imaging of the Whole Body, 4th ed, 2 vols. Haaga JR, Lanzieri CF (2003) St Louis, Mo: Mosby-Elsevier Science. ISBN-13: 9780323011334

Computed Tomography and Magnetic Resonance of the Thorax. 4th ed. Naidich D, Webb WR, Muller NR, Vlahos I, Krinsky GA (2007) Lippincott Williams & Wilkins. ISBN-13: 9780781757652

Diagnosis and Diseases of the Chest. 4th ed. Fraser RS, Muller NL, Colman N, Paré PD (1999) Philadelphia, Pa: Saunders. ISBN-13: 9780721661940

Diffuse Lung Diseases. Maffessanti M, Dalpiaz G (2006) Springer, Berlin. ISBN-13: 9788847004290

Felson's Principles of Chest Roentgenology. 2nd ed. Goodman LR (1999) Philadelphia, Pa: Saunders. ISBN-13: 9780721676852

High-resolution CT of the Lung. 2nd ed. Webb WR, Müller NL, Naidich DP (1996) Philadelphia, Pa: Lippincott-Raven. ISBN-13: 9780781702171

Imaging of Diseases of the Chest. 4th ed. Hansell D, Armstrong P, Lynch D, McAdams HP (2005) Elsevier Mosby. ISBN-13: 9780723433231

Radiology of the Chest and Related Conditions (2002) Wright FW. London, England: Taylor & Francis. ISBN13: 9789058232298

Thoracic Imaging: Pulmonary and Cardiovascular Radiology. Higgins CB, Webb WR (2004) Philadelphia, Pa: Lippincott Williams & Wilkins. ISBN-13: 9780781741194

Web Links

http://ajronline.org
http://chestjournal.org
http://content.nejm.org
http://erj.ersjournals.com
http://jcat.org
http://radiographics.rsnajnls.org
http://radiology.rsnajnls.org
http://springerlink.com
http://thoracicrad.org
http://thorax.bmj.com

Articles

Althoff Souza C, Müller N, Flint J, Wright J, Churg A. Idiopathic pulmonary fibrosis: Spectrum of high-resolution CT findings. AJR Am J Roentgenol 2005; 185:1531–1539

Blachere H, Latrabe V, Montaudon M, Valli N, Couffinhal T, Raherisson C, Leccia F, Laurent F. Pulmonary embolism revealed on helical CT angiography: comparison with ventilation-perfusion radionuclide lung scanning. AJR Am J Roentgenol 2000; 174:1041–1047

Boiselle PM, Patz EF, Vining DJ, Weissleder R, Shepard JA, McLoud TC. Imaging of mediastinal lymph nodes: CT, MR, and FDG PET. Radiographics 1998; 18:1061–1069

Brown K, Mund DF, Aberle DR, Batra P, Young DA. Intrathoracic calcifications: radiographic features and differential diagnoses. Radiographics 1994; 14:1247–1261

Burk DL, Brunberg JA, Kanal E, Latchaw RE, Wolf GL. Spinal and paraspinal neurofibromatosis: surface coil MR imaging at 1.5 T1. Radiology 1987; 162:797–801

Carpenter BL, Merten DF. Radiographic manifestations of congenital anomalies affecting the airway. Radiol Clin North Am 1991; 29:219–240

Cartier Y, Kavanagh PV, Johkoh T, Mason AC, Muller NL. Bronchiectasis: accuracy of high-resolution CT in the differentiation of specific diseases. AJR Am J Roentgenol 1999; 173:47–52

Chong S, Lee KS, Chung MJ, Han J, Kwon OJ, Kim TS. Pneumoconiosis: comparison of imaging and pathologic findings. Radiographics 2006; 26:59–77

Chooi WK, Matthews S, Bull MJ, Morcos SK. Multislice helical CT: the value of multiplanar image reconstruction in assessment of the bronchi and small airways disease. Br J Radiol 2003; 76:536–540

Coche E, Verschuren F, Keyeux A, Goffette P, Goncette L, Hainaut P, Hammer F, Lavenne E, Zech F, Meert P, Reynaert MS. Diagnosis of acute pulmonary embolism in outpatients: Comparison of thin-collimation multi-detector row spiral CT and planar ventilation-perfusion scintigraphy. Radiology 2003; 229:757–765

Corcoran HL, Renner WR, Milstein MJ. Review of high-resolution CT of the lung. Radiographics 1992; 12:917–939

Crow J, Slavin G, Kreel L. Pulmonary metastases: a pathologic and radiologic study. Cancer 1981; 47:2595–2602

Cymbalista M, Waysberg A, Zacharias C, Ajavon Y, Riquet M, Rebibo G, Grenier P. CT demonstration of the 1996 AJCC-UICC regional lymph node classification for lung cancer staging. Radiographics 1999; 19:899–900

Davis SD. CT evaluation for pulmonary metastases in patients with extrathoracic malignancy. Radiology 1991; 180:1–12

Erasmus JJ, Connolly JE, McAdams HP, Roggli VL. Solitary pulmonary nodules: Part I. Morphologic evaluation for differentiation of benign and malignant lesions. Radiographics 2000; 20:43–58

Erasmus JJ, McAdams HP, Patz EF, Goodman PC, Coleman RE. Thoracic FDG PET: state of the art. Radiographics 1998; 18:5–20

Fishman EK, Kuhlman JE, Jones RJ. CT of lymphoma: spectrum of disease. Radiographics 1991; 11:647–669

Fedullo PF, Tapson VF. Clinical practice: the evaluation of suspected pulmonary embolism. N Engl J Med 2003; 349(13):1247–1256

Fortman BJ, Kuszyk BS, Urban BA, Fishman EK. Neurofibromatosis type 1: A diagnostic mimicker at CT. Radiographics 2001; 21:601–612

Foster WL, Gimenez EI, Roubidoux MA, Sherrier RH, Shannon RH, Roggli VL, Pratt PC. The emphysemas: radiologic-pathologic correlations. Radiographics 1993; 13:311–328

Franquet T, Giménez A, Rosón N, Torrubia S, Sabaté JM, Pérez C. Aspiration diseases: findings, pitfalls, and differential diagnosis. Radiographics 2000; 20:673–685

Fraser RS, Muller NL, Colman N, Paré PD. Diagnosis and diseases of the chest. 4th ed. Saunders, 1999

Frazier AA, Galvin JR, Franks TJ, Rosado-de-Christenson ML. From the archives of the AFIP: Pulmonary vasculature: hypertension and infarction. Radiographics 2000; 20:491–524

Ghaye B, Ghuysen A, Bruyere PJ, D'Orio V, Dondelinger RF. Can CT pulmonary angiography allow assessment of severity and prognosis in patients presenting with pulmonary embolism? What the radiologist needs to know. Radiographics 2006; 26:23–39

Giménez A, Franquet T, Erasmus JJ, Martínez S, Estrada P. Thoracic complications of esophageal disorders. Radiographics 2002; 22:247–258

Grippi MA. Clinical aspects of lung cancer. Semin Roentgenol 1990; 25:5–11

Goodman LR. Felson's Principles of Chest Roentgenology. Philadelphia, Pa: Saunders, 1999

Gross BH, Glazer GM, Bookstein FL. Multiple pulmonary nodules detected by computed tomography: diagnostic implications. J Comput Assist Tomogr 1985; 9:880–885

Gross TJ, Hunninghake GW. Medical progress: Idiopatic pulmonary fibrosis. N Engl J Med 2001; 345:517–525

Haaga JR, Lanzieri CF, Gilkeson RC. CT and MR imaging of the whole body. 4th ed, 2 vols. St Louis, Mo: Mosby–Elsevier Science, 2003

Han D, Lee KS, Franquet T, Muller NL, Kim TS, Kim H, Kwon OJ, Byun HS. Thrombotic and nonthrombotic pulmonary arterial embolism: Spectrum of imaging findings. Radiographics 2003; 23(6):1521–1539

Hansell D, Armstrong P, Lynch D, McAdams HP. Imaging of diseases of the chest. Elsevier Mosby 2005

Harisinghani MG, McLoud TC, Shepard JA, Ko JP, Shroff MM, Mueller PR. Tuberculosis from head to toe. Radiographics 2000; 20:449–470

Hartman TE, Primack SL, Lee KS, Swensen SJ, Muller NL. CT of bronchial and bronchiolar diseases. Radiographics 1994; 14:991–1003

Hayashi K, Aziz A, Ashizawa K, Hayashi H, Nagaoki K, Otsuji H. Radiographic and CT appearances of the major fissures. Radiographics 2001; 21:861–874

Halvorsen RA, Fedyshin PJ, Korobkin M, Foster WL, Thompson WM. Ascites or pleural effusion? CT differentiation; four useful criteria. Radiographics 1986; 6:135–149

Helbich TH, Heinz-Peer G, Eichler I, Wunderbaldinger P, Götz M, Wojnarowski C, Brasch RC, Herold CJ. Cystic fibrosis: CT assessment of lung involvement in children and adults. Radiology 1999; 213:537–544

Hunninghake GW, Lynch DA, Galvin JR, et al. Radiologic findings are strongly associated with a pathologic diagnosis of usual interstitial pneumonia. Chest 2003; 124:1215–1223

Isabela C, Silva S, Colby TV, Müller NL. Asthma and associated conditions: High-resolution CT and pathologic findings. AJR Am J Roentgenol 2004; 183:817–824

Jeung MY, Gasser B, Gangi A, Bogorin A, Charneau D, Wihlm JM, Dietemann JL, Roy C. Imaging of cystic masses of the mediastinum. Radiographics 2002; 22:79–93

Jong PA, Muller NL, Pare PD, Coxson HO. Computed tomographic imaging of the airways: relationship to structure and function. Eur Respir J 2005; 26(1):140–152

Jung JI, Kim HH, Park SH, Song SW, Chung MH, Kim HS, Kim KJ, Ahn MI, Seo SB, Hahn ST. Thoracic manifestations of breast cancer and its therapy. Radiographics 2004; 24:1269–1285

Kawashima A, Fishman EK, Kuhlman JE, Nixon MS. CT of posterior mediastinal masses. Radiographics 1991; 11:1045–1067

Kazama T, Faria SC, Varavithya V, Phongkitkarun S, Ito H, Macapinlac HA. FDG PET in the evaluation of treatment for lymphoma: Clinical usefulness and pitfalls. Radiographics 2005; 25:191–207

Kazerooni EA. High-resolution CT of the lungs. AJR Am J Roentgenol 2001; 177:501–519

Kim EA, Lee KS, Primack SL, Yoon HK, Byun HS, Kim TS, Suh GY, Kwon OJ, Han J. Viral pneumonias in adults: Radiologic and pathologic findings. Radiographics 2002; 22:137–149

Kim HY, Song KS, Goo JM, Lee JS, Lee KS, Lim TH. Thoracic sequelae and complications of tuberculosis. Radiographics 2001; 21:839–858

Kuhlman JE, Deutsch JH, Fishman EK, Siegelman SS. CT features of thoracic mycobacterial disease. Radiographics 1990; 10:413–431

Kuhlman JE, Singha NK. Complex disease of the pleural space: radiographic and CT evaluation. Radiographics 1997; 17:63–79

Koh DM, Burke S, Davies N, Padley SPG. Transthoracic US of the chest: Clinical uses and applications. Radiographics. 2002; 22:e1

Koyama T, Ueda H, Togashi K, Umeoka S, Kataoka M, Nagai S. Radiologic manifestations of sarcoidosis in various organs. Radiographics 2004; 24:87–104

Leung AN, Muller NL, Miller RR. CT in differential diagnosis of diffuse pleural disease. AJR Am J Roentgenol 1990; 154:487–492

Lucidarme O, Coche E, Cluzel P, Mourey-Gerosa I, Howarth N, Grenier P. Expiratory CT scans for chronic airway disease: correlation with pulmonary function test results. AJR Am J Roentgenol 1998; 170:301–307

Lynch D, Travis WD, Müller NL, Galvin JR, Hansell DM, Grenier PA, King TE. Idiopathic interstitial pneumonias: CT Features. Radiology 2005; 236:10–21

Maffessanti M, Dalpiaz G. Diffuse lung diseases. Springer 2006

McAdams HP, Erasmus J, Winter JA. Radiologic manifestations of pulmonary tuberculosis. Radiol Clin North Am 1995; 33:655–678

McAdams HP, Samei E, Dobbins J, Tourassi GD, Ravin CE. Recent advances in chest radiography. Radiology 2006 241:663–683

McCarville MB, Lederman HM, Santana VM, Daw NC, Shochat SJ, Li CS, Kaufman RA. Distinguishing benign from malignant pulmonary nodules with helical chest CT in children with malignant solid tumors. Radiology 2006; 239:514–520

McGuinness G, Naidich DP. CT of airways disease and bronchiectasis. Radiol Clin North Am 2002; 40:1–19

Meziane MA, Hruban RH, Zerhouni EA, Wheeler PS, Khouri NF, Fishman EK, Hutchins GM, Siegelman SS. High resolution CT of the lung parenchyma with pathologic correlation. Radiographics 1988; 8:27–54

Miller BH, Rosado-de-Christenson ML, Mason AC, Fleming MV, White CC, Krasna MJ. From the archives of the AFIP. Malignant pleural mesothelioma: radiologic-pathologic correlation. Radiographics 1996; 16:613–644

Miller WT, Miller WT Jr. Tuberculosis in the normal host: radiological findings. Semin Roentgenol 1993; 28:109–118

Milne EN, Pistolesi M, Miniati M, Giuntini C. The radiologic distinction of cardiogenic and noncardiogenic edema. AJR Am J Roentgenol 1985; 144:879–894

Mitlehner W, Friedrich M, Dissman W. Value of computed tomography of the lung in the management of primary spontaneous pneumothorax. Am J Surg 1991; 162:39–42

Morgan-Parkes JH. Metastases: mechanisms, pathways, and cascades. AJR Am J Roentgenol 1995; 164:1075–1082

Mueller-Mang C, Grosse C, Schmid K, Stiebellehner L, Bankier A. What every radiologist should know about idiopathic interstitial pneumonias. Radiographics 2007; 27:595–615

Müller NL, Colby TV. Idiopathic interstitial pneumonias: high resolution CT and histologic findings. Radiographics 1997; 17:1016–1022

Munk PL, Muller NL, Miller RR, Ostrow DN. Pulmonary lymphangitic carcinomatosis: CT and pathologic findings. Radiology 1988; 166:705–709

Naidich DP, Webb WR, Müller NL, Vlahos I, Krinsky GA, Kim EE. Computed tomography and magnetic resonance of the thorax. J Nucl Med 2007; 48(12):2088

Nishino M, Ashiku SK, Kocher ON, Thurer RL, Boiselle PM, Hatabu H. The thymus: A comprehensive review. Radiographics 2006; 26:335–348

Noh HM, Fishman EK, Forastiere AA, Bliss DF, Calhoun PF. CT of the esophagus: spectrum of disease with emphasis on esophageal carcinoma. Radiographics 1995; 15:1113–1134

Patel S, Kazerooni EA. Helical CT for the evaluation of acute pulmonary embolism. AJR Am J Roentgenol 2005; 185:135–149

Raoof S, Amchentsev A, Vlahos I, Goud A, Naidich DP. Pictorial essay: Multinodular disease: a high-resolution CT scan diagnostic algorithm. Chest, Mar 2006; 129:805–815

Reed JC. Plain film patterns and differential diagnosis. Chest Radiology: 5th ed. Philadelphia, Pa: Elsevier Science, 2003

Remy-Jardin M, Remy J, Farre I, Marquette CH. Computed tomographic evaluation of silicosis and coal worker's pneumoconiosis. Radiol Clin North Am 1992; 30:1155–1176

Ribet ME, Cardot GR. Neurogenic tumors of the thorax. Ann Thorac Surg 1994; 58:1091–1095

Roach HW, Davies GJ, Attanoos R, Crane M, Adams H, Phillips S. Asbestos: when the dust settles an imaging review of asbestos-related disease. Radiographics 2002; 22:167–184

Rosado-de-Christenson ML, Templeton PA, Moran CA. Bronchogenic carcinoma: radiologic-pathologic correlation. Radiographics 1994; 14:429–446

Rosado-de-Christenson ML, Abbott GF, Kirejczyk WM, Galvin JR, Travis WD. From the archives of the AFIP: thoracic carcinoids: Radiologic-pathologic correlation. Radiographics 1999; 19:707–736

Rosen MJ. Chronic cough due to bronchiectasis: ACCP evidence-based clinical practice guidelines. Chest 2006; 129:122S–131S

Schoder H, Gonen MJ. Screening for cancer with PET and PET/CT: Potential and limitations. Nucl Med 2007; 48:4S–18S

Schoepf UJ, Bruening RD, Hong C, Eibel R, Aydemir S, Crispin A, Becker C, Reiser MF. Multislice helical CT of focal and diffuse lung disease: Comprehensive diagnosis with reconstruction of contiguous and high-resolution CT sections from a single thin-collimation scan. AJR Am J Roentgenol 2001; 177:179–184

Seo JB, Im JG, Goo JM, Chung MJ, Kim MY. Atypical pulmonary metastases: Spectrum of radiologic findings. Radiographics 2001; 21:403–417

Sharma A, Fidias P, Hayman LA, Loomis SL, Taber KH, Aquino SL. Patterns of lymphadenopathy in thoracic malignancies. Radiographics 2004; 24:419–434

Sider L, Weiss AJ, Smith MD, VonRoenn JH, Glassroth J. Varied appearance of AIDS-related lymphoma in the chest. Radiology 1989; 171:629–632

Sider L, Gabriel H, Curry DR, Pham MS. Pattern recognition of the pulmonary manifestations of AIDS on CT scans. Radiographics 1993; 13:771–784

Sivit CJ, Schwartz AM, Rockoff SD. Kaposi's sarcoma of the lung in AIDS: radiologic-pathologic analysis. AJR Am J Roentgenol 1987; 148:25–28

Sokhandon F, Sparschu RA, Furlong JW. Best cases from the AFIP: Bronchogenic squamous cell carcinoma. Radiographics 2003; 23:1639–1643

Stein MG, Mayo J, Muller N, Aberle DR, Webb WR, Gamsu G. Pulmonary lymphangitic spread of carcinoma: appearance on CT scans. Radiology 1987; 162:371–375

Stern EJ, Frank MS. CT of the lung in patients with pulmonary emphysema: diagnosis, quantification, and correlation with pathologic and physiologic findings. AJR Am J Roentgenol 1994; 162:791–798

Sullivan EJ. Lymphangioleiomyomatosis: a review. Chest 1998; 114:1689–1703

Tateishi U, Gladish GW, Kusumoto M, Hasegawa T, Yokoyama R, Tsuchiya R, Moriyama N. Chest wall tumors: Radiologic findings and pathologic correlation: Part 1. benign tumors. Radiographics 2003; 23:1477–1490

Tocino IM, Miller MH, Fairfax WR. Distribution of pneumothorax in the supine and semirecumbent critically ill adult. AJR Am J Roentgenol 1985; 144:901–905

Van Hise ML, Primack SL, Israel RS, Muller NL. CT in blunt chest trauma: indications and limitations. Radiographics 1998; 18:1071–1084

Wang ZJ, Reddy GP, Gotway MB, et al. Malignant pleural mesothelioma: Evaluation with CT, MR imaging, and PET. Radiographics 2004; 24:105–119

Wernecke K, Diederich S. Sonographic features of mediastinal tumors. AJR Am J Roentgenol 1994; 163:1357–1364

Whitten CR, Khan S, Munneke GJ, Grubnic S. A diagnostic approach to mediastinal abnormalities. Radiographics 2007; 27:657–671

Winer-Muram HT. The solitary pulmonary nodule. Radiology 2006; 239: 34–49

Wittram C, Mark E, McLoud T. CT-histologic correlation of the ATS/ERS 2002 classification of idiopathic interstitial pneumonias. Radiographics 2003; 23:1057–1071

Wittram C, Maher MM, Yoo AJ, Kalra MK, Shepard JAO, McLoud TC. Angiography of pulmonary embolism: Diagnostic criteria and causes of misdiagnosis. Radiographics 2004; 24(5):1219–1238

Gastrointestinal System and Disorders of the Liver, Pancreas, Spleen, and Biliary System

4

Antonio Luna Alcala, Lidia Alcala Mata, and Ramon Ribes

Introduction

The peritoneum is a complex serous membrane that divides the abdomen into multiple potential spaces communicating with one another. Some of the abdominal viscera are completely covered by peritoneum, as is the case of the liver and most of the gastrointestinal tract, while other viscera, such as the spleen, kidneys, adrenal glands and pancreas, have a retroperitoneal location. It is of the utmost importance for radiologists to know the complex anatomy and dynamic relationships between the different peritoneal spaces and abdominal systems. The entire hepatobiliopancreatic system and much of the gastrointestinal system are located in the upper abdomen, and in many clinical circumstances they are involved in the same differential diagnoses.

This complexity makes it necessary to fit the imaging procedure to the clinical pattern on an individual case-oriented basis. For example, in cases of acute pain in the right hypochondrium, ultrasound is the most appropriate procedure to rule out a gallstone, biliary obstruction, or acute pancreatitis; however, if a hiatal hernia or peptic ulcer is suspected, an upper gastrointestinal barium study should be performed. Therefore, a wide range of imaging techniques is useful in the study of the abdomen. The role of the different imaging procedures in abdominal radiology can be simply summarized as:

- Abdominal X-ray: to rule out gastrointestinal obstruction and to detect radiopaque stones within the gallbladder and urinary system
- Barium swallow and upper gastrointestinal series: to study the esophagus, stomach, and duodenum. It is most commonly used in cases of ulcer or gastric reflux
- Barium enema: to study the rectum and colon. It is most commonly indicated to study a change in bowel habits, nonspecific abdominal pain, rectal bleeding, or if a colonic mass or polyp is suspected
- Abdominal ultrasound (US): usually a first-step imaging procedure, US is able to adequately study the liver, pancreas and biliary system, and spleen.
- Computed tomography (CT): usually a second-step procedure, performed to study a specific problem, although it is also an excellent imaging screening test and especially useful in the emergency room because it can rapidly examine most of the different systems of the abdomen at the same time
- Magnetic resonance (MR): of increasing importance in recent years, it has the advantage of not use ionizing radiation. Its great flexibility makes it suitable for studying most of the abdominal systems and for solving specific diagnostic problems. It is especially useful in the study of the biliary system using MR cholangiopancreatography techniques (MRCP)

In conclusion, abdominal radiology teams need expertise in a wide variety of techniques as well as extensive knowledge about a vast range of diseases that can affect the different organs and systems in the abdomen. Abdominal radiology is one of the fastest growing and most dynamic fields in radiology and has much to offer adventurous residents and young radiologists who are not afraid to face challenging diagnostic problems.

Case 1

Acute Cholecystitis and Choledocholithiasis with Secondary Pancreatitis and Hepatic Abscess

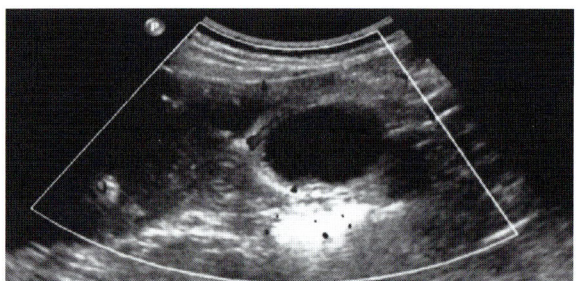

Fig. 4.1.1

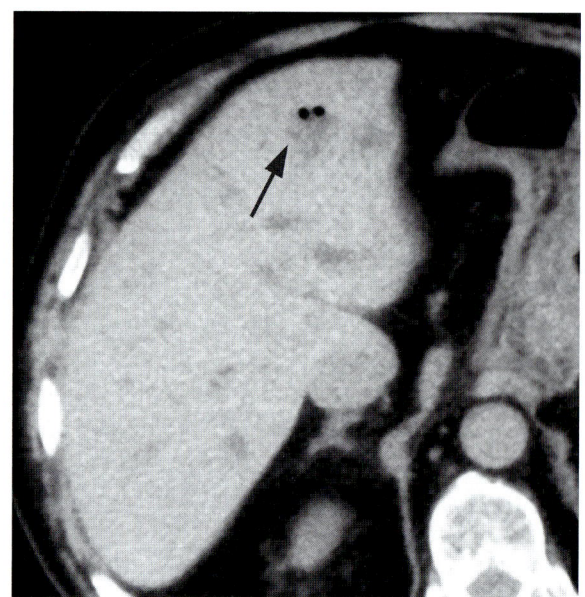

Fig. 4.1.2

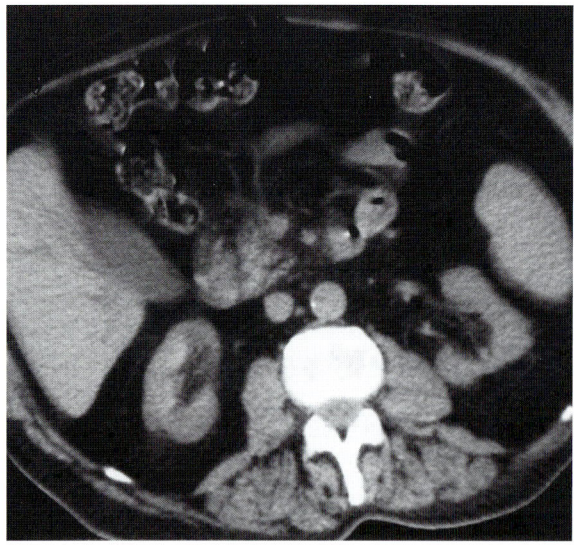

Fig. 4.1.3

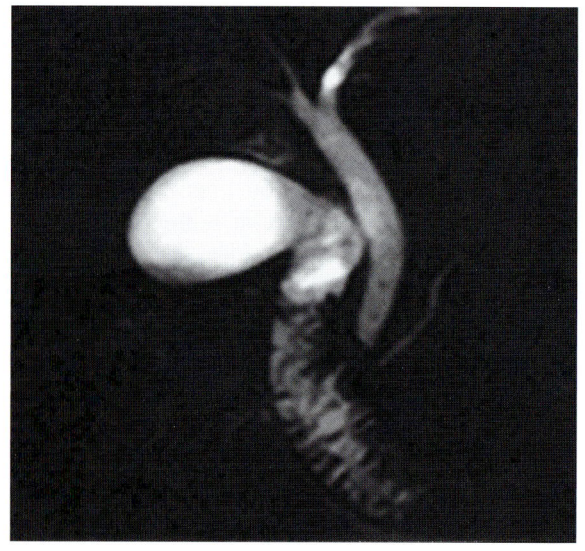

Fig. 4.1.4

An 83-year-old man presented at the emergency room with right upper quadrant pain, fever, and progressive vomiting in the previous 48 hours. At physical examination, Murphy's sign was positive. Blood test revealed leukocytosis with left shift and biochemical markers of cholestasis.

Acute cholecystitis is the most common cause of acute pain in the right upper quadrant. It occurs in one of every three patients with cholelithiasis and is usually caused by cystic duct obstruction by impacted calculus (95%). The pathogenic mechanism is increased internal pressure in the gallbladder secondary to obstruction, with chemical irritation from concentrated bile and wall ischemia, and finally associated bacterial infection. Complications of acute cholecystitis are: gangrene, perforation, and gallbladder empyema. As in this case, its association to choledocholithiasis and acute pancreatitis is common. Pyogenic hepatic abscesses are most commonly due to ascending cholangitis from obstructive biliary tract disease, as is shown in this case.

The most sensitive and specific imaging method for the detection of acute cholecystitis is ultrasound. It is used routinely in the clinical work-up of acute cholecystitis to establish the diagnosis. The triad of cholelithiasis, gallbladder wall thickening, and positive sonographic Murphy sign (focal tenderness over the gallbladder) is almost pathognomonic. Additional signs are: hazy delineation of the gallbladder wall, edema of the gallbladder wall, striated wall thickening, gallbladder hydrops, pseudomembranes, sludge, crescent-shaped pericholecystic fluid, and increased peripheral flow (visualization of the cystic artery) in color Doppler ultrasound.

It is more complicated to choose an imaging method for the study of ascending cholangitis secondary to choledocholithiasis. Conventional cholangiography is the most specific technique for visualizing the cause of obstruction. In recent years, MR-cholangiography has become the most useful imaging technique for the noninvasive detection of cholelithiasis. Ultrasound and CT are also able to detect stones in the common bile duct, although these techniques are less sensitive. All three of these noninvasive techniques are accurate in the visualization of bile duct dilatation, although MR-cholangiography again yields the best results.

In acute pancreatitis, imaging is necessary for staging and determining the prognosis. CT is the most accurate imaging technique to evaluate acute pancreatitis, although US and MR can also provide valuable information. In almost a third of cases of acute pancreatitis, the pancreas appears normal. CT is able to accurately detect areas of necrosis or hemorrhage within the pancreas. Other signs to look for are: enlargement of the pancreas with convex margins, parenchymal inhomogeneity, thickening of anterior pararenal fascia, peripancreatic fat stranding, peripancreatic fluid and fluid collection, and pseudocyst formation.

Comments

Abdominal ultrasound demonstrated clear signs of acute cholecystitis: cholelithiasis, striated wall thickening, positive sonographic Murphy's sign, and increased peripheral vascularization in color Doppler ultrasound (Fig. 4.1.1). Moderate bile duct dilatation and a focal lesion in the left liver lobe with "comet-tail artifact" were additional findings. CT and MR cholangiography were performed to further investigate these features. Unenhanced CT revealed a hepatic abscess with internal air bubbles in segment 3 (Fig. 4.1.2, *arrow*) and peripancreatic fat streaking, a sign of mild acute pancreatitis (Fig. 4.1.3). MR cholangiography demonstrated the presence of three gallstones in the common bile duct (Fig. 4.1.4).

Imaging Findings

Case 2
■
Cirrhosis with Portal Hypertension

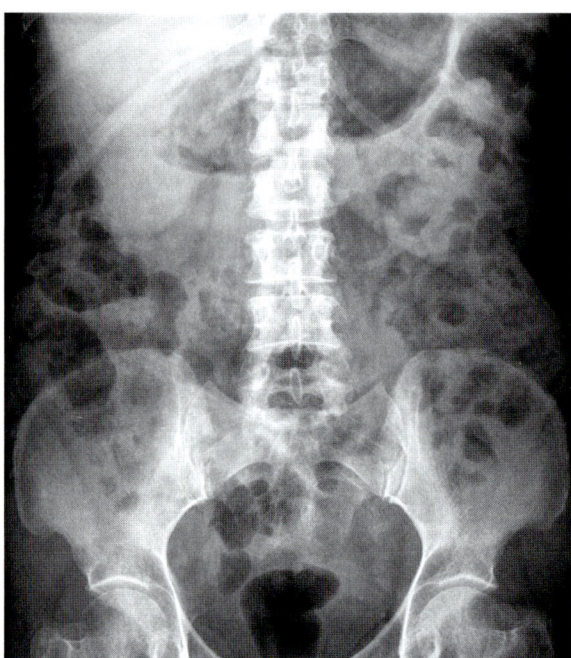

Fig. 4.2.1

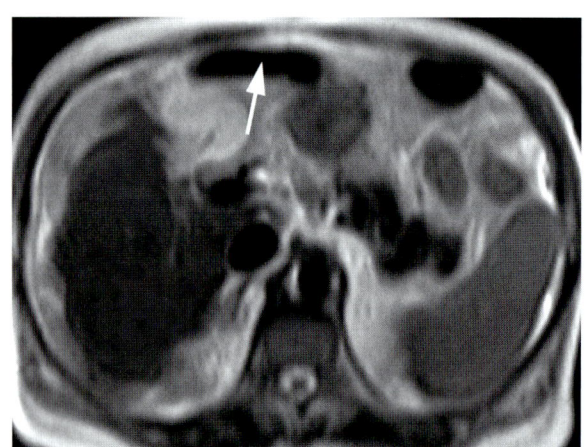

Fig. 4.2.3

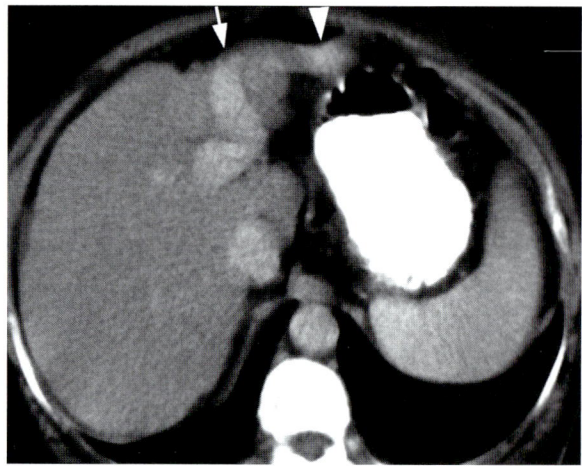

Fig. 4.2.2

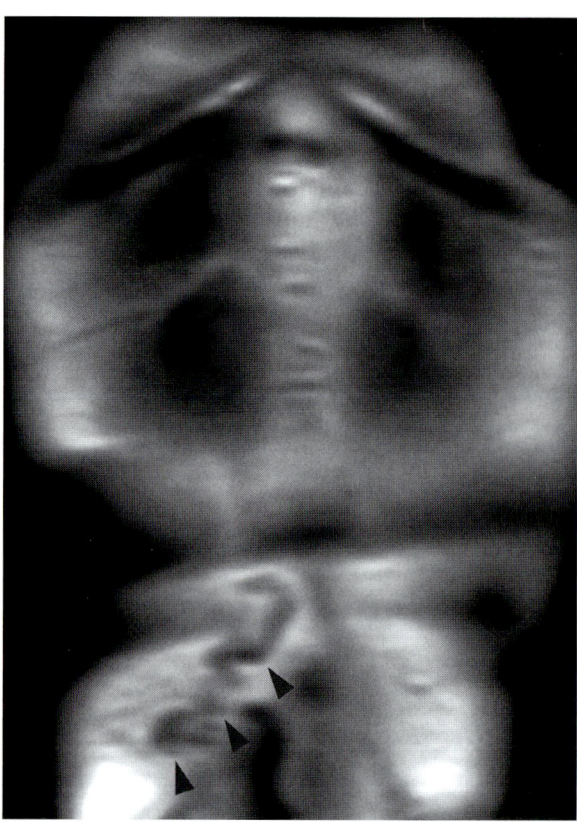

Fig. 4.2.4

A 45-year-old woman presented with progressively increased waist size, abdominal fullness, and shortness of breath in the previous two months. Laboratory tests showed a significant hepatic enzymes elevation and alteration of coagulation parameters. At physical examination, there were signs of ascites and caput medusae (collateral superficial veins in the anterior abdominal wall).

Comments

Cirrhosis is a chronic liver disease characterized by diffuse parenchymal destruction, fibrosis, and nodular regeneration with abnormal reconstruction of preexisting lobular architecture. The prevalence of cirrhosis in autopsy series has been estimated at 5 to 10%. The most common causes of cirrhosis are alcohol consumption and viral hepatitis, although there are other many possible causes. Morphologically, cirrhosis can be classified as macronodular (alcoholism), macronodular (hepatitis B), or mixed (bile duct obstruction).

Portal hypertension is commonly associated to advanced cirrhosis and occurs despite the formation of portal collateral vessels. Signs of portal hypertension are: dilatation of portal and splanchnic veins, portal vein thrombosis, cavernomatous transformation of the portal vein, portosystemic collaterals, Cruveilhier-von Baumgarten syndrome (recanalized paraumbilical vein), splenomegaly, Gamna-Gandy nodules (microhemorrhages within the spleen), and ascites.

Radiological signs of cirrhosis are: enlarged (early stage) or shrunken (late stage) liver, caudate lobe hypertrophy, shrinkage of the right lobe, peripheral liver nodularity, fatty infiltration, thickening of fissures and porta hepatis, ascites, splenomegaly, and signs of portal hypertension. Ultrasound, CT, or MR can accurately demonstrate the presence of all these signs. Ultrasound is most commonly used as a first-step technique in the evaluation of cirrhosis. Doppler ultrasound is very valuable in the assessment of portal hypertension and portal vein thrombosis. Dynamic enhanced CT or MR are preferable for the depiction and characterization of focal liver lesions in cirrhotic patients, especially to confirm or rule out hepatocellular carcinoma, which has a greatly increased prevalence in advanced cirrhosis.

Imaging Findings

Abdominal X-ray (Fig. 4.2.1) showed moderate distension of small bowel loops, which were predominantly centrally located, a signs of ascites. Contrast-enhanced abdominal CT confirmed the presence of ascites and also revealed additional signs of cirrhosis and portal hypertension (Fig. 4.2.2, axial enhanced CT in the portal phase demonstrates peripheral nodularity of hepatic parenchyma, splenomegaly, and spontaneous shunt between the left portal (*arrow*) and paraumbilical veins (*arrowhead*)). MR study ruled out the presence of focal liver lesions and confirmed the presence of cirrhosis with severe portal hypertension. The signs of portal hypertension seen at MR were (Figs. 4.2.3 and 4.2.4, axial and coronal HASTE): ascites, splenomegaly, paraumbilical vein recanalization (*arrow*), and collateral vessels in splenic vein territory and in the subcutaneous fat (*arrowheads*) of the anterior abdominal wall. Liver biopsy showed that the cirrhosis was caused by the hepatitis C virus.

Case 3
■
Hepatic Metastases

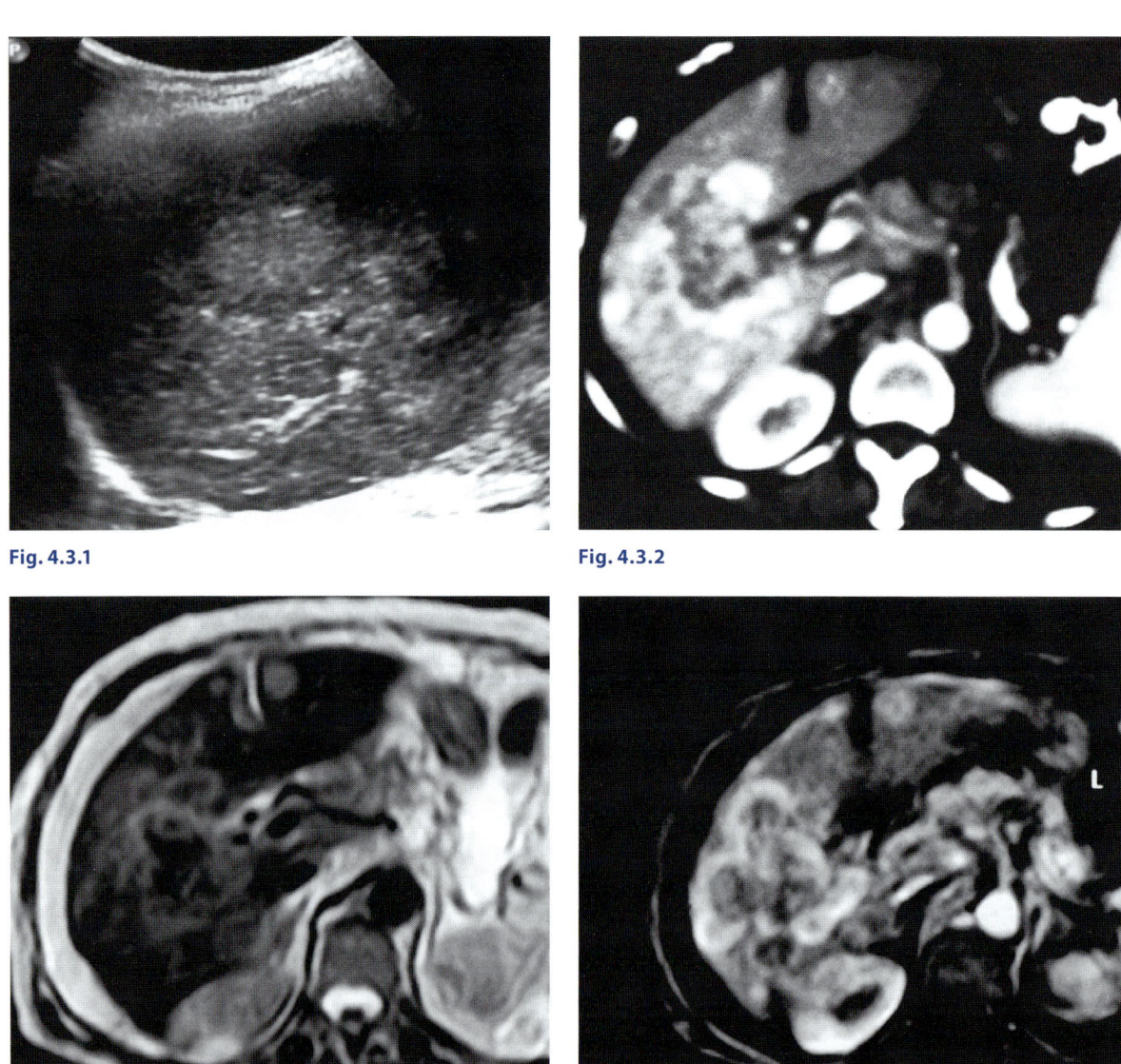

Fig. 4.3.1

Fig. 4.3.2

Fig. 4.3.3

Fig. 4.3.4

A 63-year-old woman with a history of sigmoid colon carcinoma operated on 4 years before presented with right upper quadrant abdominal pain, fever, and increased hepatic enzyme levels.

Comments

Hepatic metastases are multifocal in more than 90% of cases. Occasionally, hepatic metastasis may be solitary or confined to one segment or lobe. The most common liver metastases originate from lung, colon, pancreas, breast, or stomach carcinomas, and the most common tumors developing hepatic metastases are colorectal, uveal melanoma, neuroendocrine, and gastrointestinal tumors.

Imaging has different roles in the diagnosis and management of hepatic metastases. First of all, cross-sectional imaging techniques are able to detect them and to determine their extension. Differentiation from hepatocellular carcinoma may be challenging, although it is often possible using dynamic enhanced CT or MR. Percutaneous biopsy can resolve uncertain cases. After detection and characterization, it is also important to determine the extension and number of lesions. Limited extension to one segment or lobe and absence of vascular structures compromise would make curative surgical resection possible. Imaging is also a key factor in monitoring the response to treatment.

Imaging options in the study of focal liver lesions are multiple. Ultrasound is the most common first-step technique. The ultrasound features of hepatic metastases are varied and nonspecific. ^{18}F-FDG positron emission tomography (PET), which is very commonly used in oncologic staging, is able to detect hepatic metastases. CT and MR are the preferred techniques to confirm the presence of hepatic nodules and to determine their nature and extension. Percutaneous biopsy may be necessary in cases where the diagnosis is uncertain or when a definitive diagnosis is necessary.

It is difficult to determine the primary tumor on the basis of the imaging characteristics of the hepatic metastasis, although some patterns may help resolve this issue. The size, number, presence of necrosis, and behavior of the lesions in a dynamic enhanced series are key factors in the characterization of the metastases and in determining their origin. However, these patterns usually change after treatment, especially after chemotherapy.

Imaging Findings

Liver US (Fig. 4.3.1) showed multiple focal hyperechoic nodules throughout the liver. CT and MR were performed for further characterization. Enhanced CT in the portal phase (Fig. 4.3.2) showed the presence of ascites and multiple hepatic nodules with different degrees of enhancement. Smaller nodules were hypervascular and larger masses demonstrated peripheral enhancement with central hypovascular areas representing necrosis and/or fibrosis. The MR study (Fig. 4.3.3, axial HASTE and Fig. 4.3.4 axial dynamic enhanced fat-suppressed GE T1-weighted sequence in the portal phase) confirmed the features visualized on CT and revealed the presence of additional nodules.

Case 4
■ Pancreatic Insulinoma

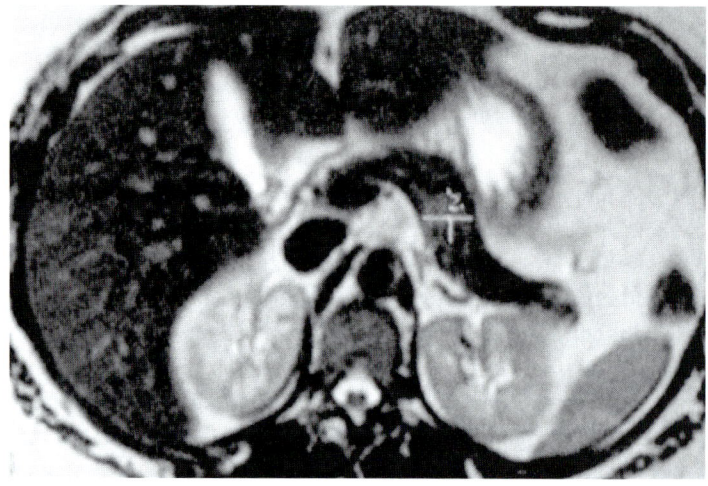

Fig. 4.4.1

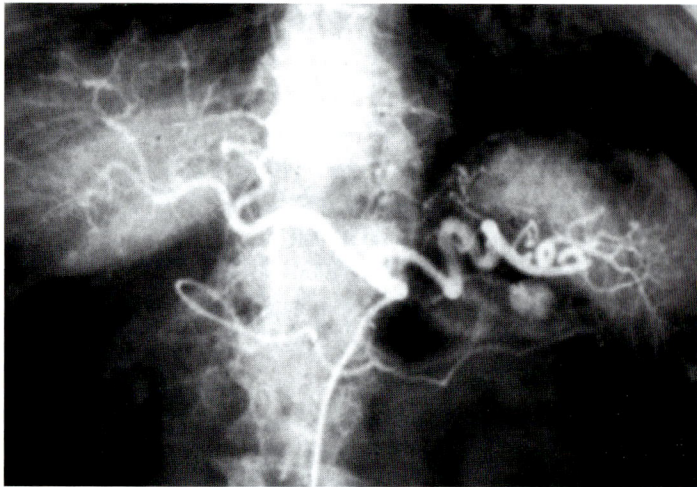

Fig. 4.4.2

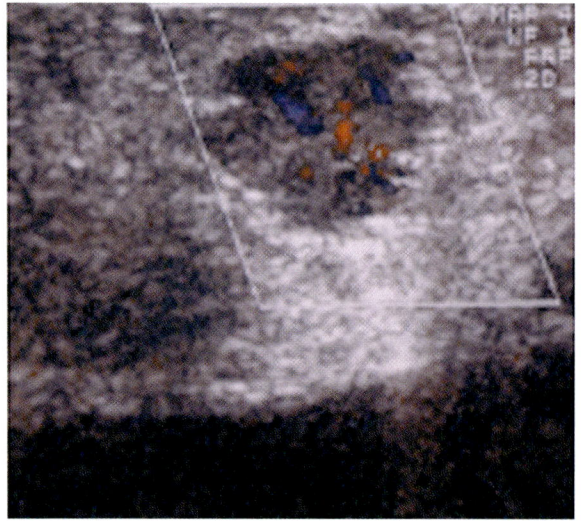

Fig. 4.4.3

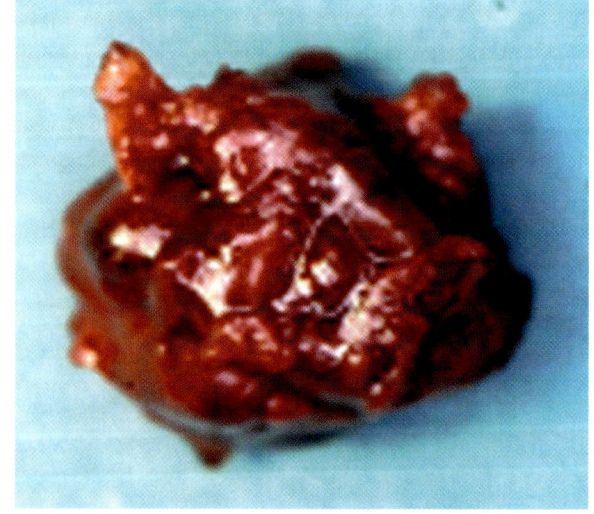

Fig. 4.4.4

A 32-year-old woman presented with recurrent crises of hypoglycemia and biochemically confirmed endogenous overproduction of insulin.

Insulinoma is a benign functioning islet cell tumor. These tumors are a complex group of endocrine neoplasms. Their origin is controversial – some believe that they belong to the group of apudomas (tumors derived from amine precursor uptake and decarboxylation (APUD) cells), while for others they arise from multipotential cells of the pancreatic ductal epithelium. The incidence of islet cell tumors is around one case per million population per year. Insulinoma is the most common islet cell tumor, followed by gastrinoma. On a clinical basis, they are separated in two different groups:

functioning islet cell tumors (FICT), i.e. those with clinically evident endocrine syndrome, and nonfunctioning islet cell tumors (NFICT), which are clinically silent tumors

FICT are named according to the active hormone responsible for the clinical syndrome. These tumors are usually homogeneous masses detected when still small, since the clinical effects of the excess hormone production appears early in their natural course. On the other hand, clinically silent tumors present as larger locally invasive masses or with distant metastasis. NFICT are always clinically silent at first and they are diagnosed late after local mass effect or metastatic disease develops. Therefore, clinical presentation is the determinant factor in their differentiation.

Multiple endocrine neoplasia type I (MEN I) is often associated with pancreatic islet cell tumors. This is an autosomal dominant disorder that manifests as pituitary adenoma, parathyroid hyperplasia, and pancreatic islet cell tumors (gastrinomas, or less commonly insulinomas).

Insulinomas are typically homogeneous masses <3 cm in size with non-aggressive local features. They may present as either a solitary benign adenoma or diffuse islet cell hyperplasia or even as malignant adenoma. Malignant transformation is infrequent in insulinomas (5–10%, as part of MEN I syndrome). Insulinomas are usually intrapancreatic neoplasms.

In the diagnostic work-up of insulinomas, the radiologist's role is to accurately locate the tumor. Octreotide scintigraphy is most commonly the initial imaging test. Multiphase enhanced CT or MR enables the number of nodules and their location to be determined. Pancreatic angiography is not usually necessary, due to the excellent angiographic images obtained with CT or MR. The presence of a hypervascular nodule in the pancreas in a patient with Whipple's triad (symptoms known or likely to be caused by hypoglycemia, low glucose at the time of the symptoms, and relief of symptoms when the glucose is raised to normal) is diagnostic of insulinoma. Intraoperative ultrasound and surgical palpation remains the gold standard to rule out additional nodules.

Pancreatic MR was performed to locate a suspected insulinoma. On the T2-weighted image (Fig. 4.4.1) a hyperintense nodule is seen in the distal pancreatic body. Pancreatic angiogram shows the hypervascular nature of the tumor (Fig. 4.4.2). Intraoperative color Doppler ultrasound (Fig. 4.4.3) also demonstrates the presence of internal flow. Figure 4.4.4 shows the macroscopic specimen.

Case 5
■
Splenic Lymphoma

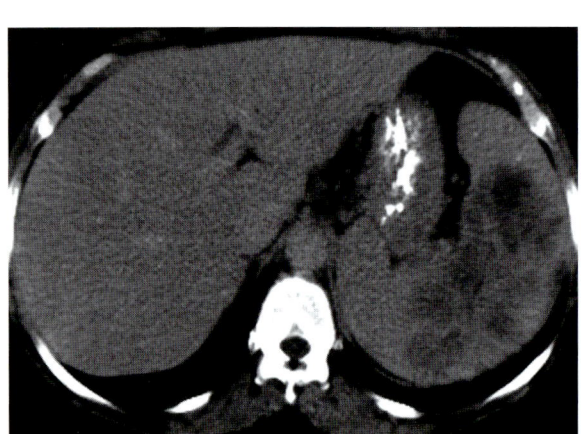

Fig. 4.5.1

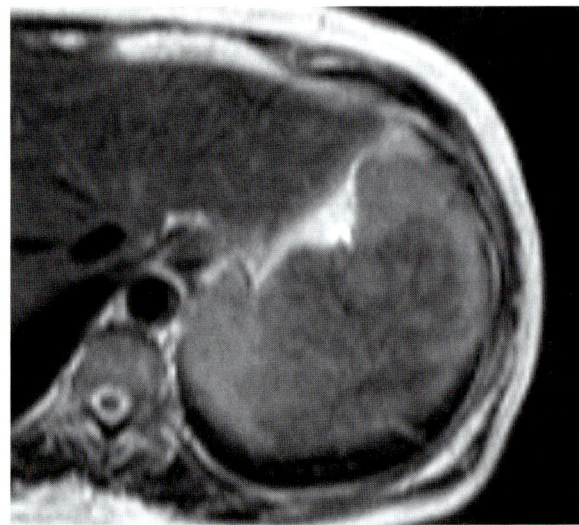

Fig. 4.5.2

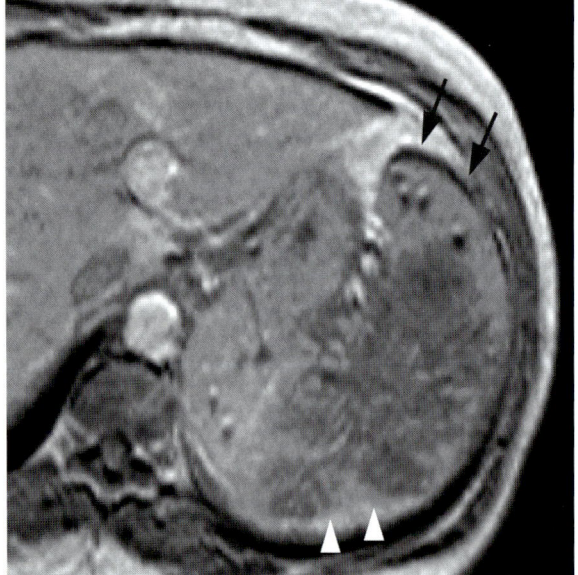

Fig. 4.5.3

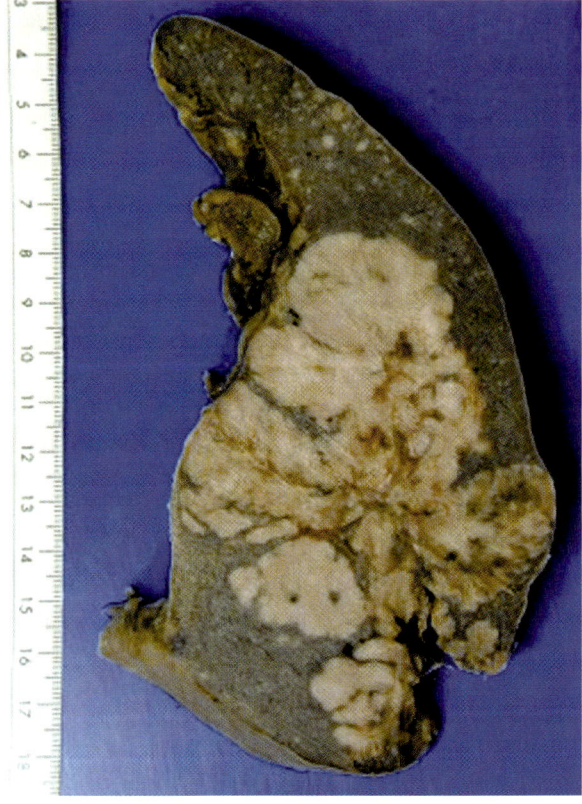

Fig. 4.5.4

A 47-year-old woman presented with left abdominal pain and weight loss over 3 months.

Lymphoma is the most common malignancy affecting the spleen. Both Hodgkin and non-Hodgkin lymphoma may present in the spleen either as a primary lesion or as a part of systemic involvement. Splenic involvement is present in up to 40% of patients with both Hodgkin and non-Hodgkin lymphoma at the time of initial diagnosis. Patients present with nonspecific clinical symptoms, usually with splenomegaly and retroperitoneal adenopathy. Pathologically, lesions range from microscopic foci involving the spleen diffusely (infiltrative pattern) to gross lesions varying in size from small miliary nodules to a single or multiple large masses.

Splenic lymphoma is difficult to diagnose with imaging techniques because of its wide spectrum of different presentations. In cases of secondary splenic lymphoma, retroperitoneal adenopathies are nearly always present and when this finding is associated to splenomegaly, it should alert the radiologist to the possibility of splenic lymphoma.

Diffuse, infiltrative splenic lymphoma is the most difficult presentation to detect by imaging. While US, CT, and MR can all adequately detect solitary or multinodular focal disease, CT and MR are superior to US in both the detection and characterization of splenic lymphoma. It is very important to perform a dynamic postcontrast series to improve the ability to detect splenic lymphoma. Acquisition of immediate post-contrast images helps to differentiate normal and abnormal splenic areas. Immediate post-contrast images demonstrate hypovascular nodules that usually become isointense/isodense to the spleen within the first minute after the injection of contrast material, although variable delayed enhancement has also been reported. In a reduced number of cases, lymphoma may present as a solitary mass.

MR is superior to CT in the distinction between splenic lymphoma and metastases, as lymphoma usually is iso- or hypo-intense on T2-weighted images and metastases are more commonly hyperintense.

Routine ultrasound study demonstrated a splenic mass (not shown). CT and MR were performed for further characterization. Contrast-enhanced CT in the equilibrium phase (Fig. 4.5.1) showed a huge hypovascular and heterogeneous mass. On the MR study, the mass was hypointense on T2-weighted images (Fig. 4.5.2) and its hypovascular nature was confirmed on a postcontrast T1-weighted gradient-echo sequence in the portal phase (Fig. 4.5.3). The MR study also revealed the spread of the tumor through the splenic capsule (*arrowheads*) and the presence of siderotic nodules (*arrows*) in the anterior pole of the spleen. Splenectomy was performed (Fig. 4.5.4). Note the close correlation between the histological and imaging findings. Histological analysis revealed a primary non-Hodgkin lymphoma.

Case 6
■
Crohn's Disease

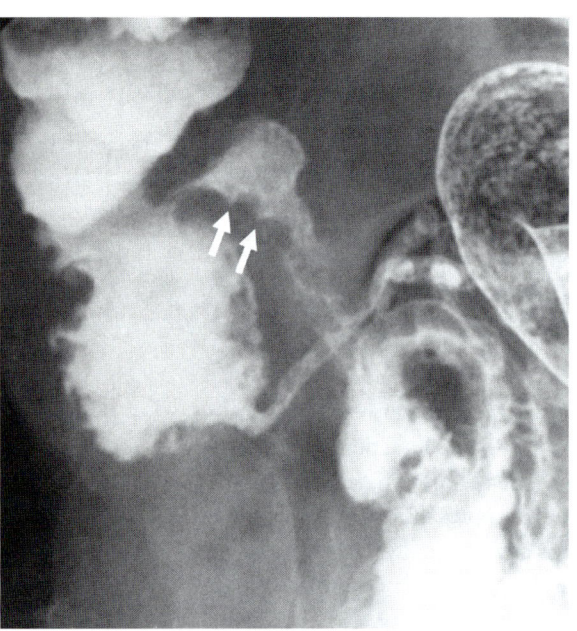

Fig. 4.6.1

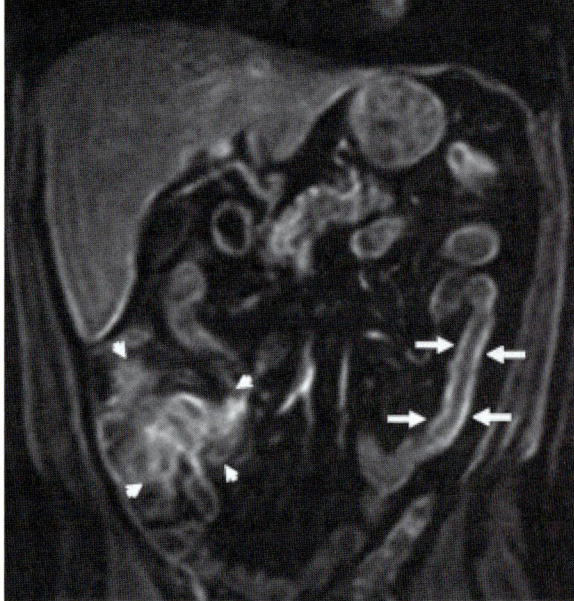

Fig. 4.6.2

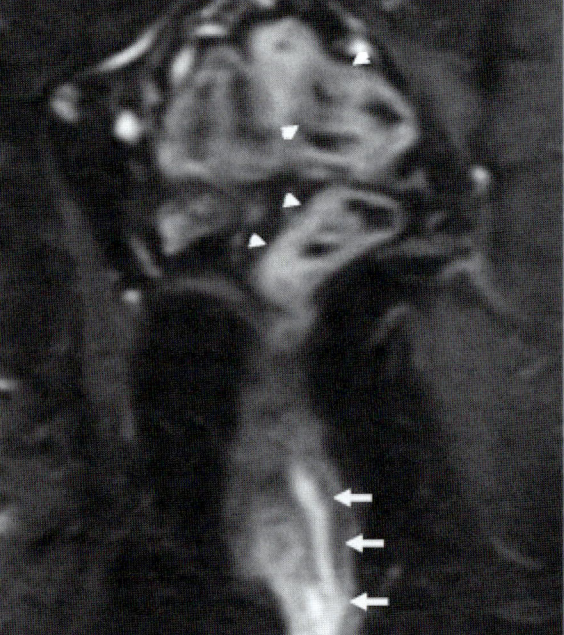

Fig. 4.6.3

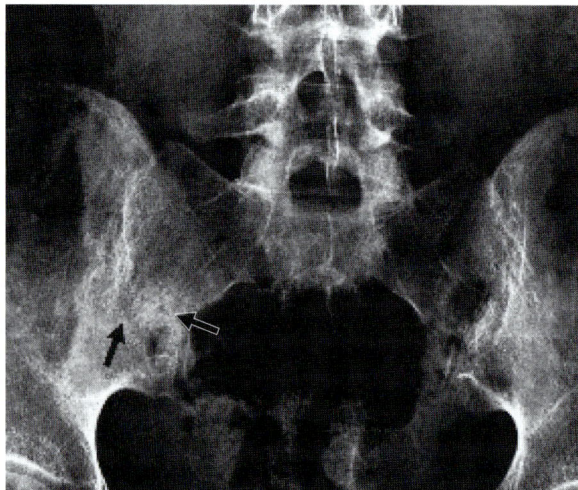

Fig. 4.6.4

A 27-year-old woman presented with recurrent episodes of diarrhea, colicky abdominal pain, and progressive weight loss. She also referred perianal discomfort and low back pain. A small bowel series performed as part of the routine diagnostic work-up demonstrated an acceleration of the intestinal transit.

Comments

The cause of Crohn's disease is unknown; it is characterized by discontinuous and asymmetric involvement of the entire gastrointestinal tract. The onset is usually before the third decade and it has no sex preference. The most common areas of gastrointestinal tract involvement are the terminal ileum (95%), small bowel (15–55%), rectum (14–50%), and colon (22–55%), although the esophagus, stomach, and duodenum can also be involved. The most common radiological findings are apthous ulcers, skip lesions, cobblestone appearance of the involved segments, pseudopolyps, and focal strictures in the late phase. Enterocolic, enterocutaneous, sinus tract, and perianal fistulas are commonly found in patients with Crohn's disease. Extraintestinal manifestations of Crohn's disease are: gallstones, sclerosing cholangitis, urolithiasis, erythema nodosum, uveitis, seronegative peripheral migratory arthritis, ankylosing spondylitis, and sacroiliitis.

In patients with diarrhea and abdominal pain, the presence of terminal ileitis suggests Crohn disease, although the differential diagnosis includes yersinia ileitis, tuberculosis, anisakiasis, lymphoma, carcinoid tumor, and eosinophilic gastroenteritis.

Crohn's disease and ulcerative colitis form part of the spectrum of inflammatory bowel disease. It is sometimes possible to differentiate between the two. Crohn's disease usually involves the terminal ileum spares different segments of the colon and small bowel. Ulcerative colitis tends to involve the entire colon. CT and MR are useful to determine the regions involved and the presence of enteric fistulas. As shown in this case, MR is the technique of choice to evaluate the presence of perianal fistulas, which are common and usually complex in Crohn's disease.

Among the extraintestinal manifestations of Crohn's disease, ankylosing spondylitis and sacroiliitis are common. This case showed unilateral sacroiliitis in a patient with negative HLA-B27.

Imaging Findings

The terminal ileum (Fig. 4.6.1) was straightened and rigid, with a severe distal stenosis and multiple ulcers (*arrows*). The diagnosis of Crohn's disease was established after a biopsy of colonic and terminal ileum mucosa. MR was also performed to study the perianal region and to determine the extent of small bowel and colonic involvement. Figures 4.6.2 and 4.6.3 are postcontrast coronal fat-suppressed T1-weighted sequences. Figure 4.6.2 shows diffuse enhancement of the terminal and distal loops of ileum, with infiltration of the adjacent fat and medial cecal involvement (*arrowheads*). Note the presence of parietal enhancement of the descendent colon indicating inflammatory activity in this segment (*arrows*). Figure 4.6.3 reveals the presence of an enhancing left transsphincteric perianal fistula (*arrows*). The enhancement of the rectal and sigmoid walls (*arrowheads*) also indicates Crohn disease involvement of these regions. An X-ray of the sacroiliac joints (Fig. 4.6.4) demonstrates loss of joint space, erosions, and reactive sclerosis in the right sacroiliac joint (*arrows*), indicative of unilateral sacroiliitis. Axial skeletal X-rays (not shown) were negative.

Case 7
■ Complicated Diverticulitis

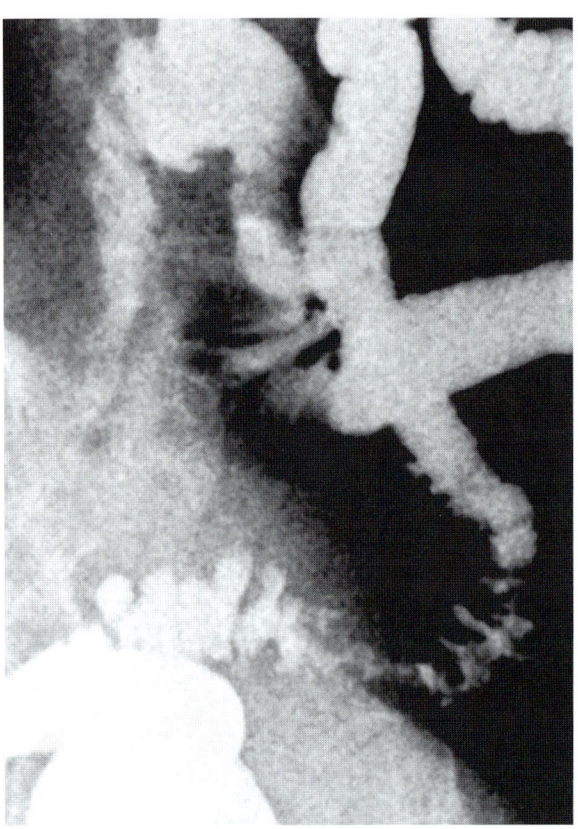

Fig. 4.7.1

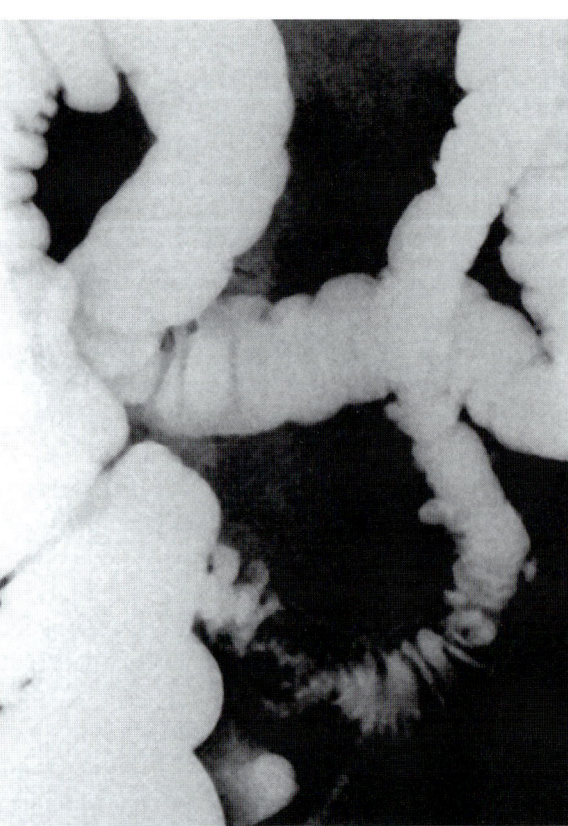

Fig. 4.7.2

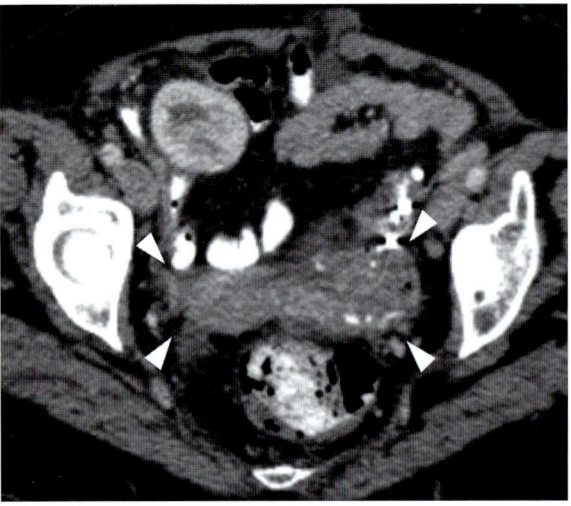

Fig. 4.7.3

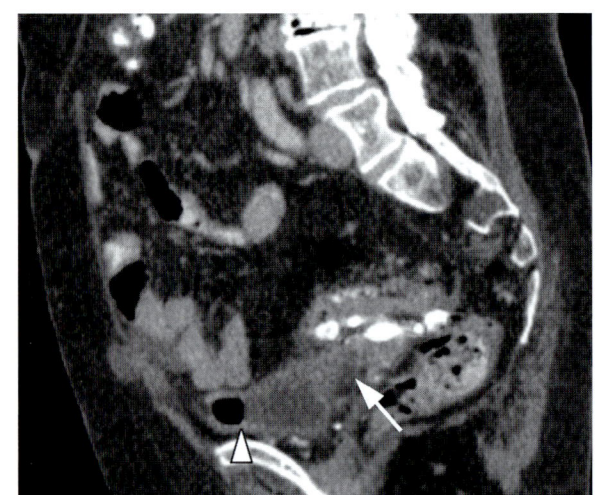

Fig. 4.7.4

A 78-year-old woman presented at the ER with left iliac fossa pain, dysuria, tenesmus, and fecal smelling urine.

The presence of diverticula or diverticulosis is very common, with an incidence of 5 to 10% in individuals over 45 years of age and of 80% in individuals over 85 years. This condition is characterized by small sacs or pouches (diverticula) in the wall of the colon. If the diverticula become inflamed, they cause a condition known as diverticulitis, which occurs in a 10 to 25% of cases of diverticular disease. Diverticula appear more commonly in the sigmoid colon, although any other colonic location is possible. Clinically, the most common symptoms are pain, local tenderness, and mass in the left lower quadrant, together with fever and leukocytosis. Common complications are perisigmoid abscess formation, colon perforation, and fistula formation (to the bladder, small bowel, or vagina).

Comments

The presence of diverticula and segmental involvement of colon are hallmarks of diverticulitis. As in other colonic inflammatory conditions, concentric wall thickening and pericolonic inflammatory changes can be visualized. The differential diagnosis includes colonic adenocarcinoma, infectious or ischemic colitis, and Crohn's colitis. Imaging evaluation enables their differentiation on many occasions. CT is the preferred imaging technique to evaluate patients over 50 years with left lower quadrant pain. CT helps to establish the diagnosis of diverticulitis, to determine its extension, and to rule out complications.

The barium contrast-enema was the classical test of choice for suspected diverticulitis, although evaluation of extraluminal changes was limited. Ultrasound has a role but CT is the most useful imaging technique in the evaluation of diverticulitis. CT allows global evaluation of the stenotic segment, pericolic inflammation, and extracolonic complications. CT is more accurate than barium enema in the detection of fistulas. MR has also shown great accuracy in the detection of colonic and small bowel fistulas thanks to its multiplanar capabilities and great sensitivity for inflammatory changes.

Barium enema detected a large stenotic segment of sigmoid colon associated to multiple diverticula (Fig. 4.7.1). A linear contrast extravasation connecting the sigmoid colon to the bladder was also observed (Fig. 4.7.2). Contrast-enhanced CT confirmed the diverticulitis associated to a colonic-bladder fistula. Figures 4.7.3 and 4.7.4 Axial and sagittal reconstructions of enhanced CT show multiple diverticula in the sigmoid colon with inflammatory changes, a complex collection (Fig. 4.7.3, *arrowheads*) in Douglas space, communication between the sigmoid colon to bladder (Fig. 4.7.4, *arrowhead*), bladder wall thickening, and an air-fluid level (Fig. 4.7.4, *arrow*) within the bladder confirming the fistula.

Imaging Findings

Case 8
■
Hiatal Hernia

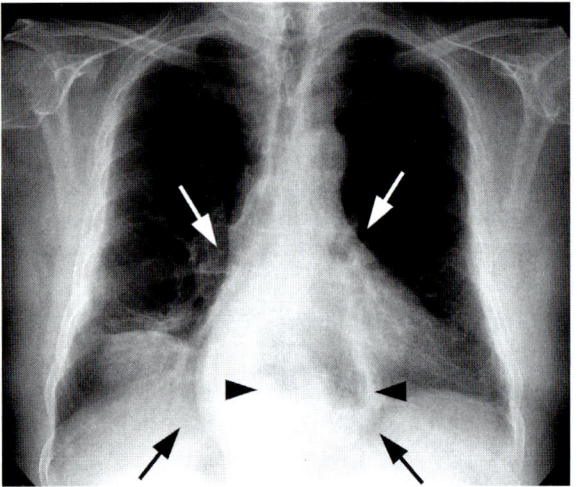

Fig. 4.8.1

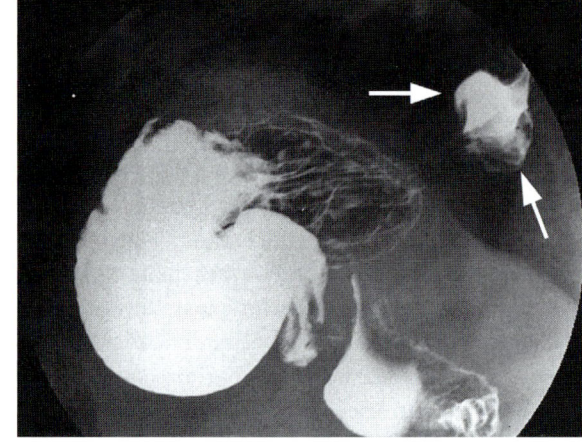

Fig. 4.8.2

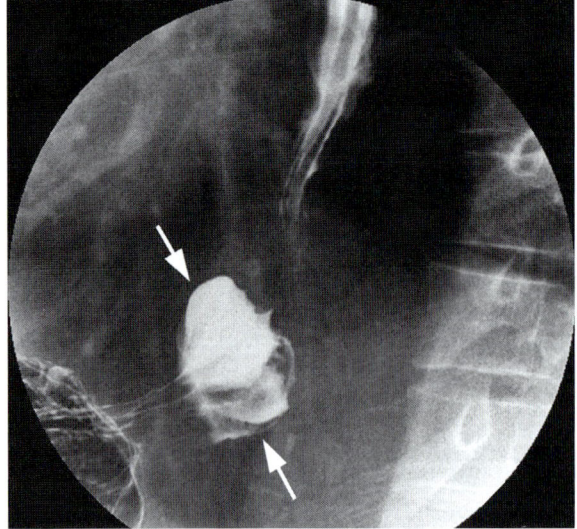

Fig. 4.8.3

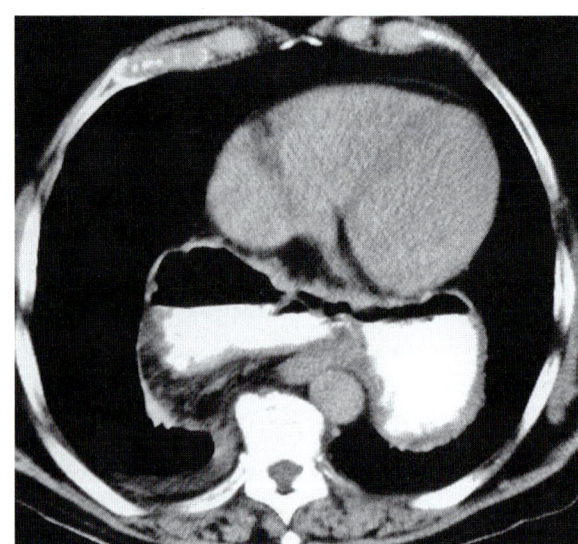

Fig. 4.8.4

A 76-year-old man presented with atypical chest pain.

Hiatal hernias are very common, affecting more than 10% of the general population. It is by far the most common type of hernia, accounting for more than 90% of all hernias. Hiatal hernia occurs when the stomach protrudes through the esophageal hiatus to the chest. It is usually asymptomatic, although a wide range of clinical manifestations is possible. Hiatal hernia can be associated to diverticulosis, reflux esophagitis, duodenal ulcer, and gallstones. Hiatal hernias can be classified as:

- Sliding hiatal hernia, also known as axial or concentric hernia. This is the most common subtype (95%). It appears in 60% of people older than 60 years of age. The esophagogastric junction remains in chest. The ascent of the fundus and cardia is due to rupture or weakness of the phrenicoesophageal membrane. It is very commonly associated to esophagogastric reflux. It may be reducible in the erect position. Surgical repairs is necessary only in symptomatic cases (severe esophagogastric reflux or advanced esophagitis)
- Paraesophageal hernia, also called parahiatal hernia (Fig. 4.8.4). Part of the stomach is displaced into the thorax, although the esophagogastric junction remains below the diaphragm. This type usually grows over time; it is commonly asymptomatic, although when large it can cause thoracic compression. It represents less than 5% of all hiatal hernias. Paraesophageal hernia is frequently non-reducible, and surgical repair is usally necessary.
- Mixed hiatal hernia, when part of the stomach and the esophagogastric junction are both located within the thorax, is a very rare type of hernia (less than 1% of all hiatal hernias). Its treatment is also surgical.

Hiatal hernias are usually detected incidentally at chest X-ray or thoracic or abdominal CT or MR. When clinically suspected, upper gastrointestinal series or esophagogastric endoscopy is necessary to establish the diagnosis. CT is used in complicated cases to delineate the topography of the hernia before surgery. CT is also useful for ruling out complications such as strangulation or incarceration of the hernia.

An epigastric mass (*arrows*) with an internal air-fluid level (*arrowheads*) was seen on a routine chest X-ray (Fig. 4.8.1). An upper gastrointestinal series carried out to rule out hiatal hernia showed the cardia and upper part of the fundus in the chest (*arrows*, Figs. 4.8.2 and 4.8.3). Associated gastroesophageal reflux was visualized during the examination and was probably the cause of the chest pain.

Case 9
■
Primary Small Bowel Lymphoma

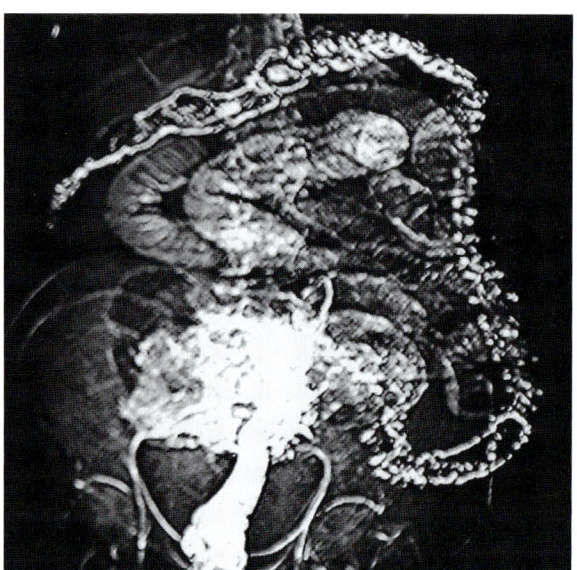

Fig. 4.9.1

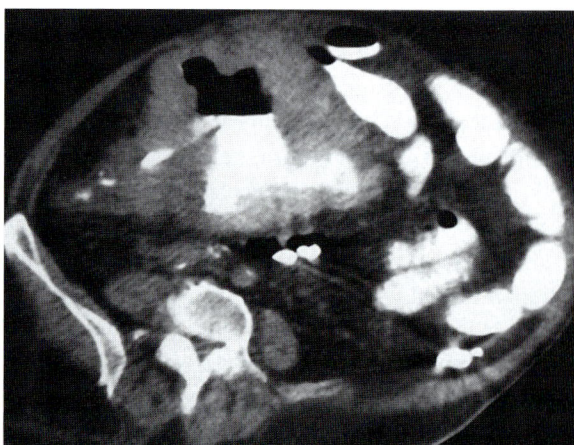

Fig. 4.9.2

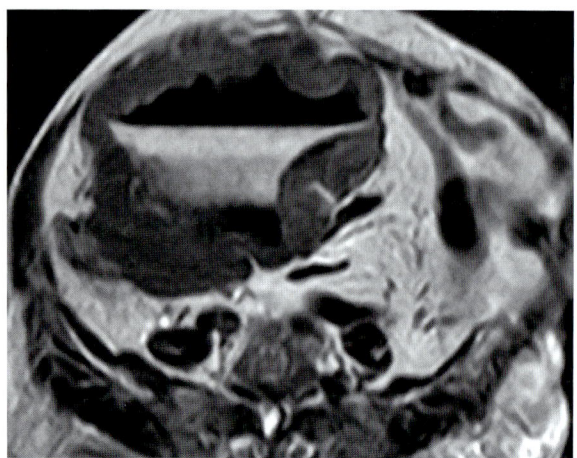

Fig. 4.9.3

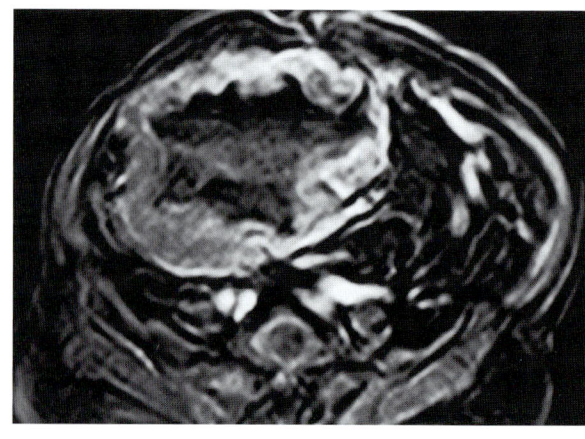

Fig. 4.9.4

An 82-year-old man presented with fever in the previous week, weight loss, and recurrent abdominal pain in the previous 3 months. Physical examination detected a mass in the right lower quadrant.

Lymphoma is the most common malignant tumor in the small bowel, accounting for approximately 25% of all malignant tumors of the small bowel. Small bowel lymphoma can be classified either as primary or secondary. Primary lymphoma can be classified as localized or diffuse. Localized primary lymphoma, as the case shown here, most commonly is a non-Hogkin lymphoma usually located in the terminal ileum. Diffuse or Mediterranean-type lymphoma is associated to parasitic infection, such as giardiasis. Secondary small bowel lymphoma forms part of a generalized systemic process.

Cross-sectional imaging techniques are the most accurate for detecting and characterizing small bowel masses. Determining the origin and associated complications (obstruction, fistulas...) helps to establish the diagnosis and therapeutic management.

Small bowel lymphoma may have different types of presentation: infiltrating lymphoma with plaque-like polypoid mass, endoexoenteric mass and mesenteric and/or retroperitoneal adenopathy. This complex range of presentations usually makes it is impossible to reach a specific diagnosis based on imaging findings, and histological analysis is usually necessary.

Small bowel lymphoma must be differentiated from other small bowel masses, such as small bowel adenocarcinoma and carcinoid tumor. Small bowel adenocarcinoma is most commonly located in the duodenum or jejunum. Carcinoid tumor is usually located in the terminal ileum; the presence of an endocrine syndrome (carcinoid syndrome), its hypervascular nature, and its peritumoral fibrotic reaction are differentiating features from intestinal lymphoma.

Imaging Findings

Abdominal CT was performed and the survey view (Fig. 4.9.1) showed an obstructive intestinal pattern with dilatation of jejunal loops. Significant contrast extravasation in the right iliac fossa and colonic diverticula were also present. CT demonstrated the presence of a cavitated mass originating in the terminal ileum (Fig. 4.9.2) with an internal air-fluid level and several fistulous tracks. The thickened walls of the mass were indicative of malignant neoplastic disease. MR confirmed the origin and characteristic of the mass (Fig. 4.9.3, axial HASTE). Intense capsular enhancement was seen (Fig. 4.9.4, axial postcontrast fat-suppressed GE T1-weighted image). After surgery, the histological analysis of the mass revealed a cavitated small bowel lymphoma.

Case 10
■
Duodenal Gallstone Ileus

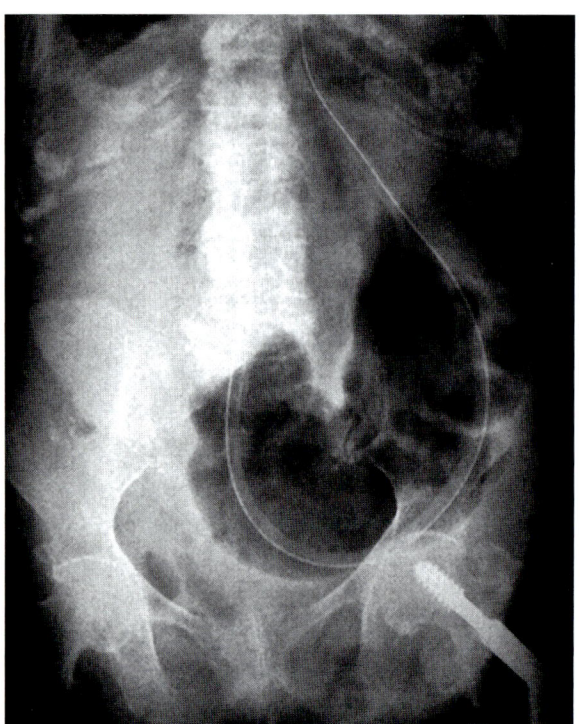

Fig. 4.10.1

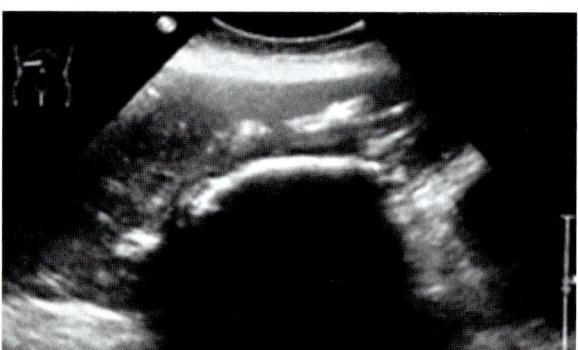

Fig. 4.10.2

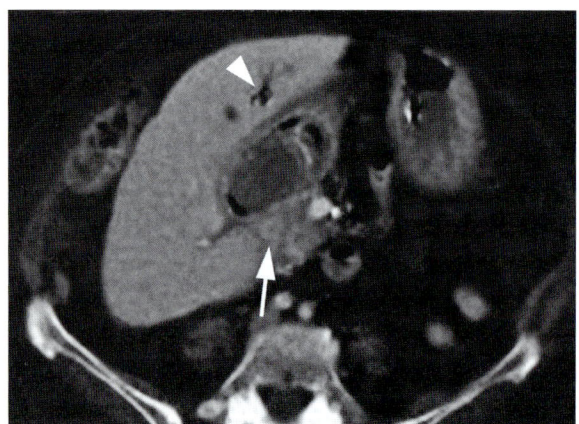

Fig. 4.10.3

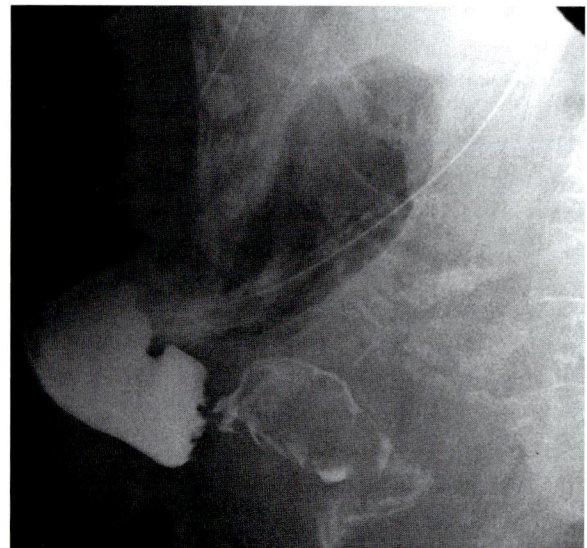

Fig. 4.10.4

An 80-year-old female presented at the ER with severe epigastralgia and incoercible vomiting in the previous week. She also presented nauseas, weight loss, and abdominal distension in the previous 3 weeks.

Comments

Cholelithiasis is a very common condition, involving up to 10% of the population. The range of clinical manifestations is very wide: it could be asymptomatic, produce biliary colic (the most common manifestation), or even cause gallstone ileus. Gallstone ileus is rare, involving less than 1% of patients with gallstones. In this condition, the most common site of obstruction is the terminal ileum, followed by the proximal ileum, distal ileum, pylorus, sigmoid, and duodenum. When the duodenum is the site of obstruction, it is called Bouveret syndrome, which represents 1 to 3% of all gallstone ileus.

In patients with epigastric pain and progressive vomiting lasting several days, it is necessary to exclude proximal obstruction. Causes that need to be considered include inflammatory duodenal conditions (duodenitis, postbulbar ulcers, duodenal Crohn involvement...), pancreatic inflammatory conditions (acute pancreatitis, pseudocysts...), pancreatic or duodenal primary or metastatic neoplasms, duodenal diverticula, duodenal hematomas, and gallstone ileus.

In the imaging diagnosis of gallstone ileus, abdominal plain films are very useful The presence of the Rigler triad (partial or complete intestinal obstruction, gas in the biliary tree, and ectopic calcified gallstone) is almost pathognomonic. On many occasions, one or more of the components of the triad are not present, and further imaging is necessary to determine the cause of obstruction. As is shown in this case, upper gastrointestinal series, ultrasound, and CT help to determine the level and cause of obstruction. Ultrasound and CT are more sensitive than plain film in detecting aerobilia. CT is probably the most accurate technique to determine the presence of partial obstruction and to identify the level and cause of obstruction. MR cholangiography is preferable to conventional cholangiography to demonstrate the chole-enteric fistula in this group of patients, who are usually old and have important surgical risk factors.

Imaging Findings

A nasogastric tube was inserted to prevent vomiting. Abdominal X-ray (Fig. 4.10.1) showed marked dilatation and ptosis of the stomach. Absence of visualization of distal gas in the stomach was suspicious of proximal obstruction. An abdominal ultrasound demonstrated a large lithiasis within the proximal duodenum (Fig. 4.10.2). Enhanced-CT confirmed the presence of a duodenal lithiasis (*arrow*) and also showed aerobilia in the left intrahepatic bile ducts (*arrowhead*), periduodenal inflammatory changes, and loss of the cleavage planes between the duodenum and gallbladder (Fig. 4.10.3). Upper gastrointestinal series confirmed the gastric dilatation and proximal duodenal obstruction (Fig. 4.10.4). The presence of proximal duodenal obstruction produced by an ectopic calcified gallstone enabled the diagnosis of Bouveret syndrome.

Further Readings

Books

Abdominal-Pelvic MRI. 2nd ed. Semelka RC (2006) Wiley-Liss, New-York. ISBN-13: 9780471692737

Advanced Imaging of the Abdomen. Skucas J (2006) Springer-Verlag, Berlin 2006. ISBN-13: 9781852339920

Clinical Imaging of the Small Intestine. 2nd ed. Herlinger H, Maglinte DDT, Birnbaum BA (2001) Springer-Verlag, Berlin. ISBN-13: 9780387953885

Computed Body Tomography with MRI Correlation. Lee JKT, Stanley RJ, Heiken JP (2005) Lippincott Williams & Wilkins ISBN-13: 9780781745260

Diagnostic Ultrasound. Rumack CM, Wilson SR, Charboneau JW (2005) Mosby. ISBN-13: 9780323020237

Double Contrast Gastrointestinal Radiology. 3rd edition. Levine MS, Rubesin SE, Laufer I (1999) W.B. Saunders Company. ISBN-13: 9780721682112

Liver MRI: Correlation with other Imaging Modalities and Histopathology. Hussain SM (2007) Springer-Verlag, Berlin. ISBN-13: 9783540255529

Medical Imaging of the Spleen. De Schepper AM; Vanhoenacker F (2000) Springer-Verlag, Berlin. ISBN-13: 9783540655350

MR Cholangiopancreatography. Atlas with Cross-Sectional Imaging Correlation. 2nd ed. Van Hoe L, Vanbeckevoort D, Mermuys K, van Steenbergen W (2006) Springer-Verlag, Berlin. ISBN-13: 9783540222699

Radiology and Imaging of the Colon. Chapman AH (2004) Springer-Verlag, Berlin. ISBN-13: 9783540435976

Radiology of the Pancreas. 2nd rev ed., Baert AL, Delorme G, Van Hoe L (1999) Springer-Verlag, Berlin. ISBN-13: 9783540634799

Web-Links

http://www.esgar.org/
http://www.sgr.org/sgr.htm
http://www.radcentral.com/
http://radiographics.rsnajnls.org/cgi/collection/gi_radiology?page=9
http://www.emedicine.com/radio/gastrointestinal.htm
http://icarus.med.utoronto.ca/imaging/residents/gi%5Fimaging/index.htm
http://www.rsna.org/Education/archive/afip.cfm#gastrointestinal
http://chorus.rad.mcw.edu/index/4.html
http://www.ctisus.com/
http://www.med-ed.virginia.edu/courses/rad/gi/index.html

Articles

Esophagus

Baker ME, Einstein DM, Herts BR, Remer EM, Motta-Ramirez GA, Ehrenwald E, Rice TW, Richter JE. Gastroesophageal Reflux Disease: Integrating the Barium Esophagram before and after Antireflux Surgery. Radiology 2007 243:329–339

Canon CL, Morgan DE, Einstein DM, Herts BR, Hawn MT, Johnson LF. Surgical Approach to Gastroesophageal Reflux Disease: What the Radiologist Needs to Know. Radiographics 2005; 25:1485–1499

Giménez A, Franquet T, Erasmus JJ, Martínez S, Estrada P. Thoracic Complications of Esophageal Disorders. Radiographics 2002; 22:247–258

Kim TJ, Lee KH, Kim YH, Sung SW, Jheon S, Cho SK, Lee KW. Postoperative Imaging of Esophageal Cancer: What Chest Radiologists Need to Know. Radiographics 2007; 27:409–429

Levine MS, Rubesin SE. Diseases of the Esophagus: Diagnosis with Esophagography. Radiology 2005 237:414–427

Luedtke P, Levine MS, Rubesin SE, Weinstein DS, Laufer I. Radiologic Diagnosis of Benign Esophageal Strictures: A Pattern Approach. Radiographics 2003; 23:897–909

Noh HM, Fishman EK, Forastiere AA, Bliss DF, CalhounPS. CT of the esophagus: spectrum of disease with emphasis on esophageal carcinoma. Radiographics 1995; 15:1113–1134

Sam JW, Levine MS, Rubesin SE, Laufer I. The "Foamy" Esophagus: A Radiographic Sign of Candida Esophagitis. AJR Am J Roentgenol 2000; 174:999–1002

Schmalfuss IM, Mancuso AA, Tart RP. Postcricoid Region and Cervical Esophagus: Normal Appearance at CT and MR Imaging. Radiology 2000; 214:237–246

Zimmerman SL, Levine MS, Rubesin SE, Mitre MC, Furth EE, Laufer I, Katzka DA. Idiopathic Eosinophilic Esophagitis in Adults: The Ringed Esophagus. Radiology 2005; 236:159–165

Stomach

An SK, Han JK, Kim YH, Kim AY, Choi BI, Kim YA, Kim CW. Gastric Mucosa-associated Lymphoid Tissue Lymphoma: Spectrum of Findings at Double-Contrast Gastrointestinal Examination with Pathologic Correlation. Radiographics 2001; 21:1491–1502

Chen CY, Hsu JS, Wu DC, Kang WY, Hsieh JS, Jaw TS, Wu MT, Liu GC. Gastric Cancer: Preoperative Local Staging with 3D Multi–Detector Row CT–Correlation with Surgical and Histopathologic Results. Radiology 2007; 242:472–482

Fishman EK, Urban BA, Hruban RH. CT of the stomach: spectrum of disease. Radiographics 1996; 16:1035–1054

Gelfand DW, Ott DJ, Chen MY. Radiologic evaluation of gastritis and duodenitis. AJR Am J Roentgenol 1999; 173:357–361

Hernanz-Schulman M, Zhu Y, Stein SM, Heller RM, Bethel LA. Hypertrophic Pyloric Stenosis in Infants: US Evaluation of Vascularity of the Pyloric Canal. Radiology 2003; 229:389–393

Kim HJ, Kim AY, Oh ST, Kim JS, Kim KW, Kim PN, Lee MG, Ha HK. Gastric Cancer Staging at Multi–Detector Row CT Gastrography: Comparison of Transverse and Volumetric CT Scanning. Radiology 2005; 236:879–885

Kim JH, Eun HW, Goo DE, Shim CS, Auh YH. Imaging of Various Gastric Lesions with 2D MPR and CT Gastrography Performed with Multidetector CT. Radiographics 2006; 26:1101–1116

Kunz P, Crelier GR, Schwizer W, Borovicka J, Kreiss C, Fried M, Boesiger P. Gastric emptying and motility: assessment with MR imaging–preliminary observations. Radiology 1998; 207:33–40

Pickhardt PJ, Asher DB. Wall Thickening of the Gastric Antrum as a Normal Finding: Multidetector CT with Cadaveric Comparison. AJR Am J Roentgenol 2003; 181:973–979

Rossi M, Broglia L, Graziano P, Maccioni F, Bezzi M, Masciangelo R, Rossi P. Local invasion of gastric cancer: CT findings and pathologic correlation using 5-mm incremental scanning, hypotonia, and water filling. AJR Am J Roentgenol 1999; 172:383–388

Small Bowel

Applegate KE, Anderson JM, Klatte EC. Intestinal Malrotation in Children: A Problem-solving Approach to the Upper Gastrointestinal Series. Radiographics 2006; 26:1485–1500

Balthazar EJ, Noordhoorn M, Megibow AJ, Gordon RB. CT of small-bowel lymphoma in immunocompetent patients and patients with AIDS: comparison of findings. AJR Am J Roentgenol 1997; 168:675–680

Furukawa A, Yamasaki M, Furuichi K, Yokoyama K, Nagata T, Takahashi M, Murata K, Sakamoto T. Helical CT in the Diagnosis of Small Bowel Obstruction. Radiographics 2001; 21:341–355

Hara AK, Leighton JA, Sharma VK, Heigh RI, Fleischer DE. Imaging of Small Bowel Disease: Comparison of Capsule Endoscopy, Standard Endoscopy, Barium Examination, and CT. Radiographics 2005; 25:697–711

Hara AK, Leighton JA, Heigh RI, Sharma VK, Silva AC, De Petris G, Hentz JG, Fleischer DE. Crohn Disease of the Small Bowel: Preliminary Comparison among CT Enterography, Capsule Endoscopy, Small-Bowel Follow-through, and Ileoscopy. Radiology 2006; 238:128–134

Kessler N, Cyteval C, Gallix B, Lesnik A, Blayac PM, Pujol J, Bruel JM, Taourel P. Appendicitis: Evaluation of Sensitivity, Specificity, and Predictive Values of US, Doppler US, and Laboratory Findings. Radiology 2004 230:472–478

Ledermann HP, Börner N, Strunk H, Bongartz G, Zollikofer C, Stuckmann G. Bowel Wall Thickening on Trans-abdominal Sonography. AJR Am J Roentgenol 2000; 174:107–115

Low RN, Sebrechts CP, Politoske DA, Bennett MT, Flores S, Snyder RJ, Pressman JH. Crohn Disease with Endoscopic Correlation: Single-Shot Fast Spin-Echo and Gadolinium-enhanced Fat-suppressed Spoiled Gradient-Echo MR Imaging. Radiology 2002 222:652–660

Macari M, Hines J, Balthazar E, Megibow A. Mesenteric Adenitis: CT Diagnosis of Primary Versus Secondary Causes, Incidence, and Clinical Significance in Pediatric and Adult Patients. AJR Am J Roentgenol 2002; 178:853–858

Maccioni F, Bruni A, Viscido A, Colaiacomo MC, Cocco A, Montesani C, Caprilli R, Marini M. MR Imaging in Patients with Crohn Disease: Value of T2- versus T1-weighted Gadolinium-enhanced MR Sequences with Use of an Oral Superparamagnetic Contrast Agent. Radiology 2005 238:517–530

Paulsen SR, Huprich JE, Fletcher JG, Booya F, Young BM, Fidler JL, Johnson CD, Barlow JM, Earnest F 4th. CT Enterography as a Diagnostic Tool in Evaluating Small Bowel Disorders: Review of Clinical Experience with over 700 Cases. Radiographics 2006; 26:641–657

Rubesin SE, Rubin RA, Herlinger H. Small bowel malabsorption: clinical and radiologic perspectives. How we see it. Radiology 1992; 184:297–305

Colon

Frank AJ, Goffner LB, Fruauff AA, Losada RA. Cecal volvulus: The CT whirl sign. Abdom Imaging 1993; 18:288–289

Geenen RW, Hussain SM, Cademartiri F, Poley JW, Siersema PD, Krestin GP. CT and MR Colonography: Scanning Techniques, Postprocessing, and Emphasis on Polyp Detection. Radiographics 2004; 24:e18

Goh V, Halligan S, Taylor SA, Burling D, Bassett P, Bartram CI. Differentiation between Diverticulitis and Colorectal Cancer: Quantitative CT Perfusion Measurements versus Morphologic Criteria – Initial Experience. Radiology 2007; 242:456–462

Hoeffel C, Crema MD, Belkacem A, Azizi L, Lewin M, Arrivé L, Tubiana JM. Multi–Detector Row CT: Spectrum of Diseases Involving the Ileocecal Area. Radiographics 2006; 26:1373-1390

Horton KM, Corl FM, Fishman EK. CT Evaluation of the Colon: Inflammatory Disease. Radiographics 2000; 20:399–418

Johnson CD, Dachman AH. CT Colonography: The Next Colon Screening Examination? Radiology 2000; 216:331–341

Oldfield AL, Wilbur AC. Retrogastric colon: CT demonstration of anatomic variations. Radiology 1993; 186:557–561

Rha SE, Ha HK, Lee SH, Kim JH, Kim JK, Kim JH, Kim PN, Lee MG, Auh YH. CT and MR Imaging Findings of Bowel Ischemia from Various Primary Causes. Radiographics 2000; 20:29–42

Silva AC, Wellnitz CV, Hara AK. Three-dimensional Virtual Dissection at CT Colonography: Unraveling the Colon to Search for Lesions. Radiographics 2006; 26:1669–1686

Tack D, Bohy P, Perlot I, De Maertelaer V, Alkeilani O, Sourtzis S, Gevenois PA. Suspected Acute Colon Diverticulitis: Imaging with Low-Dose Unenhanced Multi–Detector Row CT. Radiology 2005; 237:189–196

Urban BA, Fishman EK. Tailored Helical CT Evaluation of Acute Abdomen: (CME available in print version and on RSNA Link). Radiographics 2000; 20:725–749

Rectum and Anus

Beets-Tan RG, Beets GL. Rectal Cancer: Review with Emphasis on MR Imaging. Radiology 2004; 232:335–346

Beets-Tan RG, Beets GL, van der Hoop AG, Kessels AG, Vliegen RF, Baeten CG, van Engelshoven JM. Preoperative MR Imaging of Anal Fistulas: Does It Really Help the Surgeon? Radiology 2001; 218:75–84

Blomqvist L, Fransson P, Hindmarsh T. The pelvis after surgery and radio-chemotherapy for rectal cancer studied with Gd-DTPA-enhanced fast dynamic MR imaging. Eur Radiol 1998; 8:781–787

Buchanan GN, Halligan S, Bartram CI, Williams AB, Tarroni D, Cohen RG. Clinical Examination, Endosonography, and MR Imaging in Preoperative Assessment of Fistula in Ano: Comparison with Outcome-based Reference Standard. Radiology 2004; 233:674–681

Halligan S, Stoker J. Imaging of Fistula in Ano. Radiology 2006; 239:18–33

Iafrate F, Laghi A, Paolantonio P, Rengo M, Mercantini P, Ferri M, Ziparo V, Passariello R. Preoperative Staging of Rectal Cancer with MR Imaging: Correlation with Surgical and Histopathologic Findings. Radiographics 2006; 26:701–714

Lee JH, Lee KH, Chung WS, Hur J, Won JY, Lee DY. Transcatheter Embolization of the Middle Sacral Artery: Collateral Feeder in Recurrent Rectal Bleeding. AJR Am J Roentgenol 2004; 182:1055–1057

Pomerri F, Zuliani M, Mazza C, Villarejo F, Scopece A. Defecographic Measurements of Rectal Intussusception and Prolapse in Patients and in Asymptomatic Subjects. AJR Am J Roentgenol 2001; 176:641–645

Silva AC, Vens EA, Hara AK, Fletcher JG, Fidler JL, Johnson CD. Evaluation of Benign and Malignant Rectal Lesions with CT Colonography and Endoscopic Correlation. Radiographics 2006; 26:1085–1099

Stoker J, Rociu E, Zwamborn AW, Schouten WR, Laméris JS. Endoluminal MR Imaging of the Rectum and Anus: Technique, Applications, and Pitfalls. Radiographics 1999; 19:383–398

Liver

Annet L, Materne R, Danse E, Jamart J, Horsmans Y, Van Beers BE. Hepatic Flow Parameters Measured with MR Imaging and Doppler US: Correlations with Degree of Cirrhosis and Portal Hypertension. Radiology 2003 229:409–414

Bargalló X, Gilabert R, Nicolau C, García-Pagán JC, Bosch J, Brú C. Sonography of the Caudate Vein: Value in Diagnosing Budd-Chiari Syndrome. AJR Am J Roentgenol 2003; 181:1641–1645

Brancatelli G, Federle MP, Grazioli L, Golfieri R, Lencioni R. Large Regenerative Nodules in Budd-Chiari Syndrome and Other Vascular Disorders of the Liver: CT and MR Imaging Findings with Clinicopathologic Correlation. AJR Am J Roentgenol 2002; 178:877–883

Brancatelli G, Federle MP, Vilgrain V, Vullierme MP, Marin D, Lagalla R. Fibropolycystic Liver Disease: CT and MR Imaging Findings. Radiographics 2005; 25:659–670

Brancatelli G, Vilgrain V, Federle MP, Hakime A, Lagalla R, Iannaccone R, Valla D. Budd-Chiari Syndrome: Spectrum of Imaging Findings. AJR Am J Roentgenol 2007; 188:W168–W176

Catalano O, Nunziata A, Lobianco R, Siani A. Real-Time Harmonic Contrast Material–specific US of Focal Liver Lesions. Radiographics 2005; 25:333–349

Clark HP, Carson WF, Kavanagh PV, Ho CP, Shen P, Zagoria RJ. Staging and Current Treatment of Hepatocellular Carcinoma. Radiographics 2005; 25 (Suppl 1):S3–S23

Danet IM, Semelka RC, Leonardou P, Braga L, Vaidean G, Woosley JT, Kanematsu M. Spectrum of MRI Appearances of Untreated Metastases of the Liver. AJR Am J Roentgenol 2003; 181:809–817

Elsayes KM, Narra VR, Yin Y, Mukundan G, Lammle M, Brown JJ. Focal Hepatic Lesions: Diagnostic Value of Enhancement Pattern Approach with Contrast-enhanced 3D Gradient-Echo MR Imaging. Radiographics 2005; 25:1299–1320

Gandhi SN, Brown MA, Wong JG, Aguirre DA, Sirlin CB. MR Contrast Agents for Liver Imaging: What, When, How. Radiographics 2006; 26:1621–1636

Hamer OW, Aguirre DA, Casola G, Lavine JE, Woenckhaus M, Sirlin CB. Fatty Liver: Imaging Patterns and Pitfalls. Radiographics 2006; 26:1637–1653

Hussain SM, Terkivatan T, Zondervan PE, Lanjouw E, de Rave S, Ijzermans JN, de Man RA. Focal Nodular Hyperplasia: Findings at State-of-the-Art MR Imaging, US, CT, and Pathologic Analysis. Radiographics 2004; 24:3–17

Leslie DF, Johnson CD, Johnson CM, Ilstrup DM, Harmsen WS. Distinction between cavernous hemangiomas of the liver and hepatic metastases on CT: value of contrast enhancement patterns. AJR Am J Roentgenol 1995; 164:625–629

Mortelé KJ, Ros PR. Cystic Focal Liver Lesions in the Adult: Differential CT and MR Imaging Features. Radiographics 2001; 21:895–910

Powers C, Ros PR, Stoupis C, Johnson WK, Segel KH. Primary liver neoplasms: MR imaging with pathologic correlation. Radiographics 1994; 14:459–482

Stevens WR, Johnson CD, Stephens DH, Batts KP. CT findings in hepatocellular carcinoma: correlation of tumor characteristics with causative factors, tumor size, and histologic tumor grade. Radiology 1994; 191:531–537

Vilgrain V, Boulos L, Vullierme MP, Denys A, Terris B, Menu Y. Imaging of Atypical Hemangiomas of the Liver with Pathologic Correlation. Radiographics 2000; 20:379–397

Pancreas

Balthazar EJ. Acute Pancreatitis: Assessment of Severity with Clinical and CT Evaluation. Radiology 2002; 223:603–613

Bret PM, Reinhold C, Taourel P, Guibaud L, Atri M, Barkun AN. Pancreas divisum: evaluation with MR cholangiopancreatography. Radiology 1996; 199:99–103

Gangi S, Fletcher JG, Nathan MA, Christensen JA, Harmsen WS, Crownhart BS, Chari ST. Time Interval Between Abnormalities Seen on CT and the Clinical Diagnosis of Pancreatic Cancer: Retrospective Review of CT Scans Obtained Before Diagnosis. AJR Am J Roentgenol 2004; 182:897–903

Kawamoto S, Horton KM, Lawler LP, Hruban RH, Fishman EK. Intraductal Papillary Mucinous Neoplasm of the Pancreas: Can Benign Lesions Be Differentiated from Malignant Lesions with Multidetector CT? Radiographics 2005; 25:1451–1468

Kim YH, Saini S, Sahani D, Hahn PF, Mueller PR, Auh YH. Imaging Diagnosis of Cystic Pancreatic Lesions: Pseudocyst versus Nonpseudocyst. Radiographics 2005; 25:671–685

Lim JH, Lee G, Oh YL. Radiologic Spectrum of Intraductal Papillary Mucinous Tumor of the Pancreas. Radiographics 2001; 21:323–337

Matos C, Cappeliez O, Winant C, Coppens E, Devière J, Metens T. MR Imaging of the Pancreas: A Pictorial Tour. Radiographics 2002; 22:e2

Ros PR, Hamrick-Turner JE, Chiechi MV, Ros LH, Gallego P, Burton SS. Cystic masses of the pancreas. Radiographics 1992; 12:673–686

Semelka RC, Ascher SM. MR imaging of the pancreas. Radiology 1993; 188:593–602

Soto JA, Lucey BC, Stuhlfaut JW. Pancreas Divisum: Depiction with Multi–Detector Row CT. Radiology 2005; 235:503–508

Vaughn DD, Jabra AA, Fishman EK. Pancreatic disease in children and young adults: evaluation with CT. Radiographics 1998; 18:1171–1187

Gallblader and Biliary System

Altun E, Semelka RC, Elias J Jr, Braga L, Voultsinos V, Patel J, Balci NC, Woosley JT. Acute Cholecystitis: MR Findings and Differentiation from Chronic Cholecystitis. Radiology 2007; 244:174–183

Bloom CM, Langer B, Wilson SR. Role of US in the Detection, Characterization, and Staging of Cholangiocarcinoma. Radiographics 1999; 19:1199–1218

Fulcher AS, Turner MA, Capps GW. MR Cholangiography: Technical Advances and Clinical Applications. Radiographics 1999; 19:25–41

Lee WJ, Lim HK, Jang KM, Kim SH, Lee SJ, Lim JH, Choo IW. Radiologic Spectrum of Cholangiocarcinoma: Emphasis on Unusual Manifestations and Differential Diagnoses. Radiographics 2001; 21:97–116

Levy AD, Murakata LA, Rohrmann CA Jr. Gallbladder Carcinoma: Radiologic-Pathologic Correlation. Radiographics 2001; 21:295–314

Levy AD, Murakata LA, Abbott RM, Rohrmann CA Jr. From the Archives of the AFIP: Benign Tumors and Tumorlike Lesions of the Gallbladder and Extrahepatic Bile Ducts: Radiologic-Pathologic Correlation. Radiographics 2002; 22:387–413

Levy AD, Rohrmann CA Jr, Murakata LA, Lonergan GJ. Caroli's Disease: Radiologic Spectrum with Pathologic Correlation. AJR Am J Roentgenol 2002; 179:1053–1057

Mortelé KJ, Rocha TC, Streeter JL, Taylor AJ. Multimodality Imaging of Pancreatic and Biliary Congenital Anomalies. Radiographics 2006; 26:715–731

Park HS, Lee JM, Kim SH, Jeong JY, Kim YJ, Lee KH, Choi SH, Han JK, Choi BI. CT Differentiation of Cholangiocarcinoma from Periductal Fibrosis in Patients with Hepatolithiasis. AJR Am J Roentgenol 2006; 187:445–453

Park MS, Yu JS, Kim YH, Kim MJ, Kim JH, Lee S, Cho N, Kim DG, Kim KW. Acute cholecystitis: comparison of MR cholangiography and US. Radiology 1998; 209:781–785

Park MS, Yu JS, Kim KW, Kim MJ, Chung JP, Yoon SW, Chung JJ, Lee JT, Yoo HS. Recurrent Pyogenic Cholangitis: Comparison between MR Cholangiography and Direct Cholangiography. Radiology 2001; 220:677–682

Rizzo RJ, Szucs RA, MA Turner MA. Congenital abnormalities of the pancreas and biliary tree in adults. Radiographics 1995; 15:49–86

Rosenthal SJ, Cox GG, Wetzel LH, Batnitzky S. Pitfalls and differential diagnosis in biliary sonography. Radiographics 1990; 10:285–311

Soto JA, Alvarez O, Lopera JE, Múnera F, Restrepo JC, Correa G. Biliary Obstruction: Findings at MR Cholangiography and Cross-sectional MR Imaging. Radiographics 2000; 20:353–366

Vitellas KM, Keogan MT, Freed KS, Enns RA, Spritzer CE, Baillie JM, Nelson RC. Radiologic Manifestations of Sclerosing Cholangitis with Emphasis on MR Cholangiopancreatography. Radiographics 2000; 20:959–975

Spleen

Abbott RM, Levy AD, Aguilera NS, Gorospe L, Thompson WM. From the Archives of the AFIP: Primary Vascular Neoplasms of the Spleen: Radiologic-Pathologic Correlation. Radiographics 2004; 24:1137–1163

Elsayes KM, Narra VR, Mukundan G, Lewis JS Jr, Menias CO, Heiken JP. MR Imaging of the Spleen: Spectrum of Abnormalities. Radiographics 2005; 25:967–982

Freeman JL, Jafri SZ, Roberts JL, Mezwa DG, Shirkhoda A. CT of congenital and acquired abnormalities of the spleen Radiographics 1993; 13:597–610

Levy AD, Abbott RM, Abbondanzo SL. Littoral Cell Angioma of the Spleen: CT Features with Clinicopathologic Comparison. Radiology 2004; 230:485–490

Luna A, Ribes R, Caro P, Luna L, Aumente E, Ros PR. MRI of Focal Splenic Lesions Without and With Dynamic Gadolinium Enhancement. AJR Am J Roentgenol 2006; 186:1533–1547

Megremis SD, Vlachonikolis IG, Tsilimigaki AM. Spleen Length in Childhood with US: Normal Values Based on Age, Sex, and Somatometric Parameters. Radiology 2004; 231:129–134

Minami M, Itai Y, Ohtomo K, Ohnishi S, Niki T, Kokubo T, Yoshikawa K, Iio M. Siderotic nodules in the spleen: MR imaging of portal hypertension. Radiology 1989; 172:681–684

Mortelé KJ, Mortelé B, Silverman SG. CT Features of the Accessory Spleen. AJR Am J Roentgenol 2004; 183:1653–1657

Thompson WM, Levy AD, Aguilera NS, Gorospe L, Abbott RM. Angiosarcoma of the Spleen: Imaging Characteristics in 12 Patients. Radiology 2005 235:106–115

Urrutia M, Mergo PJ, Ros LH, Torres GM, Ros PR. Cystic masses of the spleen: radiologic-pathologic correlation. Radiographics 1996; 16:107–129

Genitourinary, Gynecological, and Obstetrical Imaging

5

Antonio Luna Alcala, Marcelo Potolicchio, and Lidia Alcala Mata

The role of the radiologist in both genitourinary and gynecological-obstetrical imaging has dramatically evolved in recent years. In most centers, urologists, gynecologists, and obstetricians are responsible for imaging procedures such as ultrasound, urography, imaging-guided biopsy, and hysterosalpingography. However, radiologists should collaborate in these techniques as their skills and specific training in imaging can add significant value to these procedures. Additionally, the advent of cross-sectional imaging techniques has widened the field of application of imaging in these areas.

In gynecology, ultrasound is the most common imaging technique for evaluating the cervix, uterus, and adnexa. Thanks to its increased spatial resolution, transvaginal ultrasound has increased the applications of ultrasound even more. Magnetic resonance (MR) is widely used for local staging of gynecological malignancies, to characterize adnexal masses, and to exclude recurrence of treated gynecological cancers. Computed tomography and PET-CT are used for distant staging of gynecologic tumors.

Imaging in obstetrics is also based on ultrasound. As MR does not use ionizing radiation, it has a role in the evaluation of gynecological or abdominal masses discovered in the mother during pregnancy. MR also complements ultrasound in the detection and management of fetal anomalies.

Genitourinary and retroperitoneal imaging examines different organs such as the kidneys, excretory system, prostate, bladder, testicles, and penis. The great diversity of pathologies in these organs means that all the available imaging techniques have their uses. Ultrasound is very useful in the evaluation of the kidneys, prostate, bladder, testicles, and penis. The excretory system is studied by conventional urography or the newer CT or MR urography. Accurate evaluation of the retroperitoneum needs cross-sectional imaging techniques, such as CT or MR. These techniques are also used to stage malignancies of all the organs of the genitourinary system.

Introduction

Case 1
■
Adrenal Myelolipoma

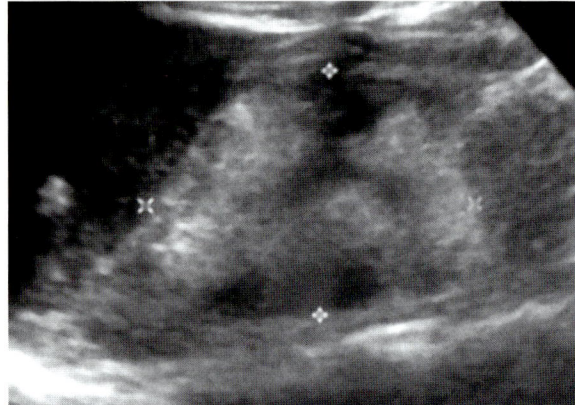

Fig. 5.1.1

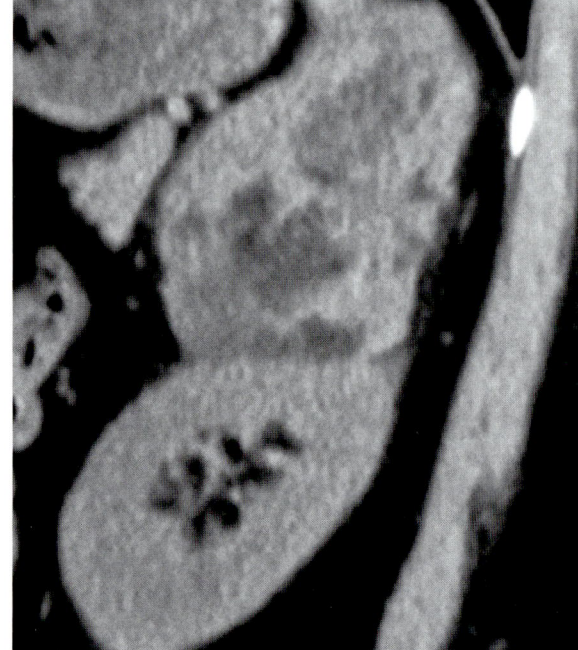

Fig. 5.1.2

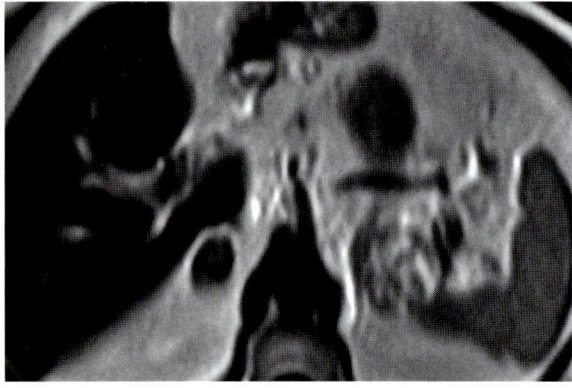

Fig. 5.1.3

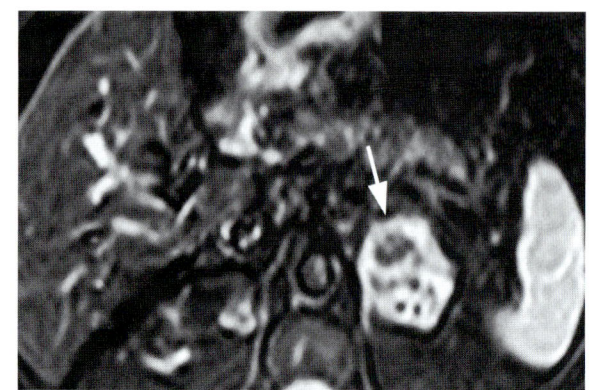

Fig. 5.1.4

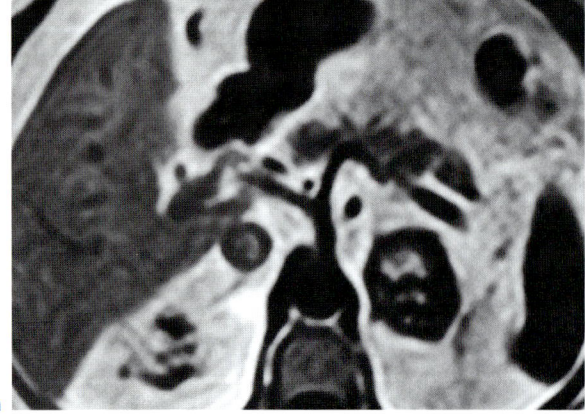

a

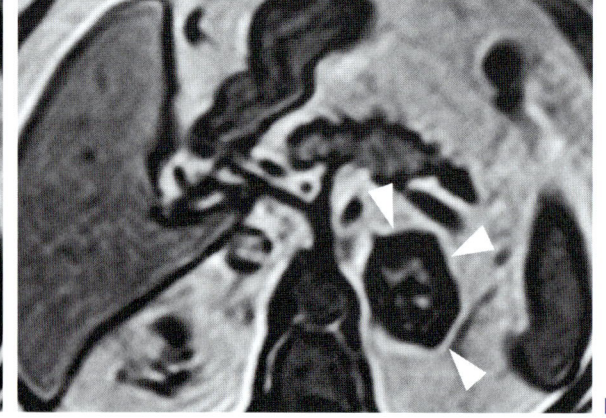

b

Fig. 5.1.5

An asymptomatic 54-year-old woman was referred for clinical suspicion of splenomegaly on physical examination. Her blood count was normal.

Myelolipomas are rare benign tumors, composed of fat and myeloid tissue (bone marrow elements). They are most commonly unilateral and small. They are usually asymptomatic, although they can bleed and cause pain. Intralesional fat is nearly diagnostic, so CT or MT can characterize these lesions and determine their adrenal origin. Percutaneous biopsy may be necessary to exclude malignancy in complicated myelolipomas with hemorrhage or infarction if small areas of fat within the tumor cannot be detected. Other adrenal lesions that can contain fat are lipoma and liposarcoma; neighboring extraadrenal lesions that can be confused with adrenal myelolipoma are retroperitoneal lipoma, liposarcoma, and renal angiomyolipoma. First, cross-sectional imaging is necessary to confirm the origin of adrenal myelolipoma in the adrenal gland. If the mass is large, sagittal or coronal acquisitions or reconstructions may be useful to exclude a renal or retroperitoneal origin. The demonstration of macroscopic fat is almost diagnostic of myelolipoma in cases of an adrenal mass, as adrenal lipomas or liposarcomas are exceedingly rare. The detection of small intratumoral areas with negative densitometric values (especially values below -20 Hounsfield units) on unenhanced CT indicates the presence of macroscopic fat deposits. Because of intermixed hematopoietic tissue, the attenuation is usually higher than that of retroperitoneal fat. MR is probably superior to CT in the detection of intratumoral fat. Areas isointense to retroperitoneal fat in all T1-weighted, T2-weighted, frequency-selective fat-suppressed, and fat-saturated images is diagnostic of intratumoral macroscopic fat.

Special caution is necessary in the differentiation between adenomas and myelolipomas. Adenomas most commonly demonstrate intratumoral microscopic fat, which can be detected using chemical-shift MR. This technique uses a double-echo acquisition, because in areas where water and fat are in similar proportions (ex: microscopic fat in adrenal adenomas), the signal from water and fat signal may be additive (in-phase acquisition) or cancelled (opposed-phase acquisition), depending on the echo time. Using this sequence, adenomas characteristically show a drop in signal greater than 20% in areas of microscopic fat. Myelolipomas can also show microscopic fat, although macroscopic fat, which will not show signal loss on chemical-shift MR, is diagnostic of myelolipomas.

Abdominal ultrasound showed a well-defined heterogeneous mass immediately inferior to the spleen and superior to the left kidney (Fig. 5.1.1). The mass was predominantly hyperechoic and measured approximately 11 cm. Unenhanced CT demonstrated the adrenal origin of the mass, which was predominantly solid with areas of intralesional fat (Fig. 5.1.2, sagittal reconstruction of unenhanced CT). Adrenal MR confirmed the diagnosis of adrenal myelolipoma. On HASTE images the mass was heterogeneous with a peripheral solid component and central areas of high signal intensity (Fig. 5.1.3). This central high signal component corresponded to macroscopic fat, as demonstrated by its suppression on STIR (short-tau inversion recovery) sequences (Fig. 5.1.4, *arrow*) and the absence of signal loss in chemical-shift imaging (Fig. 5.1.5a,b). Note the signal loss of the solid peripheral component on opposed-phase images (Fig. 5.1.5b, *arrowheads*), revealing the presence of peripheral microscopic fat (areas with similar proportions of water and fat).

Case 2
■
Complicated Cortical Renal Cyst

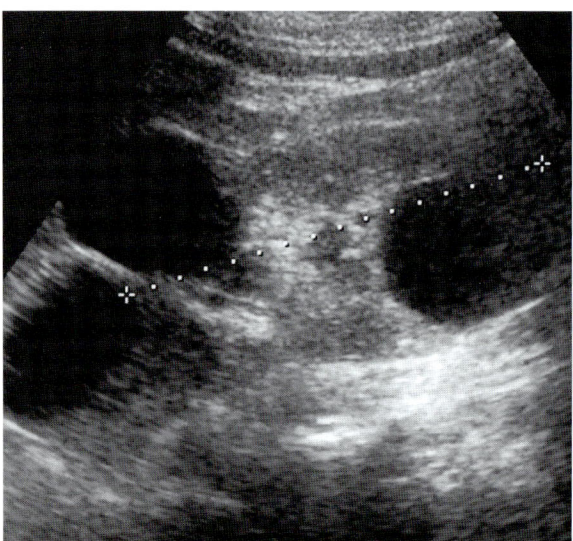

Fig. 5.2.1

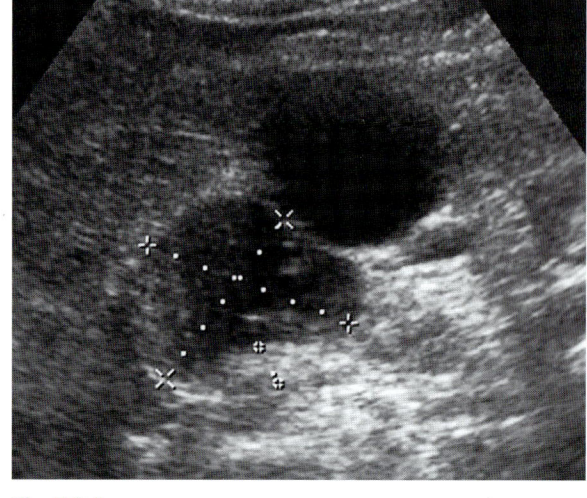

Fig. 5.2.2

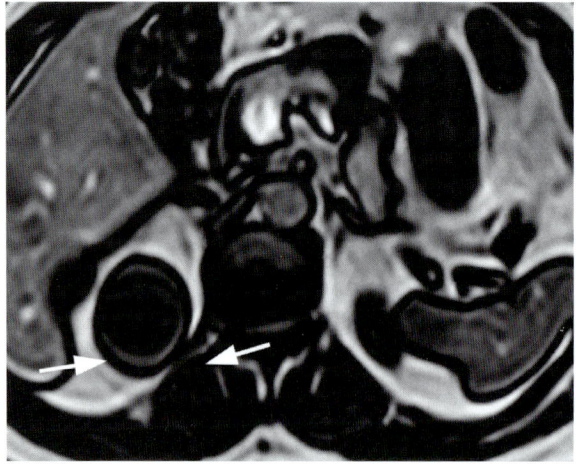

Fig. 5.2.3

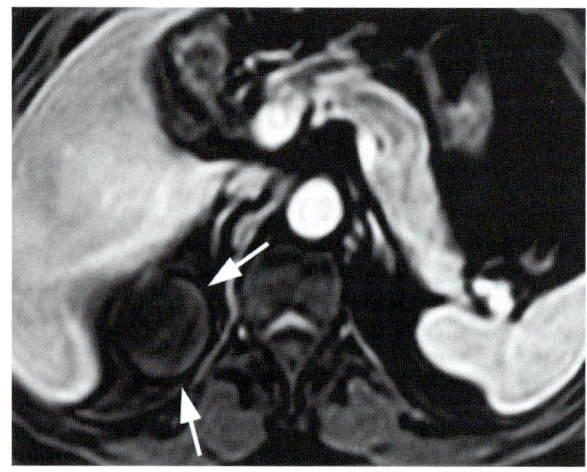

Fig. 5.2.4

A 67-year-old-man was studied for arterial hypertension of recent onset.

Renal cortical cysts are very common lesions, and their frequency increases with age. Most are asymptomatic, found incidentally during intravenous urography or renal ultrasound. Imaging criteria have been developed to establish their diagnosis. Sonographic criteria include the absence of free internal echoes, sharply defined anterior margin, and increased through-transmission of the ultrasound beam. Diagnostic CT features are homogeneous attenuation value near water density, lack of contrast enhancement, lack of measurable thickness of the cyst wall, and smooth interface with the renal parenchyma. MR diagnostic criteria are very similar to those of CT.

Cystic renal lesions with atypical features such as septa, calcifications, hemorrhagic content, debris, solid conglomerates, or irregular margins are considered complicated cysts. The management of this group of lesions is in constant evolution. They are usually classified according to Bosniak's criteria, which groups cystic lesions in 5 categories according to their complexity, from simple cyst to cystic renal neoplasm. Lesions that have all the echographic criteria of a simple cyst require no further evaluation. Indeterminate cystic lesions on ultrasound need CT or/and MR study. If a lesion has suspicious features for malignancy, surgical resection is recommended. If a true cystic lesion has indeterminate appearance on CT or MR, or it shows discordant features between different imaging modalities, follow-up imaging is the appropriate management.

Cystic renal lesions are a daily clinical problem for radiologists. The diagnosis, classification, and management of these lesions are determined by imaging criteria. Knowledge of common and atypical features of these lesions enables differentiation between simple and complicated renal cysts, as well as exclusion of other cystic renal masses, such as cystic renal carcinoma, multilocular cystic nephroma, renal artery aneurysm, renal abscess, or renal hematoma.

Renal ultrasound showed multiple bilateral renal cortical cysts (Fig. 5.2.1). One cyst, on the upper pole of the right kidney, had internal septa and hyperechoic content (Fig. 5.2.2). At MR, the lesion demonstrated typical features of a cystic lesion: it was hypointense on T1-weighted sequences and hyperintense on T2-weighted sequences, without enhancement after contrast administration. On T1-weighted images, a lineal area of peripheral hyperintensity visualized in the dependent part of the cyst revealed hemorrhagic content (Fig. 5.2.3, *arrows*, axial TSE T1-weighted image). After contrast administration, peripheral, capsular-like enhancement was detected, indicating an associated inflammatory process (Fig. 5.2.4, *arrows*, axial fat-suppressed T1-weighted GE image). These features confirmed the echographic diagnosis of complicated renal cyst, with hemorrhagic content and inflammatory changes. No signs of malignancy were demonstrated. The stability of the lesion in follow-up imaging studies confirmed its benign nature.

Case 3
■
Prostate Cancer

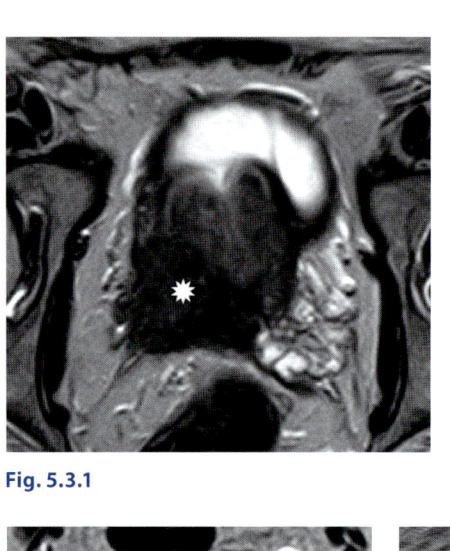

Fig. 5.3.1

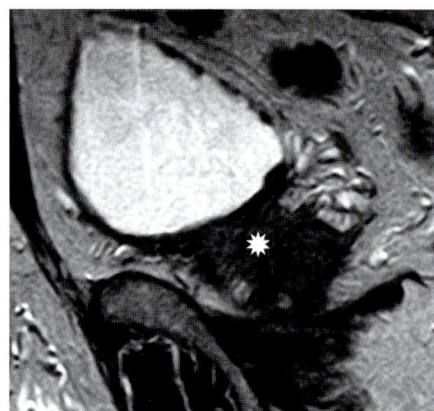

Fig. 5.3.2

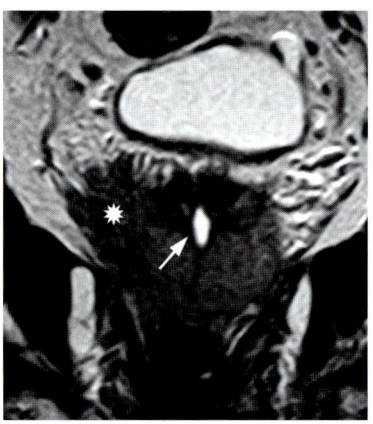

Fig. 5.3.3

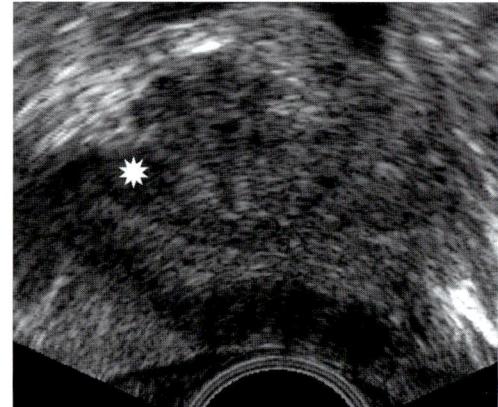

Fig. 5.3.4

Fig. 5.3.5a–c

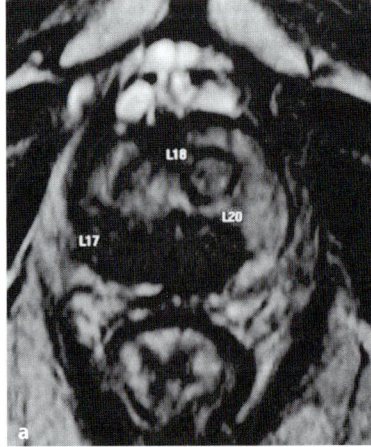

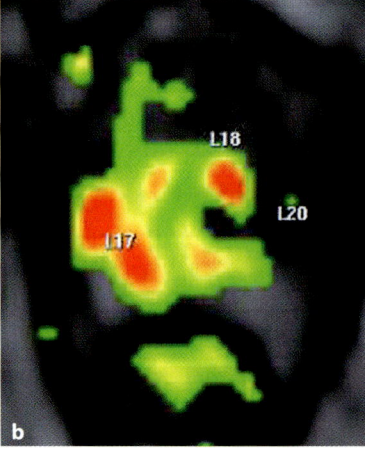

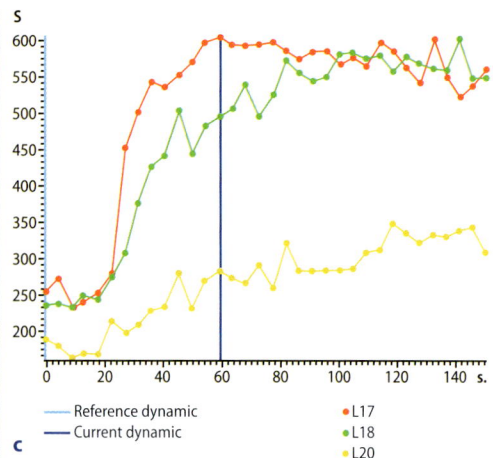

67-year-old man with confirmed prostate cancer underwent MR for local staging.

Prostate cancer is the most common malignancy in males. Diagnosis and staging are very important for appropriate management, as treatment varies according to tumor stage. The American Cancer Association recommends annual screening for all males over the age of 50 and for high risk patients over the age of 40. This screening includes a digital rectal examination and a serum prostate specific antigen (PSA) test. Tumors detected at digital rectal examination are classified as clinical prostate cancer. Occult carcinoma is found in a biopsy of a bone or lymph node metastasis in patients without symptoms of prostatic disease. PSA, an enzyme produced by epithelial cells in the prostatic ducts, is a powerful tumor marker and is crucial in prostatic cancer screening. Its normal concentration is less than 4 nanograms per millimeter and may rise as a consequence of both benign and malignant conditions. The risk of prostate cancer increases parallel to serum levels of PSA. Levels over 10 ng/ml are very suspicious and call for prostate biopsy. Clinical management of patients with serum levels between 4 and 10 ng/ml is much more controversial. Biopsy is generally advised, although imaging tests or evaluation of other serum markers such as PSA density, PSA velocity, or the ratio of free to total PSA may be considered sufficient depending on the center. In any case, close follow-up is necessary in this group of patients.

Normal findings at transrectal ultrasound do not rule out prostate cancer and biopsy should be performed if digital rectal examination findings are suspicious or PSA levels are elevated. Transrectal ultrasound only detects between 50 to 60% of all prostate cancers. Most appear as hypoechogenic nodules in the peripheral zone (Fig. 5.3.4, right longitudinal view shows a hypoechogenic nodule in the peripheral zone, *asterisk*). Around 30% of all cancers are isoechogenic to the prostate gland and thus cannot be detected. The main clinical applications of transrectal ultrasound are to guide prostate biopsy and to implant radiotherapy seeds.

MR is the technique of choice for local staging. Most tumors are hypointense nodules in the peripheral zone, although this appearance is nonspecific for cancer. MR accurately depicts invasion of the capsule, neurovascular bundle, seminal vesicles, and adjacent organs. Spectroscopy and dynamic-enhanced MR are powerful tools in the characterization of prostate nodules and in the exclusion of recurrent tumors after treatment (Fig. 5.3.5, recurrent prostate cancer (RoI number 17) after radiotherapy. A large hypointense nodule seen on T2-weighted TSE images (a) demonstrated increased vascularization compared to normal peripheral (RoI number 20) and central zones (RoI number 18) on the relative blood volume parametric map (b) and enhancement curve (c))

A low-intensity bulky mass was detected on T2-weighted images in the right peripheral zone, extending to the transition zone and central gland (Figs. 5.3.1–5.3.3, *asrerisks*). There was transcapsular extension to periprostatic fat, invading the right neurovascular bundle and both seminal vesicles (Figs. 5.3.1–5.3.3, axial, sagittal, and coronal high resolution T2-weighted TSE images). The bladder was normal. MR classified the tumor as stage C3 according to the American Urological Association System (modified Jewitt-Withmore staging system). Lymph nodes and distant metastases were ruled out by CT and scintigraphic bone scan. A midline prostatic cyst was discovered incidentally (Fig. 5.3.3, *arrow*).

Case 4
◼
Retroperitoneal Liposarcoma

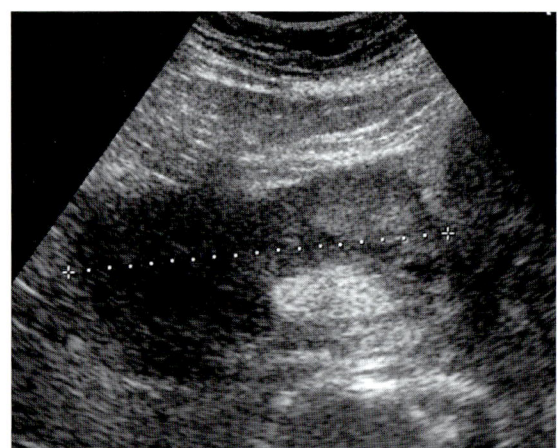

Fig. 5.4.1

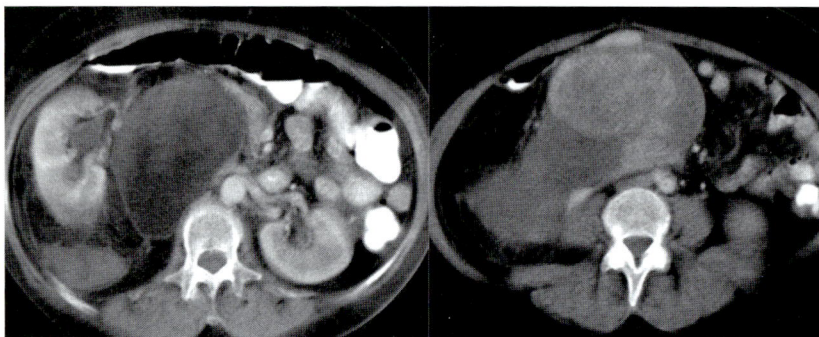

Fig. 5.4.2

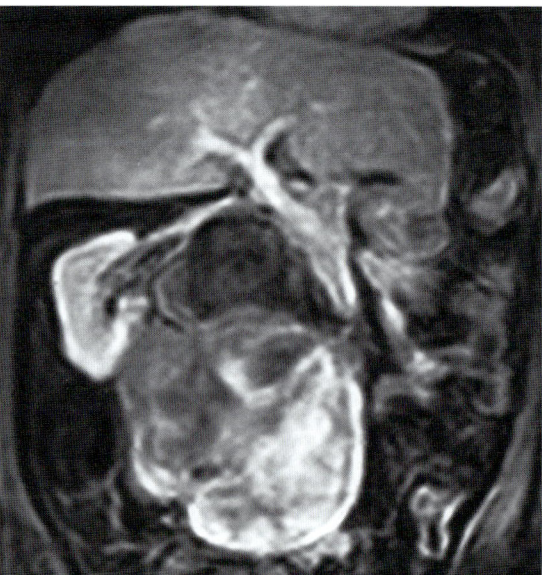

Fig. 5.4.3

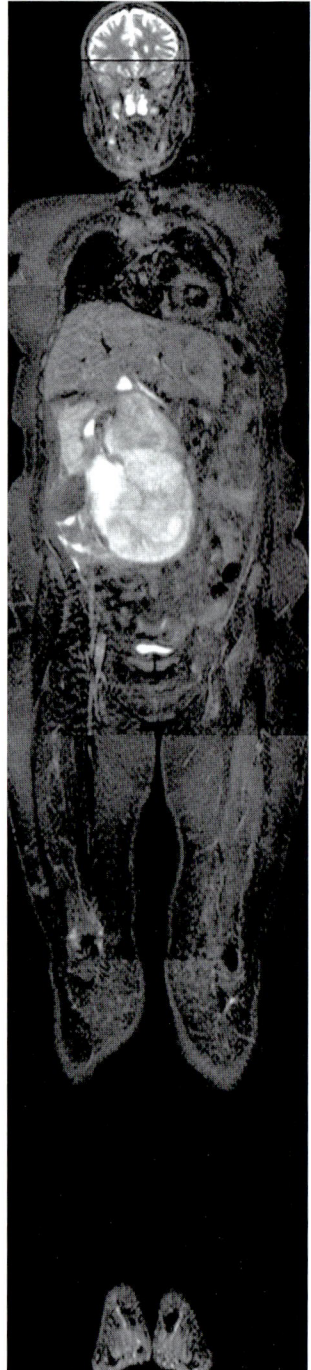

Fig. 5.4.4

A 51-year-old woman presented with increased abdominal perimeter, progressive weight loss, and fatigue.

Comments

Liposarcoma is the most common primary retroperitoneal tumor. Only around 20% of all liposarcomas are retroperitoneal. Histologically, liposarcomas can be classified, in increasing order of undifferentiation, into well-differentiated, myxoid, pleomorphic, and round-cell types. Prognosis is poorer in more aggressive tumors with high cellular undifferentiation. Most retroperitoneal liposarcomas belong to the well-differentiated or pleomorphic types. Intratumoral fat may be detected in any of these subtypes, although it is commonly observed only in well-differentiated tumors. Liposarcomas usually have a heterogeneous appearance similar to other types of sarcomas. The detection of intratumoral fat is a clue for the diagnosis, although sometimes it is present in very small proportions. Fat detection is improved with CT and especially with MR. Solid and necrotic or cystic areas are common, increasing the grade of heterogeneity parallel to the tumor undifferentiation. Calcifications are relatively common in liposarcomas.

Retroperitoneal tumors are clinically silent until they are huge; the mean size at diagnosis is 20 cm. The peak age of occurrence is between 40 to 60 years. Retroperitoneal liposarcomas are rarely infiltrating, although they displace intraabdominal organs due to their large volume. Metastases are not common.

Imaging usually detects retroperitoneal tumors in patients referred for non-specific abdominal symptoms. Knowledge of the anatomy of the retroperitoneal spaces is essential to understand the complex displacement of retro- and intra-peritoneal organs according to the location of the tumor.

Cross-sectional imaging is able to accurately determine the presence of intratumoral fat in well-differentiated liposarcomas. If fat is not present, it is very difficult to distinguish liposarcomas from other retroperitoneal tumors, such as leiomyosarcomas or malignant fibrous histiocytomas.

Imaging Findings

Abdominal ultrasound showed a complex mass with solid hypo- and hyper-echogenic areas and central cystic areas located behind the right kidney (Fig. 5.4.1). Enhanced CT performed for suspicion of a retroperitoneal tumor confirmed the retroperitoneal location of the mass, which displaced the pancreas and right kidney anteriorly (Fig. 5.4.2). Intratumoral areas with negative densitometric values corresponded to intratumoral fat and correlated well with the hyperechogenic areas visualized at ultrasound. The mass presented well-defined-borders and it was composed of fat, cystic or necrotic areas, and prominent solid enhancing components (Fig. 5.4.2). Due to the high fat content, a preoperative diagnosis of retroperitoneal liposarcoma was proposed. Abdominal MR confirmed the heterogeneous nature of the mass, with solid and fat components, and ruled out local invasion of adjacent organs (Fig. 5.4.3, coronal postcontrast fat-suppressed 3D GE sequence in the portal phase). Preoperative whole-body MR excluded distant metastases (Fig. 5.4.4, coronal whole-body STIR). Well-differentiated retroperitoneal liposarcoma was confirmed after surgery. Follow-up imaging over 2 consecutive years excluded local recurrence or metastases.

Case 5
■
Acute Obstruction by Ureteral Lithiasis

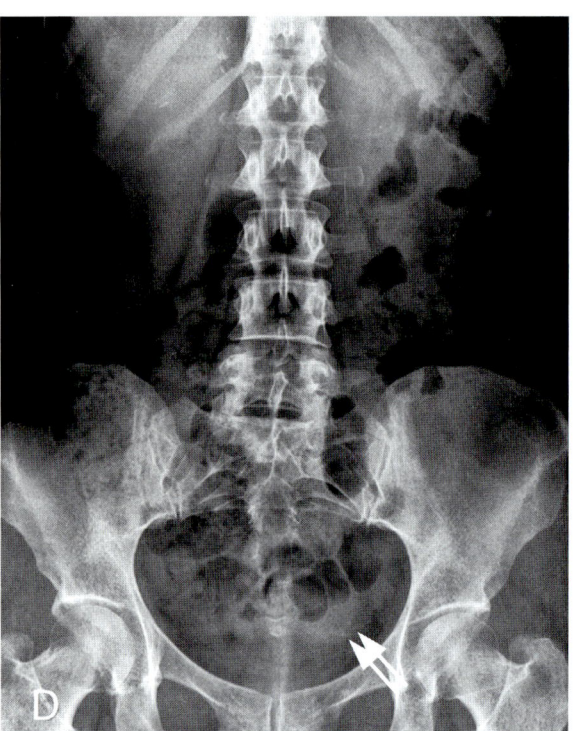

Fig. 5.5.1

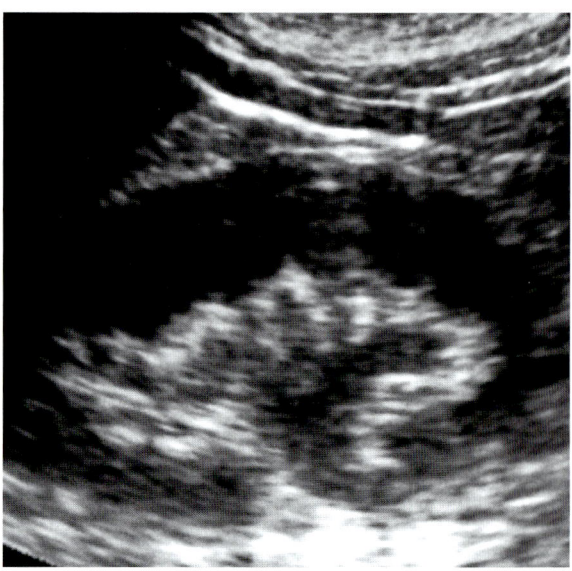

Fig. 5.5.2

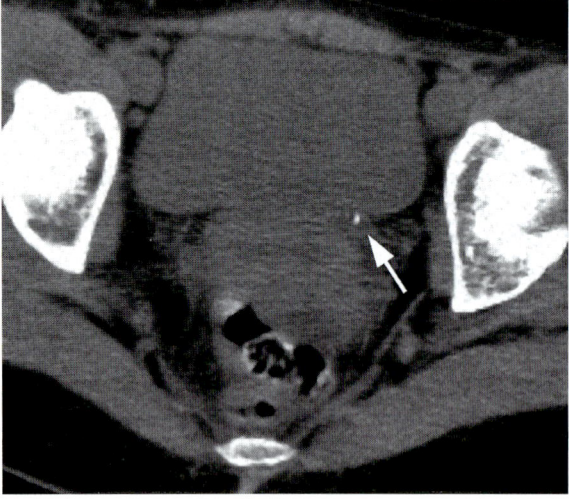

Fig. 5.5.3

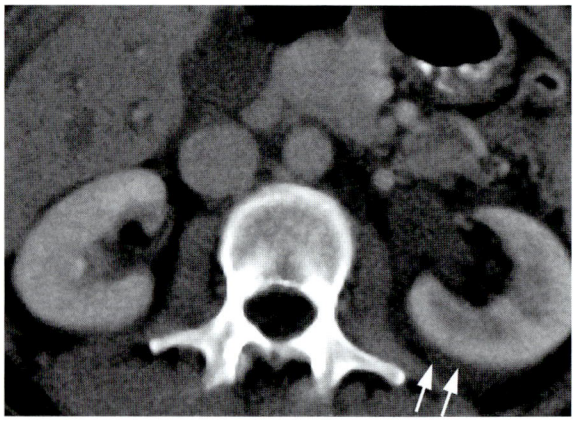

Fig. 5.5.4

A 28-year-old woman presented at the emergency room with sudden and intense left lower quadrant pain, vomiting, and fever. She had neutrophilia and microscopic hematuria.

Urolithiasis is very common; it is found in up to 50% of patients undergoing abdominal CT. Most are detected in the renal pelvis and calicel fornices. Renal calculi cause acute obstruction when they leave the kidney. Acute renal colic accounts for approximately 75% of all acute flank pain. Urolithiasis can have different mineral compositions: more than 90% are calcium stones; 3% are cystine calculi; and uric acid, xanthine, and matrix (mucoprotein /mucopolysaccharide) stones are more uncommon types of urolithiases. Calcium and cystine lithiases are radiopaque and detectable by X-ray or CT. Ultrasound can also demonstrate a proportion of ureteral lithiases, although unenhanced CT is superior in the evaluation of acute obstruction by ureteral calculi. A specific metabolic disorder is the cause of urolithiasis formation in more than 70% of cases, and the underlying disorder determines the mineral composition of the calculus. The remaining cases are usually due to urinary tract infection or are idiopathic.

Detection of unilateral pelvocaliectasis and ureteral lithiasis by imaging in a patient with acute flank pain is diagnostic of lithiasic ureteral obstruction. The diagnosis is usually established based on clinical symptoms and the presence of hematuria. Nevertheless, imaging is necessary to confirm the diagnosis, to determine the position of the ureteral calculus, and to rule out complications. Multislice CT is the imaging technique of choice in the evaluation of acute flank pain. Ultrasound also permits a comprehensive evaluation of this condition, but it fails in the direct visualization of the level of the ureteral calculus in a variable number of cases. Complications of acute lithiasic obstruction include ureterohydronephrosis, urinomas, pyelonephritis, and renal abscesses. These complications can be accurately evaluated by either CT or ultrasound. CT- and MR-urography have also substituted conventional urography in the evaluation of renal and ureteral lithiasis.

On abdominal X-ray film, two tiny calcifications were detected in the theoretical path of the left pelvic ureter (Fig. 5.5.1, *arrows*). Renal ultrasound (Fig. 5.5.2) demonstrated mild left pelvocaliectasis and dilatation of the left proximal ureter. After clinical worsening over the next two days, unenhanced CT confirmed two millimetric calculi in the distal left ureter (Fig. 5.5.3, *arrow*). Enhanced CT showed moderate left ureterohydronephrosis and signs of acute pyelonephritis secondary to ureteral lithiasis such as perirenal free fluid and delayed contrast elimination by the left kidney compared to the right one (Fig. 5.5.4, *arrows*).

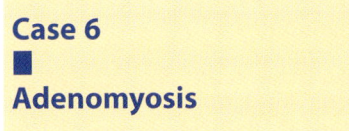

Case 6
■ Adenomyosis

A multiparous 34-year-old woman presented with hypermenor-rhea and pelvic pain of several months' evolution.

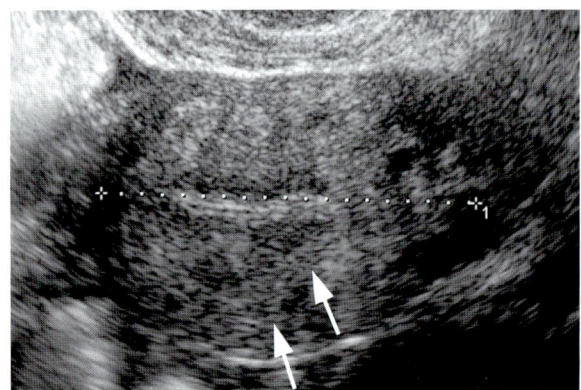

Fig. 5.6.1

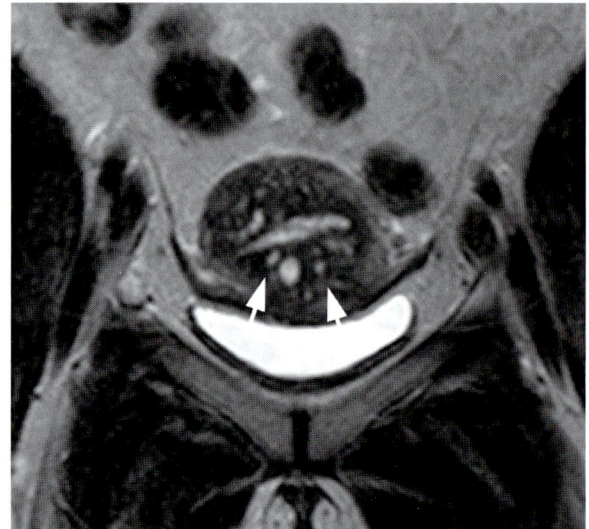

Fig. 5.6.3

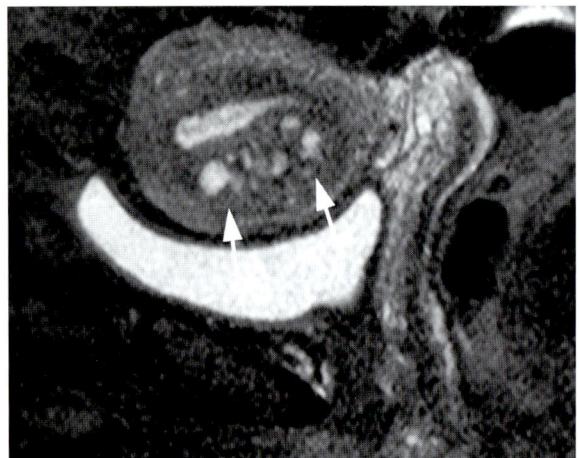

Fig. 5.6.2

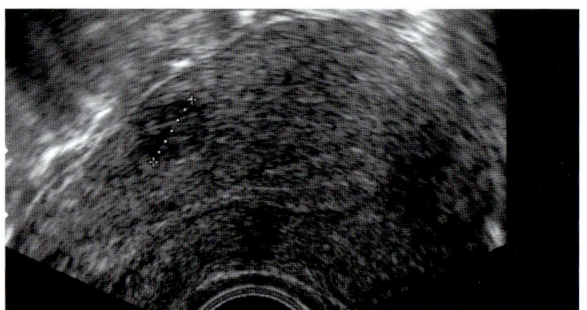

Fig. 5.6.4

Adenomyosis, also known as endometriosis interna, is a very common condition in which benign invasion of myometrium by heterotopic endometrium results in myometrial hyperplasia. Endometrial islands, including heterotopic endometrial glands and stroma, proliferate within the normal myometrium, which interdigitates with secondary hyperplastic myometrium, resulting in a diffused, ill-defined thickening of myometrium. Areas of cystic hemorrhage of the heterotopic endometrium are uncommon. Adenomyosis may be focal or diffuse. In focal adenomyosis, an oval or elongated mass with ill-defined margins and in contiguity with the junctional zone is the most common presentation (Fig. 5.6.4, endovaginal sonogram, different patient than in Figs. 5.6.1 to 5.6.3). Diffuse adenomyosis is more difficult to detect, as it usually presents as smooth uterine enlargement. It most commonly involves premenopausal, multiparous women, although it is not uncommon in postmenopausal women. Adenomyosis is usually an incidental finding in an ultrasound or MR study, as it may be completely asymptomatic. When clinically symptomatic, hypermenorrhea, pelvic pain, and uterine enlargement are classic features. It is associated to endometriosis in approximately 40% of the cases. It has classically been a controversial diagnosis. Nonspecific gynecological findings in cases of adenomyosis have often been erroneously attributed to other common gynecologic pathologies such as leiomyomas, uterine contractions, or endometriosis, which require a completely different treatment. Hysterectomy is the treatment for symptomatic adenomyosis.

Adenomyosis is difficult to diagnose with transabdominal ultrasound. The better spatial resolution of endovaginal ultrasound has led to increased diagnosis of this entity. However, MR is the imaging technique of choice for its evaluation. Diagnostic criteria of adenomyosis on MR include: on T2-weighted images, low-signal either diffuse or focal enlargement of the junctional zone invading the myometrium and/or a focal myometrial mass with ill-defined borders (adenomyoma). Junctional zone thickness greater than 12 mm is consider diagnostic for adenomyosis and thickness greater than 8 mm is suspicious when there are related clinical symptoms. Internal foci of hyperintensity on T1-weighted images, representing hemorrhage, or focal areas of hyperintensity on T2-weighted images, corresponding to hemorrhage or cystic dilatation of endometrial gland, are also common features.

The main differential diagnosis of adenomyosis is with leiomyoma and uterine contraction. As all of these conditions require different treatments, it is very important to differentiate among them. Ultrasound and especially MR are very useful for this purpose. Ill-defined borders and minimal mass effect on the endometrium relative to lesional volume are more common in adenomyomas than in leiomyomas. Sequential imaging allows myometrial contractions to be ruled out (due to their transient nature, the apparent lesion disappears or changes its appearance over time).

Endovaginal ultrasound (Fig. 5.6.1, coronal view) demonstrated an enlarged uterus and heterogeneous appearance of the myometrium, which was asymmetrically thickened. The junctional zone was also thickened inferiorly, with extension to the myometrium (*arrows*). MR was performed for further evaluation of these findings. Figures 5.6.2 and 5.6.3 (sagittal fat-suppressed T2-weighted TSE and coronal T2-weighted TSE images, respectively) confirmed the uterine enlargement and diffuse thickening of the junctional zone, mostly in its inferior face, invading the myometrium (*arrows*). There are multiple hyperintense nodules within the thickened junctional zone, representing ectopic endometrium. All these features are diagnostic of diffuse adenomyosis.

Comments

Imaging Findings

Case 7
■
Cervical Cancer

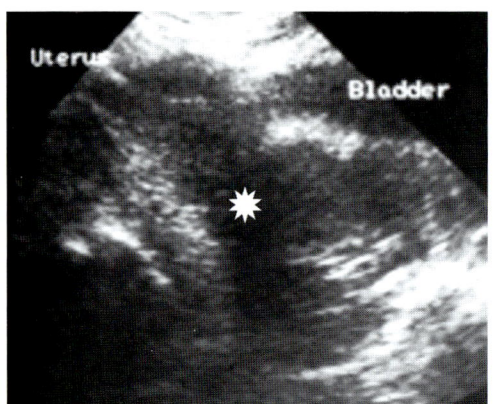

Fig. 5.7.1

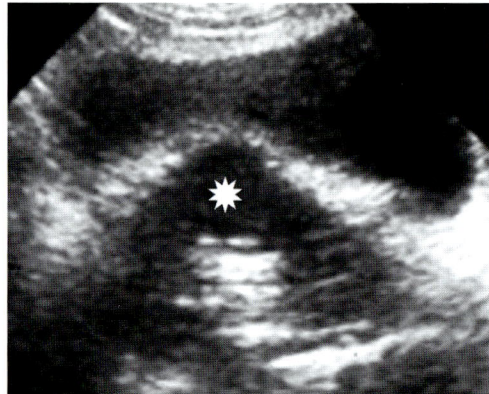

Fig. 5.7.2

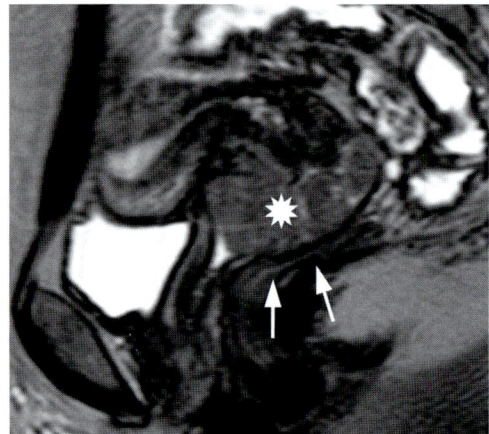

Fig. 5.7.3

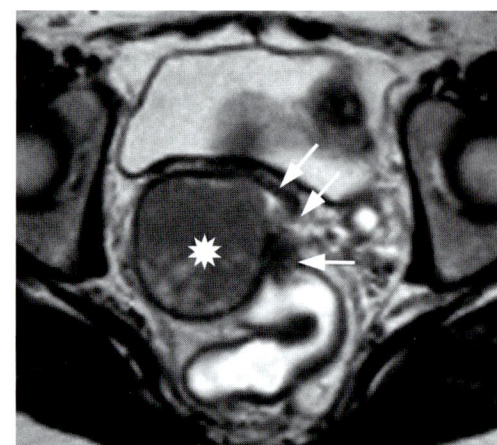

Fig. 5.7.4

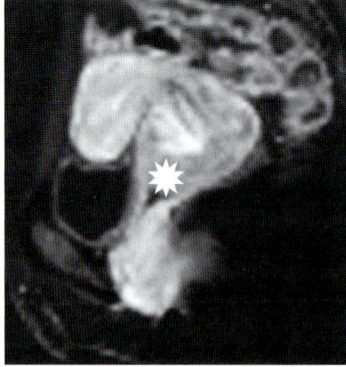

Fig. 5.7.5

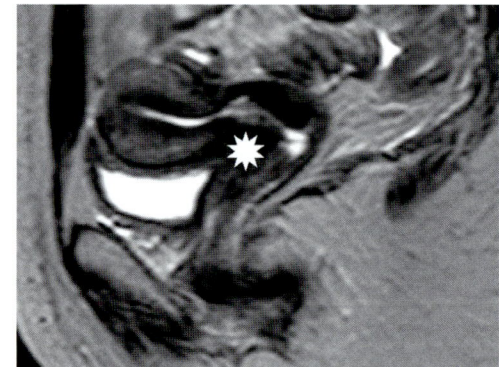

Fig. 5.7.6

A cervical mass was detected during a routine transabdominal gynecologic ultrasound in an asymptomatic 43-year-old woman.

Cervical cancer is the second most common malignancy in women. Most cases occur in women between 45 and 55 years of age. More than 95% of the tumors are squamous cell carcinomas. Due to its high incidence and mortality, screening programs have been established in women over 18 years old. The screening includes the Papanicolaou test and pelvic examination. Patients over 30 years old may be tested for the human papillomavirus, which is strongly associated with cervical cancer. The natural evolution of cervical cancer includes consecutively: cervical intraepithelial neoplasia (CIN), squamous intraepithelial lesion (SIL), carcinoma in situ, and invasive carcinoma.

Noninvasive cervical cancer is usually asymptomatic. Clinical symptoms of invasive cervical cancer include: leucorrhea, vaginal or postcoital bleeding, and metrorrhagia. After a positive Papanicolaou test, the diagnosis is confirmed with either cone biopsy or colposcopy and biopsy. After the diagnosis is made, local and distant staging is performed using CT and MR, respectively. Clinical staging is performed according to the FIGO staging system. Treatment varies according to tumor stage: carcinoma in situ or microinvasive carcinoma is treated with loop electrode excision, cryosurgery, or laser ablation; invasive carcinoma or tumors extending to the upper vagina are treated with radical hysterectomy and pelvic node dissection; – in cases of invasive tumors between 3 and 5 cm without parametrial or lower vagina invasion, radiation therapy is added after surgery; and more advanced tumors are treated with radiation therapy and chemotherapy.

Imaging is not usually important in the diagnosis of cervical cancer. In the case shown, a cervical cancer was found incidentally at routine gynecologic ultrasound, but this is an uncommon presentation. However, imaging is very useful in the local and distant staging of cervical cancer.

MR is the best imaging method for local staging of cervical carcinoma. MR is very accurate in determining tumor size, as well as stromal and parametrial invasion. MR has a high negative predictive value for parametrial invasion and stage IVa disease, so it is useful for determining whether patients should receive surgical or radiation treatment. MR is also useful in the evaluation of pregnant woman with cervical carcinoma and in the assessment of recurrent cancer in treated patients (Fig. 5.7.6, sagittal T2-weighted TSE image. Same patient as in Figs. 5.7.1 to 5.7.5. Postradiotherapy follow-up MR demonstrated a marked reduction in tumor volume. Compare to Fig. 5.7.3).

CT and more recently CT-PET are commonly used to exclude lymph node and distant metastases in patients with cervical carcinoma.

Figures 5.7.1 and 5.7.2, sagittal and axial ultrasound views. *Asterisks* indicate the cervical mass. Cone biopsy established the diagnosis of cervical cancer. MR Figures 5.7.3, 5.7.4 and 5.7.5, sagittal and axial T2-weighted TSE images and postcontrast sagittal fat-suppressed T1-weighted TSE image was performed for local staging and pre-treatment planning. *Asterisks* represent the cervical cancer. Local staging corresponded to IIb stage of the FIGO staging system (superior vaginal, Fig. 5.7.3, *arrows,* and left parametrial invasion Fig. 5.7.4, *arrows.*

Case 8
■
Endometrial Polyp

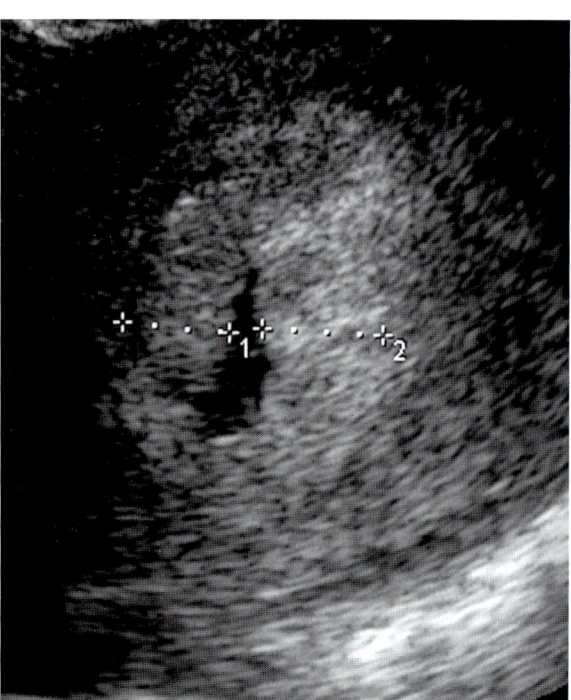

Fig. 5.8.1

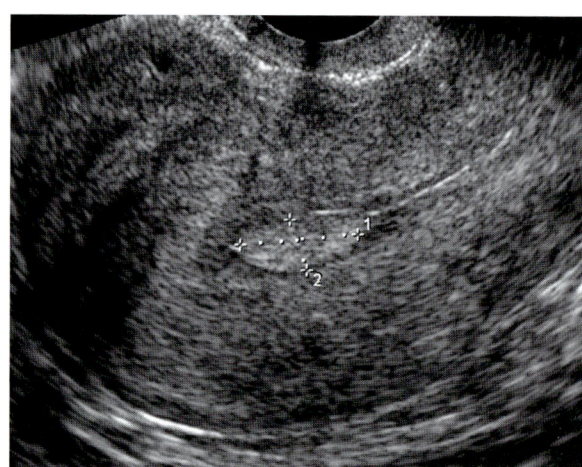

Fig. 5.8.2

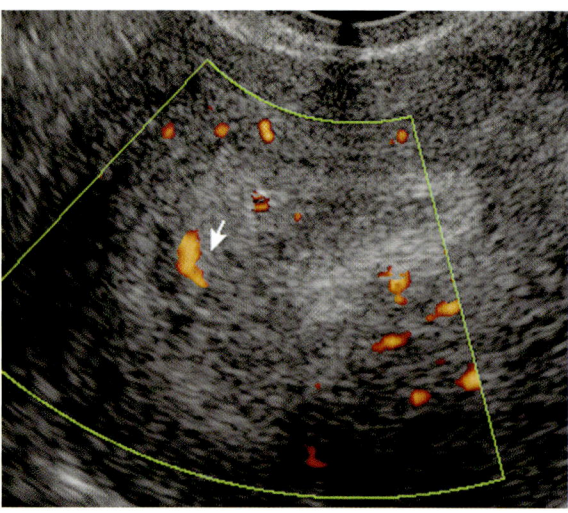

Fig. 5.8.3

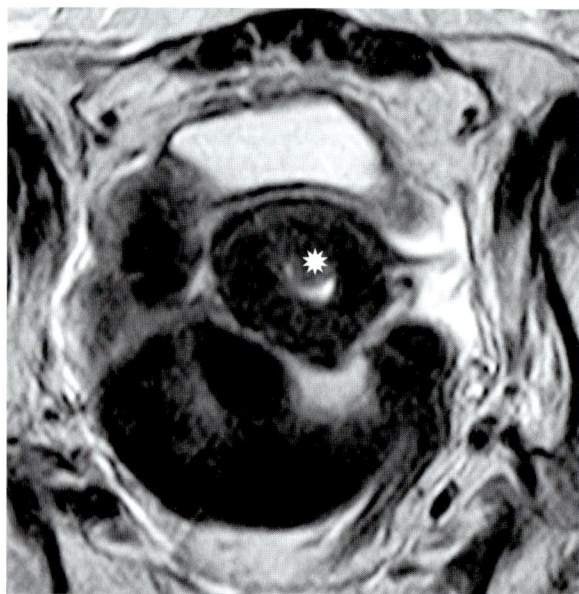

Fig. 5.8.4

A 41-year-old woman presented recurrent intermenstrual and postcoital hemorrhages.

Endometrial polyps are frequent in peri- or post-menopausal women. Their incidence increases with age until menopause and decreases after manopause. The most frequent symptom of endometrial polyps is metrorrhagia and post-menstrual spotting is also common. Endometrial polyps account for 25% of abnormal bleeding in both premenopausal and postmenopausal women. Polyps result from focal hyperplasia of the endometrial stratum basale, which contains endometrial glands and stroma covered by epithelium. Endometrial polyps may be attached to the uterine wall by either a broad peduncle (pedunculated polyps) or a thin stalk. Endometrial polyps may be mobile and invade the cervix or vagina. They rarely show malignant transformation. Hysteroscopic-guided resection is the treatment of choice, as curettage often fails to remove endometrial polyps because of their mobile bodies and tips.

Ultrasound is the imaging technique of choice in the study of postmenopausal bleeding. Endometrial polyps usually present as a hyperechogenic mass. Sonohysterography helps in their diagnosis, and it is very useful in the differentiation between endometrial polyps and submucosal fibroids. A heterogeneous appearance of the mass suggests complications such as hemorrhage or cystic degeneration. Ultrasound can demonstrate the stalk of the polyp and identify the feeding vessel within it, using color and pulsed Doppler techniques. This is a very specific finding for endometrial polyps.

MR does not have a clearly defined role in the evaluation of endometrial polyps. It helps in cases with uncertain ultrasound diagnosis and when the lesion cannot be confidently differentiated from submucosal fibroid. Endometrial polyps are usually iso- or hypo-intense compared to the normal endometrium on T2-weighted images and show enhancement after intravenous contrast administration. This last feature is helpful in distinguishing them from submucosal fibroids, which are usually hypovascular.

Transabdominal ultrasound showed a round focal echogenic mass within the endometrium (Fig. 5.8.1). Sonohysterography (transvaginal ultrasound after distension of the uterine cavity with the infusion of sterile saline through a catheter placed in the cervix) confirmed the presence of the mass and delineated its borders better (Fig. 5.8.2). Color Doppler ultrasound demonstrated a vascular pedicle within the mass (*arrow*), which is typical in endometrial polyps (Fig. 5.8.3). MR confirmed the diagnosis of endometrial polyp (Fig. 5.8.4, coronal T2-weighted TSE image shows a hypointense mass within the endometrium (*asterisk*)).

Case 9
■
Fetal Lissencephaly

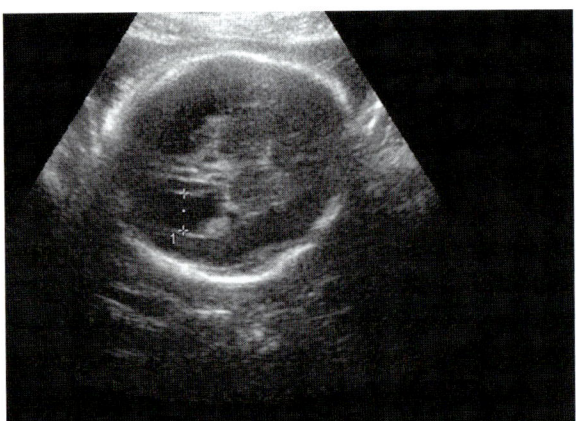

Fig. 5.9.1

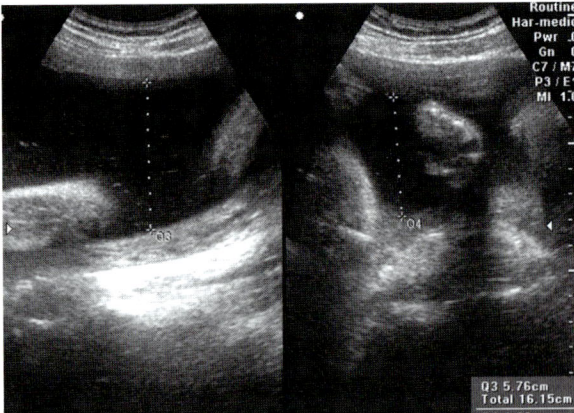

Fig. 5.9.2

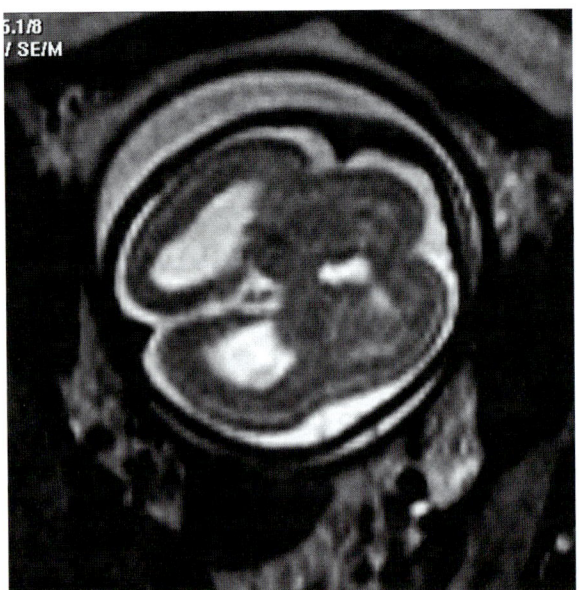

Fig. 5.9.3

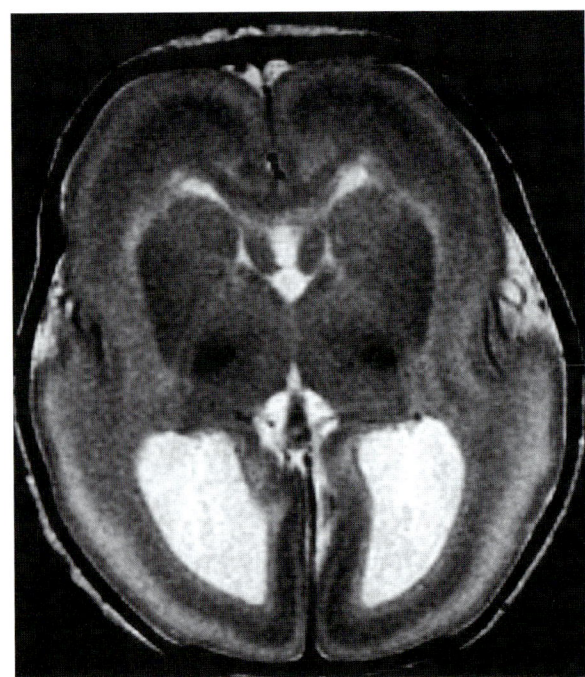

Fig. 5.9.4

A 36-year-old woman underwent routine 28 week obstetric ultrasound.

The term lissencephaly means "smooth brain". It corresponds to a severe malformation of the cerebral cortex, secondary to impaired neuronal migration between the third and fourth months of gestation. The most common findings are either the absence (agyria) or the paucity (pachygyria) of cerebral convolutions, although other cranial and extra-cranial features may be present, depending on the associated syndrome. Lissencephaly is classified in two groups: In type I, or classic lissencephaly, neurons fail to reach the cortical plate, and patients have different degrees of agyria, pachygyria, and/or subcorti-cal band heterotopia. Type I lissencephaly is most commonly associated to Miller-Dieker or Norman-Roberts syndrome. In type II, or cobblestone complex, neurons move into the subpial space. Type II lissencephaly is usually observed in some forms of congenital muscular dystrophy associated with cortical maldevelopment.

Prenatal diagnosis with ultrasound is difficult. Depending on the series, the earli-est cases are diagnosed between 23 and 31 weeks' gestation. Cases associated to Miller-Dieker (type I lissencephaly) or Walker-Warburg (type II lissencephaly) syndromes are easier to diagnose due to associated intracranial malformations. Fetal MR can detect or confirm the abnormal cortical development and associated abnormalities. Less severe types of cortical dysplasia that may not become evident on ultrasound until late in preg-nancy (if ever) are also more conspicuous on MR. An underlying genetic malformation is present in a variable rate of lissencephaly cases. If a mutation is present, early prenatal diagnosis can be achieved with DNA analysis; in these cases, fetal MR and genetic study of the mother are advised.

Obstetric ultrasound is routinely performed in almost every pregnant woman. It is a safe and accurate marker of the gestation that can detect many fetal malformations and other complications. The lack of ionizing radiation makes MR ideal for the study of the fetus. It is most commonly used after the detection of a genetic, analytical, or ultrasound abnormality to establish or rule out a suspected diagnosis. Fetal MR can evaluate not only central nervous system malformations, but also cardiac, pulmonary, genitourinary, and gastrointestinal anomalies. Prenatal MR can also be used to study gynecologic or abdominal masses or abnormalities in the mother during pregnancy.

Isolated ventriculomegaly (dilatation of the posterior horns) and polyhydramnios (Figs. 5.9.1 and 5.9.2, in the 28th week obstetric ultrasound). Previous fetal ultrasound examinations at 12 and 20th weeks' gestation were normal. No chromosomopathies were found in the amniotic fluid. Fetal MRI performed at 31 weeks' gestation revealed (Fig. 5.9.3, axial T2-weighted TSE image) confirmed the dilatation of the posterior horns and also revealed hypoplasia of the corpus callosum, delayed cerebral sulci development (corresponding to 26 weeks' gestation), agyria (absence of sulci and convolutions), and vertically oriented sylvian fissures. All these data helped establish the prenatal diag-nosis of type I lissencephaly, which was confirmed at postnatal MRI (Fig. 5.9.4, axial T2-weighted TSE image).

Case 10
■
Ovarian Serous Cystoadenocarcinoma

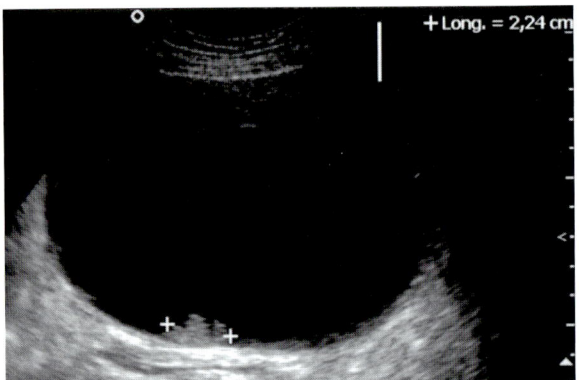

Fig. 5.10.1

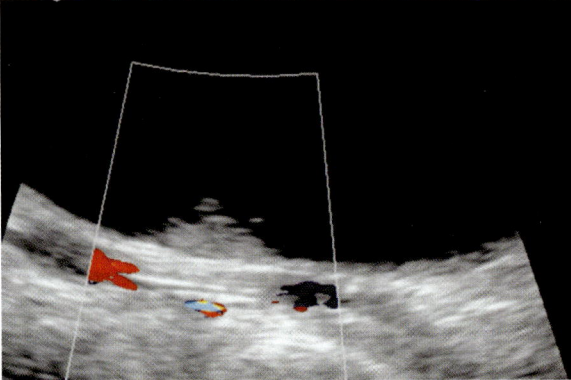

Fig. 5.10.2

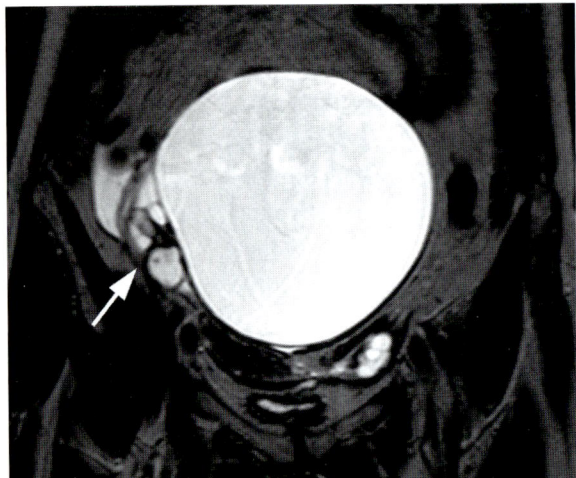

Fig. 5.10.3

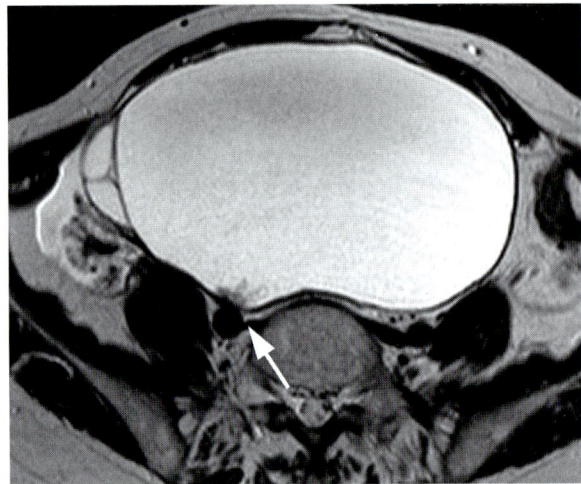

Fig. 5.10.4

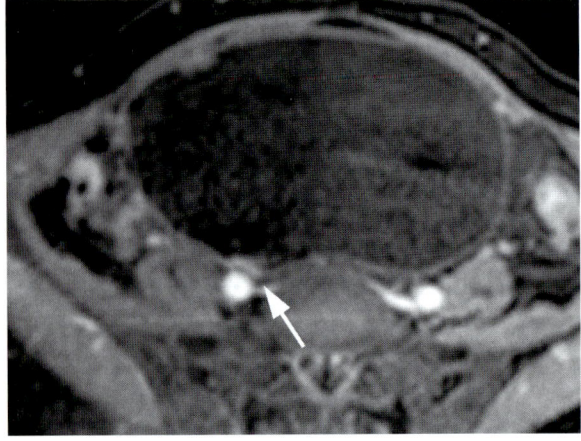

Fig. 5.10.5

A 63-year-old-woman presented with progressive increase of abdominal perimeter and weight loss in the previous three months.

Ovarian carcinoma is the leading cause of death from gynecologic cancers. More than 80% of cases occur in women over 50 years of age. These tumors are usually clinically silent until the advanced stages. Frequent clinical symptoms include pelvic pain, constipation, increase urinary frequency, early satiety, and ascites. Increased CA-125 levels are present in more than 80% of cases. Paraneoplastic hypercalcemia is not rare. Pelviabdominal spread is common at diagnosis. Most commonly, either direct spread or microscopic exfoliation of tumor cells into the peritoneal space occurs. Lymphatic or hematogenous spread is more typically seen in the late stages of the disease. Mortality is very high, increasing with stage dramatically. The overall 5 year survival rate is lower than 40% for patients with stages II to IV.

Histologically, there are four major groups of ovarian malignancies: epithelial tumors, germ-cell tumors, stromal tumors, and metastases. Tumors of surface epithelium represent 70–75% of all ovarian tumors and can be subclassified in decreasing order of frequency into: serous, mucinous, endometroid, clear-cell, Brenner, and undifferentiated tumors. Serous tumors account for 50% of all malignant ovarian masses. They are typically unilocular, cystic lesions involving only one adnexa, although with increasing undifferentiation they may show hemorrhage, solid elements, and necrosis. Either microscopic or macroscopic papillae are characteristic. Psammoma bodies are not rare. Mucinous ovarian cancer is the second most common subtype of all ovarian malignancies. These tumors are typically very large at presentation, with multiple locules delimited by internal septa and mucinous content in different proportions. Bilaterality and signs of complication of the cysts are more common in mucinous than in serous ovarian tumors.

Ultrasound is the imaging method most commonly used to detect ovarian masses. Ultrasound can usually differentiate cystic and solid masses and detect features suggestive of malignancy. MR is superior to CT in the characterization of ovarian masses and in the staging of ovarian carcinoma. Ultrasound and MR features of an ovarian mass are not characteristic of a specific histological subtype but may suggest the cell type of origin. As in the case shown, a unilateral cystic mass with internal papillae is very typical of serous tumors. Detection of microscopic peritoneal metastases is still a challenge for imaging techniques.

Gynecologic ultrasound showed a cystic pelvic mass with solid internal papillary projections (Fig. 5.10.1). These solid projections had no internal vascularization on color Doppler ultrasound (Fig. 5.10.2). MR was performed to confirm the ovarian origin of the mass. Coronal T2-weighted TSE images demonstrated a multiseptated cystic mass originating in the right adnexa (Fig. 5.10.3, *arrow*). Axial T2-weighted TSE and postcontrast fat-suppressed T1-weighted TSE images (Figs. 5.10.4 and 5.10.5) demonstrated the cystic nature of the mass and internal papillae (*arrows*), which were hypointense on T2-weighted sequences and enhanced on postcontrast images. T2-weigted images detected perilesional ascites. There were no signs of contralateral adnexal involvement or pelvic extension. The diagnosis of ovarian serous cystadenocarcinoma proposed on the basis of these imaging features was confirmed at histology.

Further Readings

Books

Clinical Gynecologic Imaging. Fleischer AC, Javitt MC, Jeffrey RB, Jones HW (1997) Lippincott Williams & Wilkins. ISBN-13: 9780397517060

Diagnostic Imaging of Fetal Anomalies. 2nd Sub ed. Nyberg DA, McGahan JP, Pretorius DH, Pilu G (2002) Lippincott Williams & Wilkins. ISBN-13: 9780781732116

Diagnostic Ultrasound. Rumack CM Wilson S, Charboneau JW, Johnson JA (2005) Mosby. ISBN-13: 9780323020237

Doppler Ultrasound in Obstetrics and Gynecology. 2nd rev. and enlarged ed. Maulik D, Zalud I (2005) Springer-Verlag, Berlin. ISBN-13: 9783540230885

Genitourinary Radiology: Radiology Requisites Series. 2nd ed. Zagoria R (2004) Mosby. ISBN-13: 9780323018425

Imaging of the Scrotum & Penis. Rifkin M, Cochlin DL (2002) Informa Healthcare. ISBN-13: 9781853175091

MRI and CT of the Female Pelvis. Hamm B, Forstner R (2007) Springer-Verlag, Berlin. ISBN: 9783540222897

Step by Step Ultrasound in Gynecology. Singh K, Malhotra N (2004) McGraw-Hill Professional. ISBN-13: 9780071446556

Step by Step Ultrasound in Obstetrics. Singh K, Malhotra N (2004) McGraw-Hill Professional. ISBN-13: 9780071446549

Textbook of Uroradiology. 3rd ed. Dunnick NR, Sandler CM, Newhouse JH, Amis ES (2001) Lippincott Williams & Wilkins. ISBN-13: 9780781723893

Web-Links

http://chorus.rad.mcw.edu/index/5.html

http://emedicine.com/radio/GENITOURINARY.htm

http://emedicine.com/radio/OBSTETRICSGYNECOLOGY.htm

http://meddean.luc.edu/lumen/medEd/urology/guimaghm.htm

http://med-ed.virginia.edu/courses/rad/abdtrauma/

http://obgyn.net/ultrasound/

http://radcentral.com/

http://rsna.org/Education/archive/afip.cfm#geni-tourinary

http://thefetus.net/index.php

http://womensimagingonline.arrs.org/item.cfm?itemID=156

Articles

Adrenal Glands

Bae KT, Fuangtharnthip P, Prasad SR, Joe BN, Heiken JP. Adrenal masses: CT characterization with histogram analysis method. Radiology 2003; 228:735–742

Bessell-Browne R, O'Malley ME. CT of pheochromocytoma and paraganglioma: risk of adverse events with IV administration of nonionic contrast material. AJR Am J Roentgenol 2007; 188:970–974

Blake MA, Kalra MK, Sweeney AT, Lucey BC, Maher MM, Sahani DV, Halpern EF, Mueller PR, Hahn PF, Boland GW. Distinguishing benign from malignant adrenal masses: Multi–detector row CT protocol with 10-minute delay. Radiology 2005 238: 578–585

Chong S, Lee KS, Kim HY, Kim YK, Kim BT, Chung MJ, Yi CA, Kwon GY. Integrated PET-CT for the characterization of adrenal gland lesions in cancer patients: Diagnostic efficacy and interpretation pitfalls. Radiographics 2006; 26:1811–1824

Doppman JL, Miller DL, Dwyer AJ, Loughlin T, Nieman L, Cutler GB, Chrousos GP, Oldfield E, Loriaux DL. Macronodular adrenal hyperplasia in Cushing disease. Radiology 1988; 166:347–352

Elsayes KM, Mukundan G, Narra VR, Lewis JS Jr, Shirkhoda A, Farooki A, Brown JJ. Adrenal masses: MR imaging features with pathologic correlation. Radiographics 2004; 24:S73–S86

Korobkin M, Brodeur FJ, Yutzy GG, Francis IR, Quint LE, Dunnick NR, Kazerooni EA. Differentiation of adrenal adenomas from nonadenomas using CT attenuation values. AJR Am J Roentgenol 1996; 166:531–536

Krebs TL, Wagner BJ. MR imaging of the adrenal gland: radiologic-pathologic correlation. Radiographics 1998; 18:1425–1440

McNicholas MM, Lee MJ, Mayo-Smith WW, Hahn PF, Boland GW, Mueller PR. An imaging algorithm for the differential diagnosis of adrenal adenomas and metastases. AJR Am J Roentgenol 1995; 165:1453–1459

Musante F, Derchi LE, Zappasodi F, Bazzocchi M, Riviezzo GC, Banderali A, Cicio GR. Myelolipoma of the adrenal gland: sonographic and CT features. AJR Am J Roentgenol 1988; 151:961–964

Kidneys

Dacher JN, Pfister C, Monroc M, Eurin D, LeDosseur P. Power Doppler sonographic pattern of acute pyelonephritis in children: comparison with CT. AJR Am J Roentgenol 1996; 166:1451–1455

Erwin BC, Carroll BA, Sommer FG. Renal colic: the role of ultrasound in initial evaluation. Radiology 1984; 152:147–150

Hattery RR, Williamson B Jr, Hartman GW, LeRoy AJ, Witten DM. Intravenous urographic technique. Radiology 1988; 167:593–599

Kawashima A, Sandler CM, Ernst RD, Tamm EP, Goldman SM, Fishman EK. CT evaluation of renovascular disease. Radiographics 2000; 20:1321–1340

Nascimento AB, Mitchell DG, Zhang XM, Kamishima T, Parker L, Holland GA. Rapid MR imaging detection of renal cysts: Age-based standards. Radiology 2001; 221:628–632

Prando A, Prando D, Prando P. Renal cell carcinoma: unusual imaging manifestations. Radiographics 2006; 26:233–244

Prasad SR, Humphrey PA, Menias CO, Middleton WD, Siegel MJ, Bae KT, Heiken JP. Neoplasms of the renal medulla: Radiologic-pathologic correlation. Radiographics 2005; 25:369–380

Rha SE, Byun JY, Jung SE, Oh SN, Choi YJ, Lee A, Lee JM. The renal sinus: Pathologic spectrum and multimodality imaging approach. Radiographics 2004; 24: S117–S131

Riccabona M, Fritz GA, Schöllnast H, Schwarz T, Deutschmann MJ, Mache CJ. Hydronephrotic kidney: Pediatric three-dimensional US for relative renal size assessment – initial experience. Radiology 2005; 236:276–283

Rothpearl A, Frager D, Subramanian A, Bashist B, Baer J, Kay C, Cooke K, Raia C. MR urography: technique and application. Radiology 1995; 194:125–130

Sheth S, Scatarige JC, Horton KM, Corl FM, Fishman EK. Current concepts in the diagnosis and management of renal cell carcinoma: role of multidetector CT and three-dimensional CT. Radiographics 2001; 21:237–254

Sheth S, Ali S, Fishman EK. Imaging of renal lymphoma: patterns of disease with pathologic correlation. Radiographics 2006; 26:1151–1168

Slywotzky CM, Bosniak MA. Localized cystic disease of the kidney. AJR Am J Roentgenol 2001; 176:843–849

Silverman SG, Pearson GD, Seltzer SE, Polger M, Tempany CM, Adams DF, Brown DL, Judy PF. Small (< or = 3 cm) hyperechoic renal masses: comparison of helical and convention CT for diagnosing angiomyolipoma. AJR Am J Roentgenol 1996; 167:877–881

Silverman SG, Mortele KJ, Tuncali K, Jinzaki M, Cibas ES. Hyperattenuating renal masses: Etiologies, pathogenesis, and imaging evaluation. Radiographics 2007; 27:1131–1143

Urinary Tract

Berrocal T, López-Pereira P, Arjonilla A, Gutiérrez J. Anomalies of the distal ureter, bladder, and urethra in children: Embryologic, radiologic, and pathologic features. Radiographics 2002; 22:1139–1164

Berrocal T, Gayá F, Arjonilla A. Vesicoureteral reflux: Can the urethra be adequately assessed by using contrast-enhanced voiding US of the bladder? Radiology 2005; 234:235–241

Dyer RB, Chen MY, Zagoria RJ. Abnormal calcifications in the urinary tract. Radiographics 1998; 18:1405–1424

Dyer RB, Chen MY, Zagoria RJ. Intravenous urography: technique and interpretation. Radiographics 2001; 21:799–821

Filgueiras MF, Lima EM, Sanchez TM, Goulart EM, Menezes AC, Pires CR. Bladder dysfunction: Diagnosis with dynamic US. Radiology 2003; 227:340–344

Gentili A, Miron SD, Adler LP, Bellon EM. Incidental detection of urinary tract abnormalities with skeletal scintigraphy. Radiographics 1991; 11:571–579

Jinzaki M, Tanimoto A, Shinmoto H, Horiguchi Y, Sato K, Kuribayashi S, Silverman SG. Detection of bladder tumors with dynamic contrast-enhanced MDCT. AJR Am J Roentgenol 2007; 188:913–918

Joffe SA, Servaes S, Okon S, Horowitz M. Multi-detector row CT urography in the evaluation of hematuria. Radiographics 2003; 23:1441–1455

Kim JK, Ahn JH, Park T, Ahn HJ, Kim CS, Cho KS. Virtual cystoscopy of the contrast material – filled bladder in patients with gross hematuria. AJR Am J Roentgenol 2002; 179:763–768

Kim JK, Kim YJ, Choo MS, Cho KS. The urethra and its supporting structures in women with stress urinary incontinence: MR imaging using an endovaginal coil. AJR Am J Roentgenol 2003; 180:1037–1044

Retroperitoneum

Amis ES Jr. Retroperitoneal fibrosis. AJR Am J Roentgenol 1991; 157:321–329

Gupta AK, Cohan RH, Francis IR, Sondak VK, Korobkin M. CT of recurrent retroperitoneal sarcomas. AJR Am J Roentgenol 2000; 174:1025–1030

Nishino M, Hayakawa K, Minami M, Yamamoto A, Ueda H, Takasu K. Primary retroperitoneal neoplasms: CT and MR imaging findings with anatomic and pathologic diagnostic clues. Radiographics 2003; 23:45–47

Steyerberg EW, Keizer HJ, Sleijfer DT, Fosså SD, Bajorin DF, Gerl A, de Wit R, Kirkels WJ, Koops HS, Habbema JD. Retroperitoneal metastases in testicular cancer: Role of CT measurements of residual masses in decision making for resection after chemotherapy. Radiology 2000; 215:437–444

Yang DM, Jung DH, Kim H, Kang JH, Kim SH, Kim JH, Hwang HY. Retroperitoneal cystic masses: CT, clinical, and pathologic findings and literature review. Radiographics 2004; 24:1353–1365

Prostate

Barozzi L, Pavlica P, Menchi I, De Matteis M, Canepari M. Prostatic abscess: diagnosis and treatment. AJR Am J Roentgenol 1998; 170:753–757

Beyersdorff D, Winkel A, Hamm B, Lenk S, Loening SA, Taupitz M. MR Imaging–guided prostate biopsy with a closed MR unit at 1.5 T: Initial results. Radiology 2005; 234:576–581

Choi YJ, Kim JK, Kim N, Kim KW, Choi EK, Cho KS. Functional MR imaging of prostate cancer. Radiographics 2007; 27:63–75

Curran S, Akin O, Agildere AM, Zhang J, Hricak H, Rademaker J. Endorectal MRI of prostatic and periprostatic cystic lesions and their mimics. AJR Am J Roentgenol 2007; 188:1373–1379

Halpern EJ, Rosenberg M, Gomella LG. Prostate cancer: Contrast-enhanced US for detection. Radiology 2001; 219:219–225

Harris RD, Schned AR, Heaney JA. Staging of prostate cancer with endorectal MR imaging: lessons from a learning curve. Radiographics 1995; 15:813–829

Littrup PJ, Lee F, McLeary RD, Wu D, Lee A, Kumasaka GH. Transrectal US of the seminal vesicles and ejaculatory ducts: clinical correlation. Radiology 1988; 168:625–628

Pretorius ES, Siegelman ES, Ramchandani P, Banner MP. MR imaging of the penis. Radiographics 2001; 21:283–298

Bertolotto M, Serafini G, Savoca G, Liguori G, Calderan L, Gasparini C, Mucelli RP. Color Doppler US of the postoperative penis: Anatomy and surgical complications. Radiographics 2005; 25:731–748

Yablon CM, Banner MP, Ramchandani P, Rovner ES. Complications of prostate cancer treatment: Spectrum of imaging findings. Radiographics 2004; 24:S181–S194

Vulva and Vagina

Brown JJ, Gutierrez ED, Lee JK. MR appearance of the normal and abnormal vagina after hysterectomy. AJR Am J Roentgenol 1992; 158:95–99

Dwarkasing S, Hussain SM, Hop WC, Krestin GP. Anovaginal fistulas: Evaluation with endoanal MR imaging. Radiology 2004; 231:123–128

Fisseha S, Mueller G. Radiology illustrated: gynecologic imaging. AJR Am J Roentgenol 2006; 186:594–595

Hahn WY, Israel GM, Lee VS. MRI of female urethral and periurethral disorders. AJR Am J Roentgenol 2004; 182:677–682

Kim CR, Eaton BA, Stevens KR Jr. Localization of the apex of the vagina: Implications for radiation therapy planning. Radiology 1999; 212:155–158

Kirks DR, Currarino G. Imperforate vagina with vaginourethral communication. AJR Am J Roentgenol 1977; 129:623–628

Siegelman ES, Outwater EK, Banner MP, Ramchandani P, Anderson TL, Schnall MD. High-resolution MR imaging of the vagina. Radiographics 1997; 17:1183–1203

Sohaib SA, Richards PS, Ind T, Jeyarajah AR, Shepherd JH, Jacobs IJ, Reznek RH. MR imaging of carcinoma of the vulva. AJR Am J Roentgenol 2002; 178:373–377

Togashi K, Nishimura K, Itoh K, Fujisawa I, Nakano Y, Torizuka K, Ozasa H, Ohshima M. Vaginal agenesis: classification by MR imaging. Radiology 1987; 162:675–677

Cervix and Uterus

Atri M, Nazarnia S, Aldis AE, Reinhold C, Bret PM, Kintzen G. Transvaginal US appearance of endometrial abnormalities. Radiographics 1994; 14:483–492

Baldwin MT, Dudiak KM, Gorman B, Marks CA. Focal intracavitary masses recognized with the hyperechoic line sign at endovaginal US and characterized with hysterosonography. Radiographics 1999; 19:927–935

Davis PC, O'Neill MJ, Yoder IC, Lee SI, Mueller PR. Sonohysterographic findings of endometrial and subendometrial conditions. Radiographics 2002; 22:803–816

Fleischer AC. Transvaginal sonography of endometrial disorders: an overview. Radiographics 1998; 18:923–930

Jeong YY, Kang HK, Chung TW, Seo JJ, Park JG. Uterine cervical carcinoma after therapy: CT and MR imaging findings. Radiographics 2003; 23:969–981

Mogavero G, Sheth S, Hamper UM. Endovaginal sonography of the nongravid uterus. Radiographics 1993; 13:969–981

Murase E, Siegelman ES, Outwater EK, Perez-Jaffe LA, Tureck RW. Uterine leiomyomas: Histopathologic features, MR imaging findings, differential diagnosis, and treatment. Radiographics 1999; 19:1179–1197

Nalaboff KM, Pellerito JS, Ben-Levi E. Imaging the endometrium: Disease and normal variants. Radiographics 2001; 21:1409–1424

Okamoto Y, Tanaka YO, Nishida M, Tsunoda H, Yoshikawa H, Itai Y. MR imaging of the uterine cervix: Imaging-pathologic correlation. Radiographics 2003; 23:425–445

Reinhold C, Tafazoli F, Mehio A, Wang L, Atri M, Siegelman ES, Rohoman L. Uterine adenomyosis: Endovaginal US and MR imaging features with histopathologic correlation. Radiographics 1999; 19:147–160

Scanlan KA, Propeck PA, Lee FT Jr. Invasive procedures in the female pelvis: Value of transabdominal, endovaginal, and endorectal US guidance. Radiographics 2001; 21:491–506

Ovary

Kim KA, Park CM, Lee JH, Kim HK, Cho SM, Kim B, Seol HY. Benign ovarian tumors with solid and cystic components that mimic malignancy. AJR Am J Roentgenol 2004; 182:1259–1265

Reviews

Brammer HM 3rd, Buck JL, Hayes WS, Sheth S, Tavassoli FA. From the archives of the AFIP. Malignant germ cell tumors of the ovary: radiologic-pathologic correlation. Radiographics 1990; 10:715–724

Hertzberg BS, Kliewer MA. Sonography of benign cystic teratoma of the ovary: pitfalls in diagnosis. AJR Am J Roentgenol 1996; 167:1127–1133

Jeong YY, Outwater EK, Kang HK. Imaging evaluation of ovarian masses. Radiographics 2000; 20:1445–1470

Jung SE, Lee JM, Rha SE, Byun JY, Jung JI, Hahn ST. CT and MR imaging of ovarian tumors with emphasis on differential diagnosis. Radiographics 2002; 22:1305–1325

Olson MC, Posniak HV, Tempany CM, Dudiak CM. MR imaging of the female pelvic region. Radiographics 1992; 12:445–465

Outwater EK, Dunton CJ. Imaging of the ovary and adnexa: clinical issues and applications of MR imaging. Radiology 1995; 194:1–18

Outwater EK, Mitchell DG. Normal ovaries and functional cysts: MR appearance. Radiology 1996; 198:397–402

Rha SE, Byun JY, Jung SE, Jung JI, Choi BG, Kim BS, Kim H, Lee JM. CT and MR imaging features of adnexal torsion. Radiographics 2002; 22:283–294

Saksouk FA, Johnson SC. Recognition of the ovaries and ovarian origin of pelvic masses with CT. Radiographics 2004; 24:S133–S146

Obstetrics

Braffman BH, Coleman BG, Ramchandani P, Arger PH, Nodine CF, Dinsmore BJ, Louie A, Betsch SE. Emergency department screening for ectopic pregnancy: a prospective US study. Radiology 1994; 190:797–802

Amin RS, Nikolaidis P, Kawashima A, Kramer LA, Ernst RD. Normal anatomy of the fetus at MR imaging. Radiographics 1999; 19:201–214

Fong KW, Toi A, Salem S, Hornberger LK, Chitayat D, Keating SJ, McAuliffe F, Johnson JA. Detection of fetal structural abnormalities with US during early pregnancy. Radiographics 2004; 24:157–174

Woodward PJ, Sohaey R, Kennedy A, Koeller KK. From the archives of the AFIP: A comprehensive review of fetal tumors with pathologic correlation. Radiographics 2005; 25:215–242

Taylor KJ, Ramos IM, Feyock AL, Snower DP, Carter D, Shapiro BS, Meyer WR, De Cherney AH. Ectopic pregnancy: duplex Doppler evaluation. Radiology 1989; 173:93–97

Musculoskeletal Imaging

6

Joan C. Vilanova and Ramon Ribes
Sandra Baleato (Contributor)

Introduction

Musculoskeletal radiology is a subspecialty which has widely expanded its scope and imaging capabilities with the advent of ultrasound, MRI, multi-detector CT, and PET. Prior to the advent of MRI, the primary tools of musculoskeletal radiologists were conventional X-rays and arthrograms. The subspecialty has progressed from primary imaging of osseous structures and indirect imaging of articular spaces to direct imaging of soft-tissue structures with direct visualization and precise depiction of musculoskeletal structures.

Specialized musculoskeletal radiology requires a sound knowledge of anatomy, pathophysiology and surgical techniques, coupled with a solid background in the imaging modalities involved in musculoskeletal radiology. Musculoskeletal (MSK) imaging involves all aspects of anatomy, function, disease states and the aspects of interventional radiology related to the musculoskeletal system. This includes imaging in orthopedics, trauma, rheumatology, metabolic and endocrine diseases as well as aspects of pediatrics, oncology and sports imaging.

Subspecialty training in MSK radiology should provide the experience necessary to ensure competence in the following techniques: plain radiography, ultrasonography, CT, MRI, nuclear medicine, bone densitometry and fluoroscopic procedures including arthrography. It is important for the musculoskeletal radiologist to be aware of the strengths and weaknesses of the different imaging methods in various pathological conditions. Furthermore, it is the role of a subspecialty expert to choose the appropriate imaging technique and/or the appropriate sequence in the investigation of specific clinical problems.

An MSK radiologist should have acquired an in-depth understanding of diseases of the MSK system and understand the role of imaging in the diagnosis and treatment of MSK disease. Moreover, due to innovations and new medical imaging modalities, clinical specialists requests are increasingly demanding. If radiologists cannot keep up with the increasing demands for musculoskeletal interpretations, clinicians will be forced to compete with radiologists in providing these interpretations.

From the beginning of the subspecialty in the 1970s with the foundation of the International Skeletal Society, many multidisciplinary or dedicated skeletal radiology societies have been founded and organized from international or national societies and continue to play an important role in the development of the subspeciality.

Case 1
Osteomyelitis

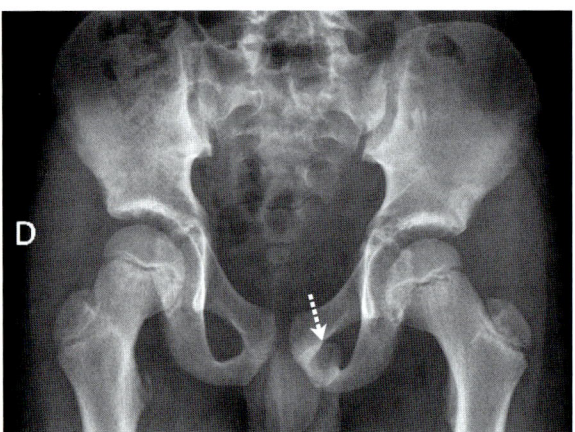

Fig. 6.1.1

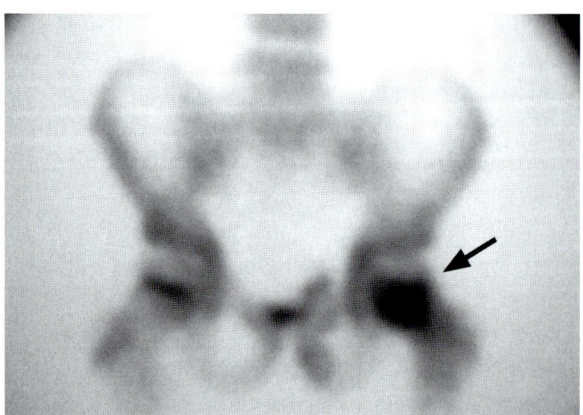

Fig. 6.1.2

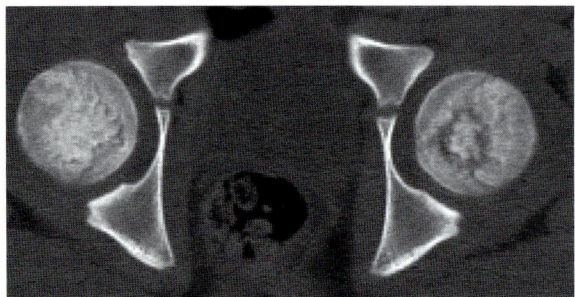

Fig. 6.1.3

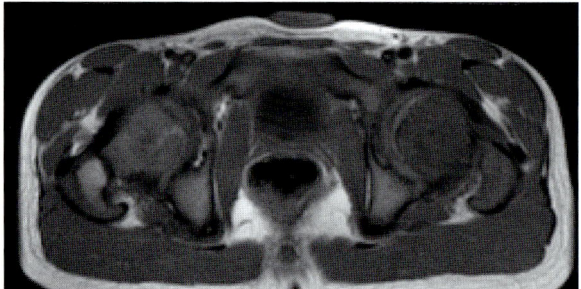

Fig. 6.1.4

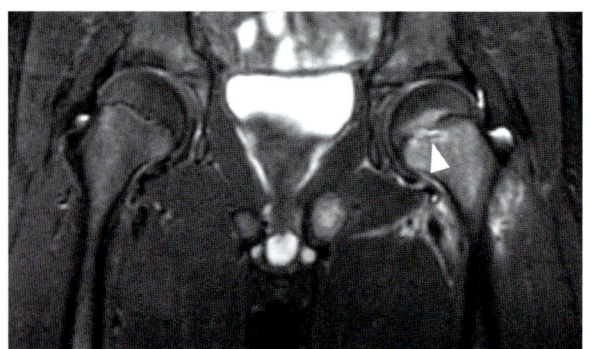

Fig. 6.1.5

A 9-year-old boy complained of left hip pain for 3 weeks. Four weeks prior, the patient had suffered from a superficial injury to his abdomen which required a subcutaneous suture. At admission the patient had intermittent elevated temperature. He was reluctant to bear weight on the left limb and had gait disturbances. Plain-film pelvic radiographs performed in the emergency room were suspicious for a bone tumor of the left ischium. CT, bone scintigraphy and an MRI examination were requested to rule out bone tumor.

Acute hematogenous osteomyelitis usually occurs during skeletal growth when the growth plate is open. Early detection of osteomyelitis is essential in order to start therapy before bone devitalization.

Hematogenous osteomyelitis may not be evident on plain films until at least 10 days after the onset of symptoms. The evolution of the infection can manifest radiographically as soft-tissue swelling with obliteration of adjacent muscle planes, subperiosteal calcification, and resorption of bony trabeculae.

Bone scintigraphy is a highly sensitive imaging procedure for the diagnosis of osteomyelitis. Bone scintigraphy scans are sensitive indicators of altered osteoblastic activity, but local disturbances in vascular perfusion, clearance rate, permeability, and chemical binding also affect imaging.

CT should be used only as a third-line technique for visualizing bony destruction, gas within the bone, or bony sequestration.

MRI is a highly sensitive technique as an indicator of disease because pathological findings are evident much earlier in the course of the disease. The MRI diagnosis of osteomyelitis is based on its capability to detect bone marrow abnormalities within the physis. Active osteomyelitis foci appear as low signal intensity areas on T1-weighted images and high signal intensity areas on T2-weighted images, fat-suppression, or STIR sequences. MRI is a unique technique for the detection of osteomyelitis and the depiction of its extent.

It is important to understand the limitations of each imaging technique to avoid delays in the diagnosis and management of osteomyelitis and prevent possible complications.

The differential diagnosis of pelvic osteomyelitis in children should include septic arthritis, Legg-Calve-Perthes disease, toxic synovitis, and less commonly, collagen-vascular diseases, neoplasms involving bone, and retroperitoneal abscess.

Plain film of the pelvis (Fig. 6.1.1) shows no pathologic findings for bone infection in the left femur. A swollen left ischiopubic synchondrosis was found incidentally (*dotted arrow*) and was at first interpreted as the reason for the patient's complaint.

Bone scintigraphy (Fig. 6.1.2) scan shows increased uptake within the left femoral head (*arrow*) and slight uptake on the left ischiopubic synchondrosis (*open arrowhead*).

CT (Fig. 6.1.3) shows a round annular area in the left femoral head corresponding to the focal site of infection.

Axial T1-weighted MRI (Fig. 6.1.4) shows diffuse low signal intensity within the proximal metaphysis of the left femur. Coronal STIR MRI (Fig. 6.1.5) reveals high signal intensity in the bone marrow of the femur proximal growth plate, with edema in the surrounding soft tissues. Note the hypertrophy of the ischiopubic synchondrosis (*arrowhead*).

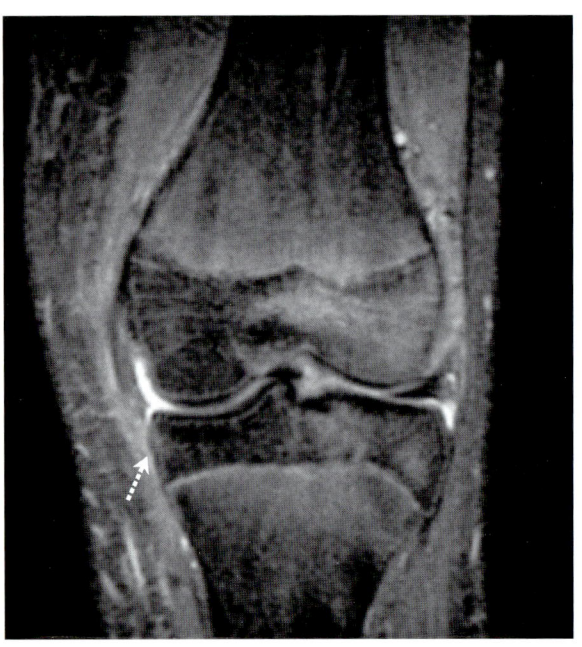

Fig. 6.2.1

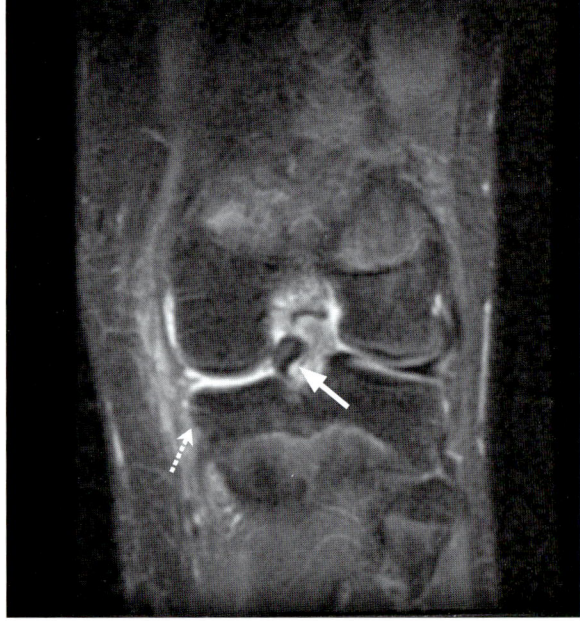

Fig. 6.2.2

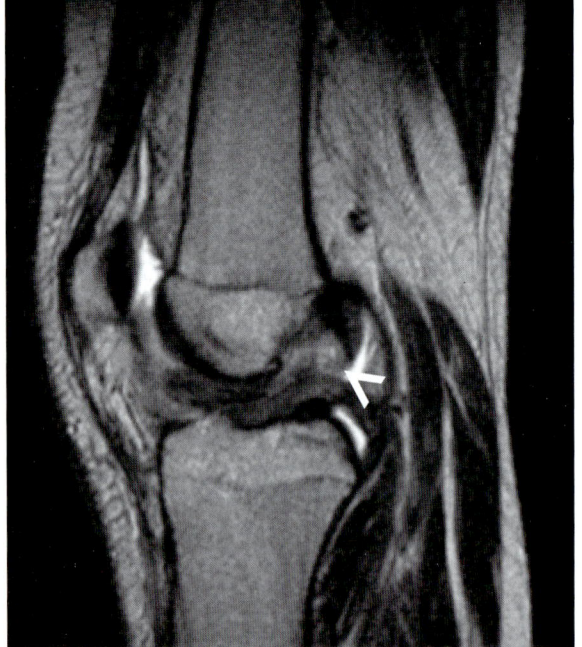

Fig. 6.2.3

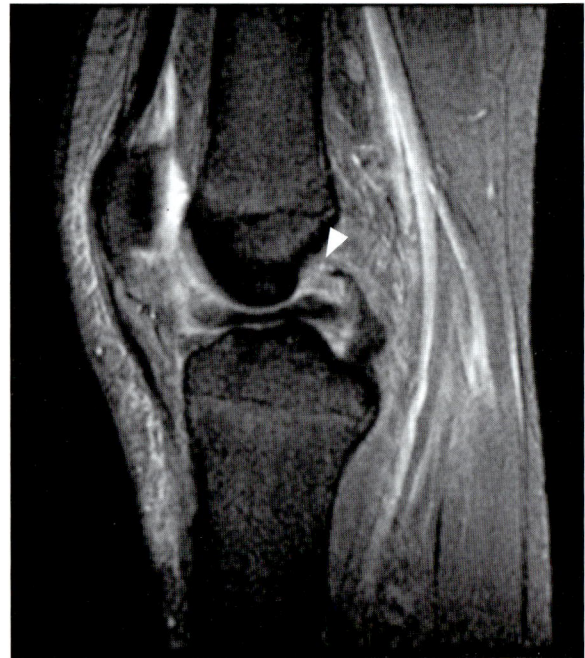

Fig. 6.2.4

A 15-year-old male suffered an acute traumatic injury 6 weeks prior to imaging and continued to have pain in the left knee.

Comments

Complex injuries of the knee are common after accidents or sports-related injuries. MRI is the preferred imaging technique to assess joint injuries. These lesions occur as a result of multiple forces (varus, valgus, rotation, and hyperextension) applied to the joint. Depending on the injury mechanism different patterns can be recognized. The normal anterior cruciate ligament (ACL) is a straight, taut structure that runs parallel to the roof of the intercondylar notch. ACL tears occur more frequently (70%) in the middle aspect of the ligament. Sagittal T2-weighted images are recommended to depict the ACL. Different signs reveal ACL injuries. Primary signs involve the absence of the normal dark band of the ACL. Secondary signs are bone-related injuries due to the indirect mechanism of the traumatic event (microfracture of the posterolateral aspect of the tibial plateau and lateral femoral condyle) and soft-tissue signs secondary to the anterior translation of the tibia. These indirect signs have a low sensitivity but a high specificity.

The posterior cruciate ligament (PCL) appears as a low signal structure in the intercondylar notch, gently curving between the posterior aspect of the proximal tibia and the distal femur. The majority of PCL tears are incomplete and intrasubstance and are best seen on sagittal images. Isolated PCL injuries make up only 30% of cases.

The medial collateral ligament (MCL) originates on the medial aspect of the distal femur and inserts on the medial aspect of the proximal tibia. MRI shows the MCL as a thin dark band. MCL injuries are revealed on fluid-sensitive coronal sequences and their treatment with either immobilization or surgery depends on the presence or absence of meniscal tear or ACL injuries.

The menisci are fibrocartilaginous structures attached to the superior aspect of the tibial plateau. MRI is the best imaging modality for the evaluation of meniscal trauma. The normal meniscus is devoid of signal on all sequences, but linear images are seen within the menisci when they are torn. Medial meniscus tears are associated with MCL rupture in almost 70% of cases. Meniscal tears are described as horizontal, vertical, radial, and longitudinal. A different type of meniscal tear is the bucket handle tear (BHT) which tends to involve the medial meniscus. BHT is a longitudinal vertical tear with unstable displaced inner fragment that can usually be found in the intercondylar notch. The presence of the displaced fragment within the intercondylar notch is known as the "double PCL" sign and can be seen in sagittal images.

Imaging Findings

Coronal T2-weighted fat-suppression FSE MR images (Figs. 6.2.1 and 6.2.2) reveal increased signal in the distal insertion of the MCL (*dotted arrow*) and a bucket handle tear of the medial meniscus with a fragment displaced into the notch (*arrow*). Edema on the lateral condyle of the femur is an indirect sign for the rupture of the ACL (Fig. 6.2.1).

Sagittal T2-weighted FSE (Fig. 6.2.3) and GRE (Fig. 6.2.4) MR images through the intercondylar notch show the absence of the ACL (*open arrowhead*) without clearly identifiable fibers. The PCL shows increased signal with surface disruption on its proximal insertion (*arrowhead*). A small joint effusion is present.

Case 3
■
Radius Fracture

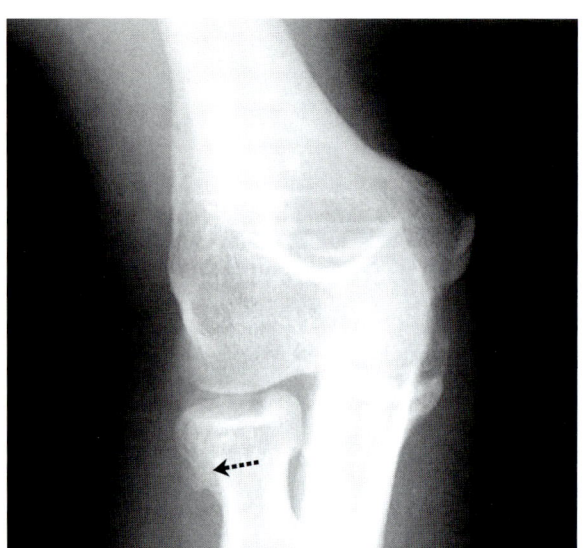

Fig. 6.3.1

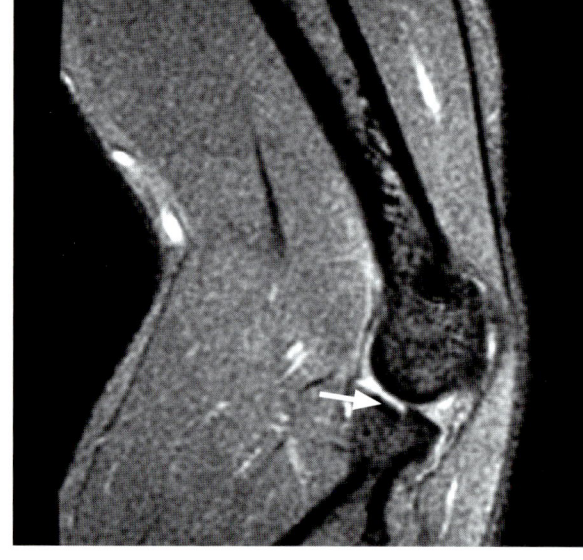

Fig. 6.3.2

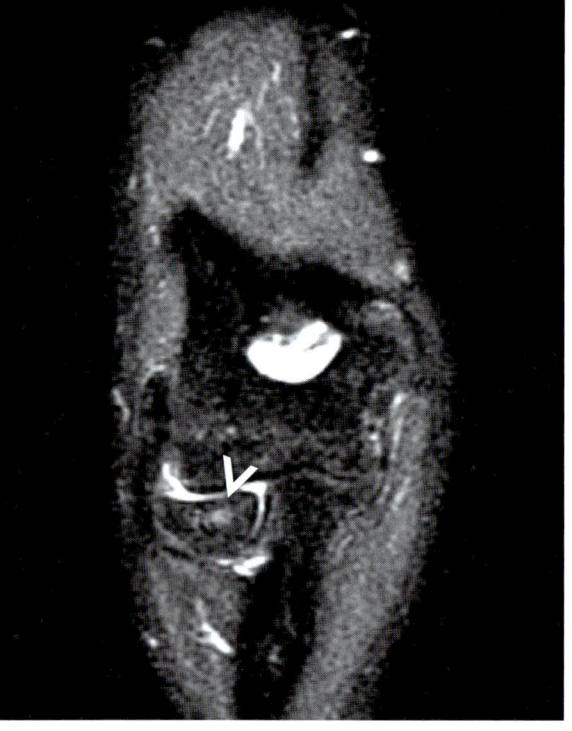

Fig. 6.3.3

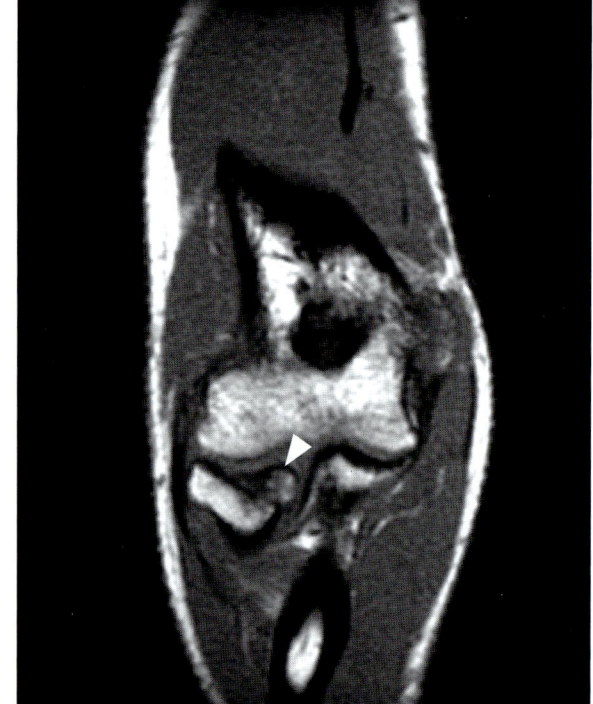

Fig. 6.3.4

A 29-year-old man complained of pain in the right elbow after a motorcycle accident 4 months prior. His ability to flex, extend, and rotate the elbow and forearm was limited

Elbow trauma is very common. Elbow fractures most commonly involve the head of the radius (60%), followed by the distal humerus (30%) and the coronoid process (5%). Standard radiographs usually reveal the abnormality. In some cases, however, particularly if a radial head or coronoid process fracture is not displaced or if it is minimally displaced, it may not be apparent on routine examination.

In the management of elbow fractures, especially of the head of the radius and the capitellum, the correct diagnosis is fundamental not only for deciding whether or not to operate, but also for deciding on the type of surgical procedure. Radiographically occult or equivocal fractures of the elbow may be assessed with MR imaging.

MR imaging is useful for the detection and characterization of radial head fractures and is also helpful in the exclusion of associated collateral ligament injuries that may contribute to instability. The integrity of the medial collateral ligament (MCL) is especially important if excision of the radial head is considered. When there is ligamentous disruption and instability, displaced fractures of the radial head are best treated with internal fixation.

On MR images, radial head fractures are indicated by linear decreased signal intensity within the radial head surrounded by edema.

Anteroposterior radiograph of the elbow shows a non-displaced fracture (*dotted arrow*) of the radial head (Fig. 6.3.1). Oblique sagittal T2-weighted GRE MR image reveals a fracture of the radial head (*arrow*) as linear discontinuity of the articular surface (Fig. 6.3.2)

Coronal STIR MR image reveals a minimal joint effusion with slight bone marrow edema (*open arrowhead*) (Fig. 6.3.3).

Coronal T1-weighted SE MR image shows the intraarticular fracture with the cortical disruption (*arrowhead*) and mild compression of the radial surface.

Case 4
■
Ewing Sarcoma

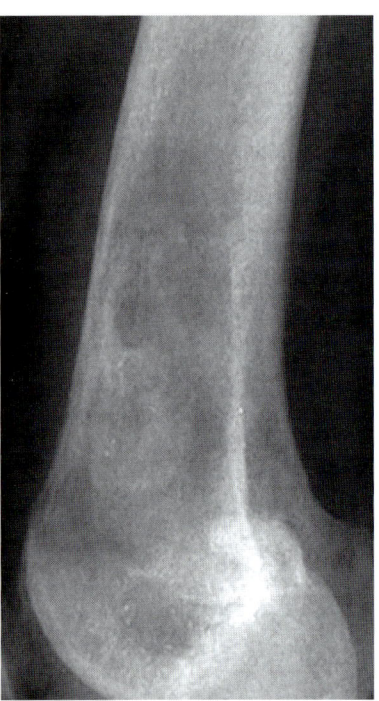

Fig. 6.4.1

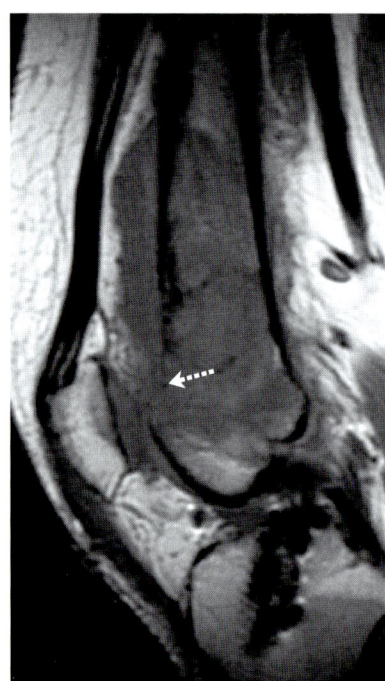

Fig. 6.4.2

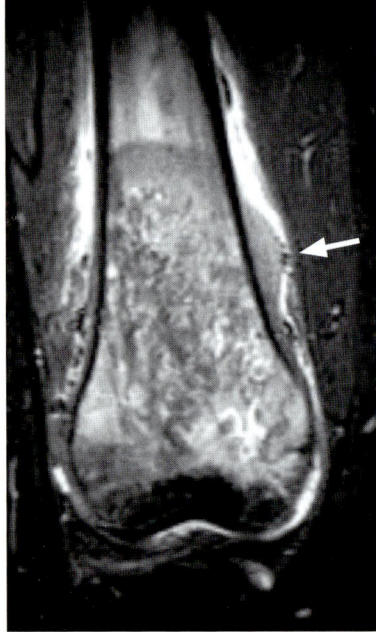

Fig. 6.4.3

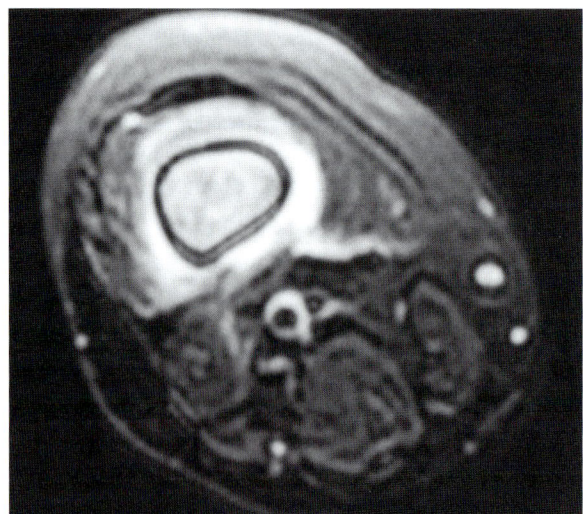

Fig. 6.4.4

A 22-year-old man presented with pain in his right knee one year after anterior cruciate ligament reconstruction with a patellar tendon autograft.

Ewing's sarcoma is the sixth most common malignant tumor, accounting for approximately 11–12% of all malignant bone tumors. The tumor is derived from red bone marrow.

Ewing's sarcoma usually occurs in young people (4–25 years) and the mean age of presentation is 13 years. The tumor has a decisively male predominance. Patients typically present systemic symptoms (fever, anemia, and leukocytosis) and a painful mass.

Ewing's sarcoma can occur in both long (60%) and flat (40%) bones. The long bones are more commonly affected in younger patients. The most common sites are the femur, tibia and humerus. The most commonly affected flat bones (typically in older patients) are the pelvis and the ribs. In the long bones, the tumor almost always affects the metaphysis or the diaphysis.

Although Ewing's sarcoma presents multiple radiological appearances, it is typically based within the medullary cavity, metadiaphyseal in location and poorly delineated, with aggressive periosteal reaction and a large associated soft-tissue mass. Commonly there is a permeative lytic pattern.

MRI is essential to evaluate the bone marrow and soft-tissue extent of the tumor. The typical MRI appearance of Ewing's sarcoma includes low signal on T1-weighted sequences, high signal on T2-weighted sequences, and heterogeneous contrast enhancement.

MRI provides useful information for preoperative planning and posttreatment follow-up.

The differential diagnosis should include osteomyelitis, lymphoma, chondrosarcoma, Langerhans cell granuloma, and osteosarcoma. It is important to remember that age is the most important factor for narrowing the differential diagnosis for bone tumors.

Plain lateral radiograph of the distal femur (Fig. 6.4.1) shows a permeative lytic pattern of bone destruction.

Sagittal T1-weighted MRI demonstrates the intraosseous and extraosseus extent of the tumor and the disruption of the cortex (*dotted arrow*) (Fig. 6.4.2). The tumor has lower signal intensity than normal marrow fat in this pulse sequence. Notice the hyperintensity of the patellar tendon from which the ACL plastia was taken.

Coronal T2-weighted fat-suppression MRI shows a heterogeneous high signal intensity lesion within the medullar cavity with a soft-tissue mass (*arrow*) (Fig. 6.4.3).

Axial T2-weighted fat-suppression MRI (Fig. 6.4.4) reveals the intramedullary lesion and the soft-tissue mass extending to the cortex.

Case 5
Schwannoma

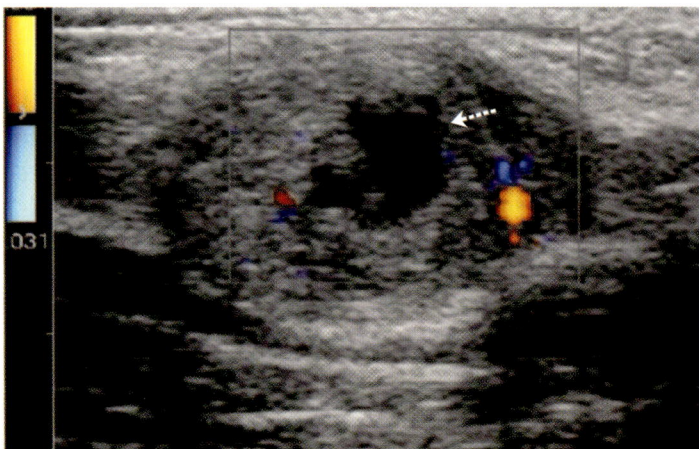

Fig. 6.5.1

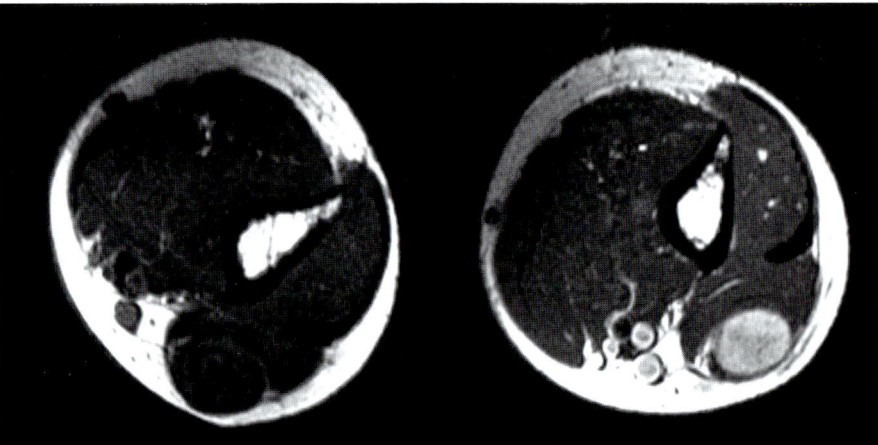

Fig. 6.5.2

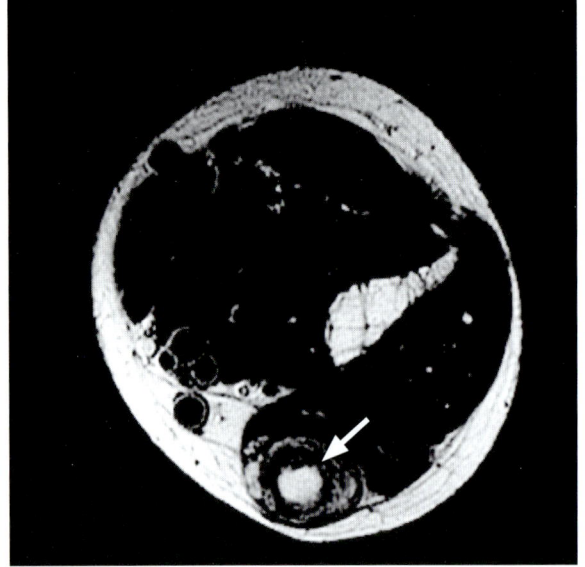

Fig. 6.5.3

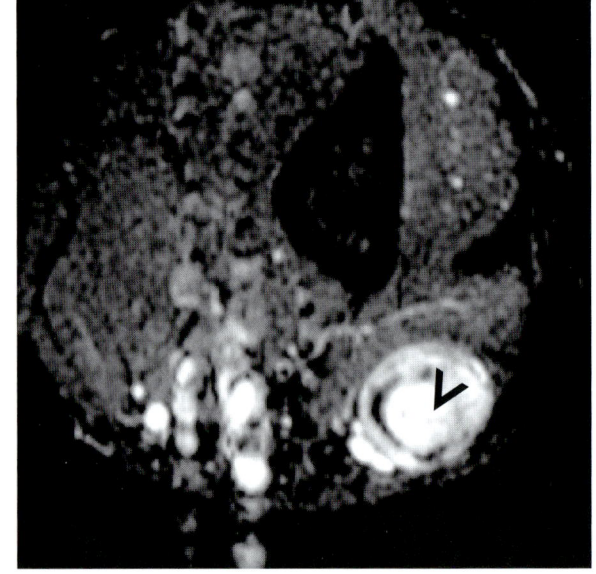

Fig. 6.5.4

A 27-year-old man presented with a painful palpable mass in the left elbow after a recent traumatic event.

Solitary benign peripheral nerve sheath tumors are divided into two major groups: schwannoma (neurilemmoma, neurinoma) and neurofibroma. Both schwannomas and neurofibromas contain cells that are closely related to normal schwann cells.

Schwannoma most frequently affects patients aged 20–30 and constitutes approximately 5% of all benign soft-tissue neoplasms. Men and women are affected equally. Commonly involved sites include the spinal and sympathetic nerve roots of the head and neck, as well as nerves in the flexor surfaces of the upper and lower extremities. The posterior mediastinum and retroperitoneum can also be affected.

Neurilemmomas are usually solitary, with nonaggressive features, including slow growth and small size. Pain and neurologic symptoms are unusual except in large tumors. Schwannoma is rarely multiple, and multiple neurilemmomas in association with neurofibromatosis 1 (NF1) are apparent in only about 5% of the cases.

Radiologic features of schwannoma are an eccentric mass relative to and separable from the nerve, with well-circumscribed margins. Heterogeneous signal intensity may be seen in schwannomas, especially in larger lesions, reflecting hypo- or hyper-cellularity, xanthomatous changes, cystic degeneration, necrosis, or hemorrhage. The target sign (low signal intensity centrally and high signal intensity peripherally) corresponds to central fibrous components and myxomatous elements and appears in 50% of schwannomas. The target sign is more common in neurofibromas and a heterogeneous target sign might be observed in cases with hemorrhage. Another key to differentiating schwannomas from neurofibromas is that, unlike neurofibromas, schwannomas are eccentric and separable from normal nerve.

Neurilemmomas are usually treated by surgical excision. The affected nerve is usually separable from the neoplasm after incision of the epineurium, allowing the native nerve and its function to be preserved. Recurrence is unusual.

US shows a well-circumscribed fusiform mass with an anechoic central area (dotted *arrow*) and appreciable vascularity (Fig. 6.5.1).

Axial T1-weighted SE MR image shows the lesion in the posterior cubital region, which is predominantly isointense to skeletal muscle. After contrast administration, marked enhancement within the mass is seen (Fig. 6.5.2).

Axial T2-weighted FSE MR image (Fig. 6.5.3) shows a well-defined mass, mildly heterogeneous with central high signal intensity due to the hemorrhagic component and a thin hypointense peripheral rim due to hemosiderin (*arrow*).

On the axial STIR MR image, the mass shows a markedly hyperintense central target sign (*open arrowhead*) (Fig. 6.5.4).

Case 6

■

Soft-Tissue Liposarcoma

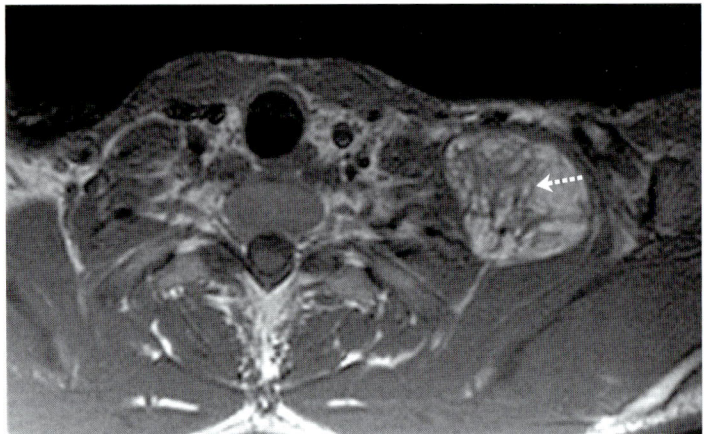

Fig. 6.6.1

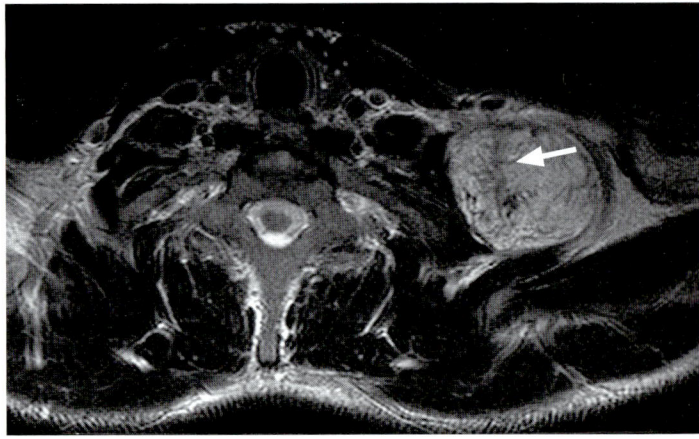

Fig. 6.6.2

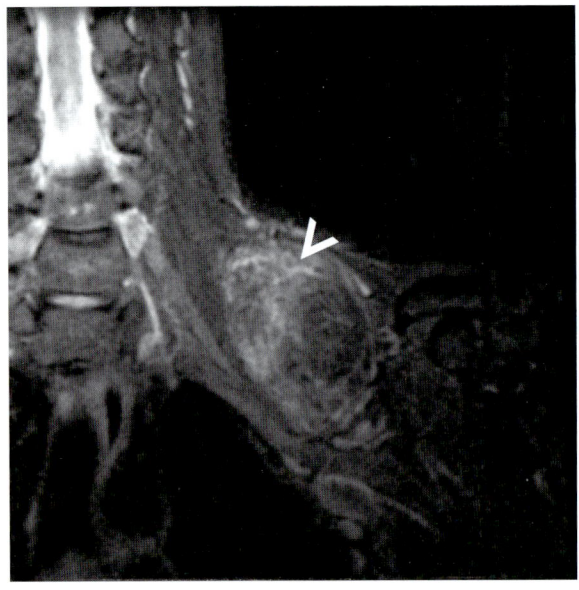

Fig. 6.6.3

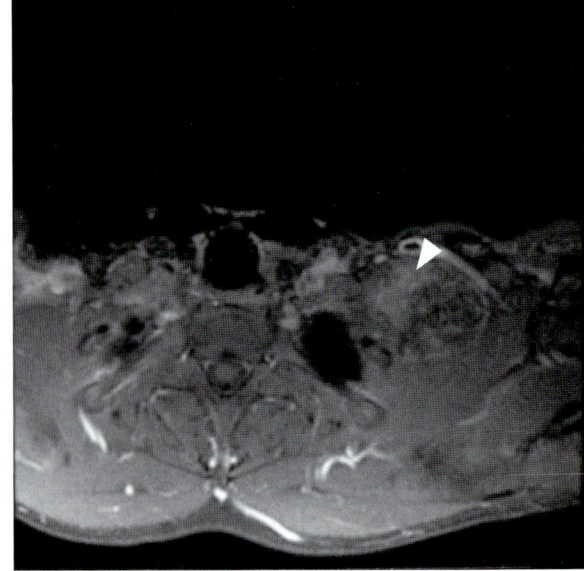

Fig. 6.6.4

A 22-year-old man presented with a painless, tender mass in the upper left supraclavicular region.

Liposarcoma is a malignant tumor of mesenchymal origin. The term liposarcoma does not imply that the tumor is derived from fat, but rather that the tumor tissue contains differentiated adipose tissue. Liposarcoma is the second most common soft-tissue sarcoma seen in adults (10–18%) after malignant fibrous histiocytoma. Liposarcomas are classified into four histologic subtypes: well differentiated, myxoid, round cell, and pleomorphic. Well-differentiated liposarcoma is synonymous with atypical lipoma. Between 40 and 65% of liposarcomas of the extremities occur in the thigh. Other common sites, in the order of descending frequency, are the upper arm and shoulder, popliteal fossa and lower leg, buttocks, and forearm. Clinically, these tumors manifest as painless masses.

The radiological features of a liposarcoma depend on the histological type and tend to reflect its degree of differentiation. CT or MRI findings for well-differentiated liposarcomas closely resemble those of subcutaneous fat or a simple lipoma. They are frequently composed of more than 75% fat, while the other types usually have less than 25%.

On CT a well-differentiated liposarcoma may appear as a well-delineated mass, with attenuation values equal to those of simple fat, mimicking a benign lipomatous tumor.

On MRI a well-differentiated liposarcoma shows some thickened linear or nodular soft-tissue septa that enhance after intravenous administration of contrast material. These small nonlipomatous components are of low signal intensity on T1-weighted images and increased signal intensity on T2-weighted images with fat suppression.

Features for discriminating a well-differentiated liposarcoma from a simple lipoma include a deep (intramuscular) rather than subcutaneous location, a size of more than 10 cm in maximum diameter, the presence of nodular nonadipose components or thick septa, high signal intensity of septa or nodular soft-tissue areas on T2-weighted fat suppression or STIR images, and contrast-enhancement of nonadipose components (best seen on fat-suppressed T1-weighted images)

MRI is the most specific modality for diagnosing liposarcoma. Figure 6.6.1 shows an axial T1-weighted image of a large mass located in the left supraclavicular region, posterior to the sternocleidomastoideus muscle and medial to the scalene muscles and brachial plexus. The tumor is predominantly isointense to subcutaneous fat. Multiple thickened septa extend throughout the tumor (dotted *arrow*).

On axial T2-weighted MR image the signal intensity of the tumor is similar to that of subcutaneous fat (Fig. 6.6.2) with thick, low signal intensity septa (*arrow*).

Coronal STIR MR (Fig. 6.6.3) shows the nonadipose areas with increased signal intensity relative to fat (*open arrowhead*).

Axial T1-weighted fat-suppression MR image (Fig. 6.6.4) obtained after contrast administration shows moderate heterogeneous enhancement of the nonadipose areas (*arrowhead*).

Case 7
■
Chordoma

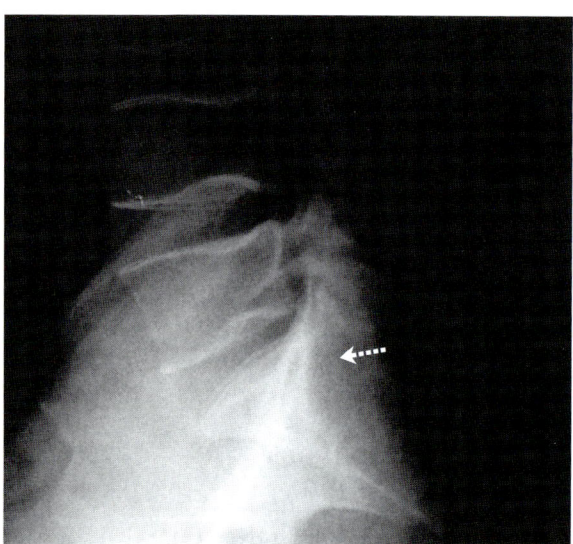

Fig. 6.7.1

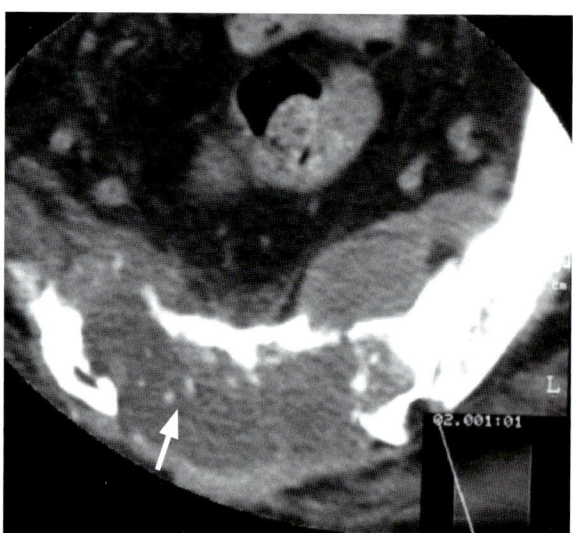

Fig. 6.7.2

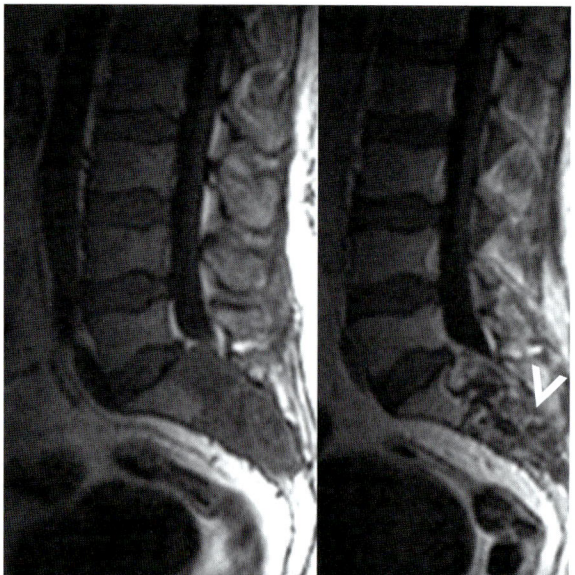

Fig. 6.7.3

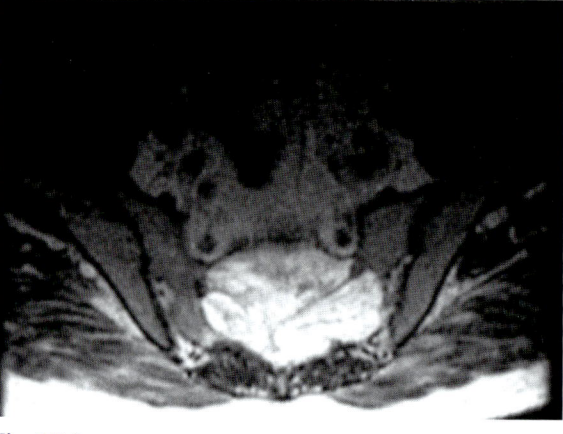

Fig. 6.7.4

A 54-year-old man had severe low back pain of several weeks' duration. The pain radiated to both legs. The medical history and physical examination were unremarkable.

Chordoma is the most common primary malignant sacral tumor and accounts for 2–4% of malignant osseous neoplasms. Chordomas arise from the fetal notochord, which is normally replaced by mesodermal tissue by the 7th week of development. Scattered vestiges of notochord may be found in the nucleus pulposus and can be present at any level from the skull base to the coccyx. Fifty to 60% of chordomas develop in the sacrococcygeal region. These tumors are found at all ages. The mean age at diagnosis is the 6th decade. Chordoma is more common in males by a 2:1 ratio.

The classic appearance of chordoma is a destructive, lytic lesion, commonly with internal calcifications (30%). A large presacral soft-tissue component is usually present. These tumors are capable of extending across the adjacent disk space and the sacroiliac joint. Chordoma shows heterogeneous low signal intensity on T1-weighted images and prominent heterogeneous increased signal intensity on T2- weighted MR images, reflecting the high water content of the lesions. Contrast enhancement at MR imaging is common.

The differential diagnosis includes other primary tumors (sarcoma, giant-cell tumor, and, rarely, ependymoma). Metastases are the most common sacral neoplasm.

The treatment of chordoma is surgical. Total surgical resection provides the best hope for cure. MR imaging has proven highly accurate for evaluating the extent of disease. The majority of patients succumb to locally recurrent tumor because chordoma is relatively radioresistant, although patients with chordoma often survive many years after surgery. The 5-year survival in patients treated with radiation therapy is 50%.

Plain radiography of the sacrum is nonspecific and might reveal a lytic lesion, with obliteration of the cortex (dotted *arrow*) (Fig. 6.7.1).

CT is useful to detect the internal calcifications (*arrow*) (Fig. 6.7.2) and the extent of the destructive soft-tissue mass within the sacrum. In this case, the mass extends across the sacral canal and the anterior neuronal foramina.

MRI is the best imaging technique, showing on sagittal T1-weighted images low signal intensity, and marked enhancement after contrast administration with a peripheral septal pattern (*open arrowhead*) (Fig. 6.7.3). T2-weighted MR image (Fig. 6.7.4) shows a heterogeneously (due to the presence of septa) hyperintense sacral mass with a presacral and soft-tissue component within the canal.

Case 8
Osteonecrosis

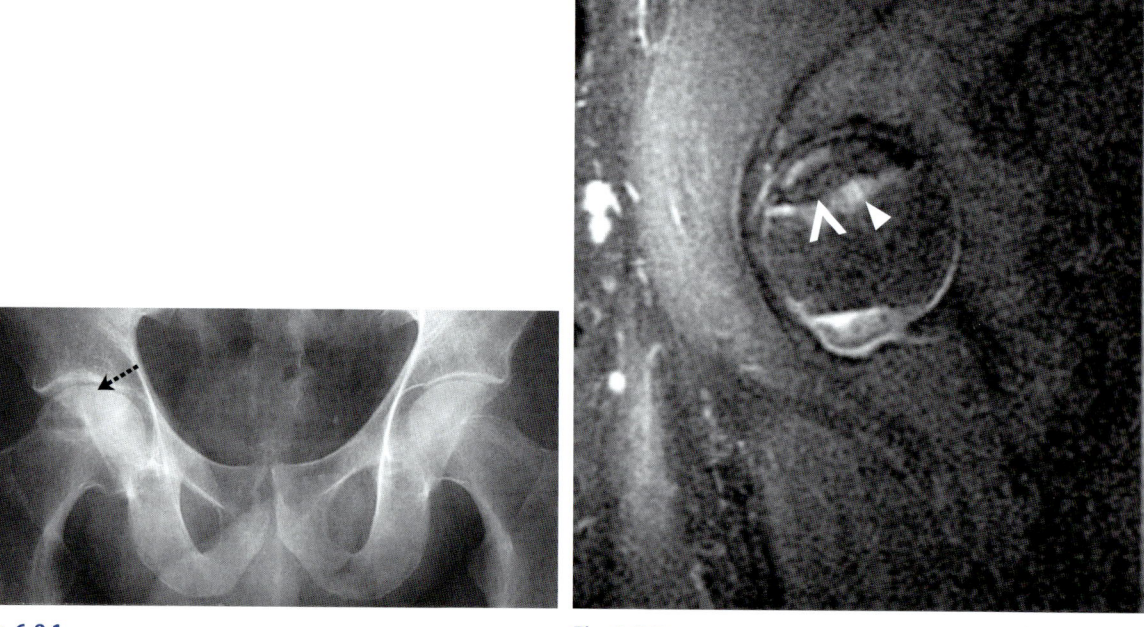

Fig. 6.8.3

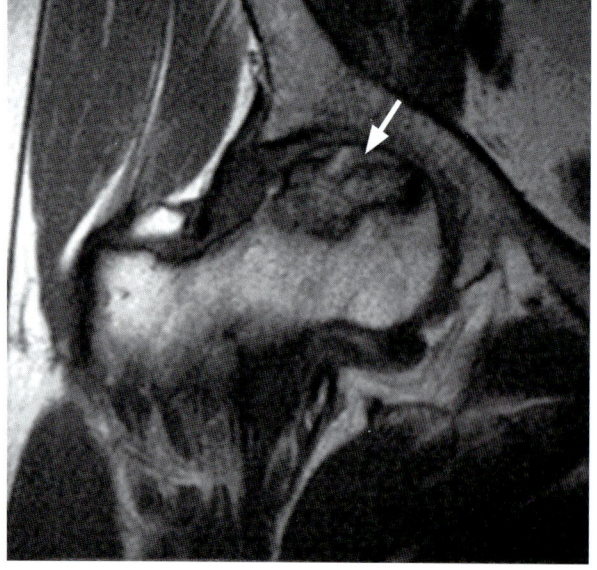

Fig. 6.8.1

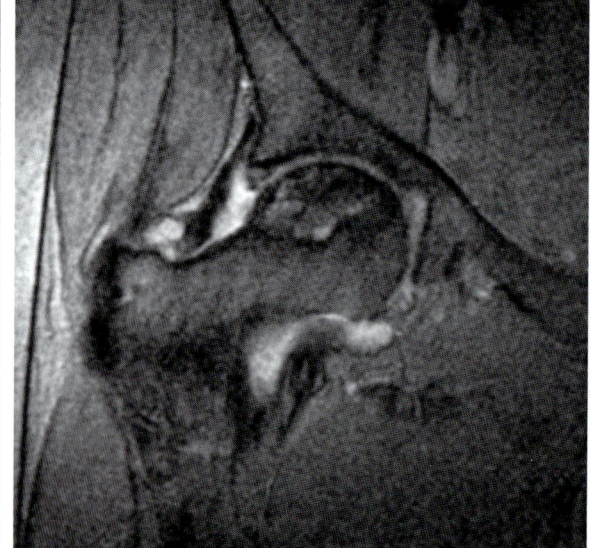

Fig. 6.8.2

Fig. 6.8.4

A 41-year-old man on chronic steroid therapy suffered right hip pain and disabled joint function.

Avascular necrosis of the femoral head appears in a wide spectrum of clinical conditions: corticoid steroid therapy, alcohol abuse, idiopathic, Gaucher disease, lupus, coagulopathies, hyperlipidemia, organ transplantation, and thyroid disorders. Osteonecrosis may be caused by emboli or increased bone marrow pressure and subsequent decreased blood flow, anoxia, and eventual death of trabecular bone.

Avascular necrosis is bilateral in 40% of hips; therefore, it is essential to image both hips.

Diagnosis by conventional radiography is difficult in the early stages of osteonecrosis.

MR imaging is the most sensitive method to detect the presence of early femoral head osteonecrosis and provides information regarding articular cartilage, marrow conversion, joint fluid, and associated insufficiency fractures. On MRI, ischemic necrosis leads to abnormal geographic areas of low signal intensity with different patterns: homogeneous or inhomogeneous areas, marginal line of low signal intensity with higher signal intensity centrally, subchondral fractures, and cortical collapse.

The Ficat grading system classifies the radiographic findings as: grade 0, no pain and no radiological findings; grade I, pain, negative X-ray and positive MRI and bone scan; grade II, positive X-ray (sclerosis-lucency), without subchondral fracture on MRI; grade III, crescent sign on X-ray and subchondral collapse on MRI; and grade IV, joint space narrowing and osteoarthritis.

Early diagnosis and treatment of the femoral head osteonecrosis improves the prognosis, often preventing significant disability.

Positive findings on plain radiography (dotted *arrow*) indicate at least stage II osteonecrosis (Fig. 6.8.1). MRI is the most specific and sensitive technique to evaluate osteonecrosis. Oblique coronal T1-weighted MR image of the right hip shows a subchondral lesion with mixed signal intensity (*arrow*), involving approximately 45% of the femoral head (Fig. 6.8.2).

Oblique sagittal STIR MR image reveals an area of low signal intensity with a marginal hypointense line (*open arrowhead*). High signal intensity edema is seen in the subchondral area (*arrowhead*) and also bordering the marginal low signal intensity line; without subchondral fracture (Fig. 6.8.3).

Oblique coronal T2-weighted GRE MR image demonstrates stage II osteonecrosis with slight hip joint effusion (Fig. 6.8.4).

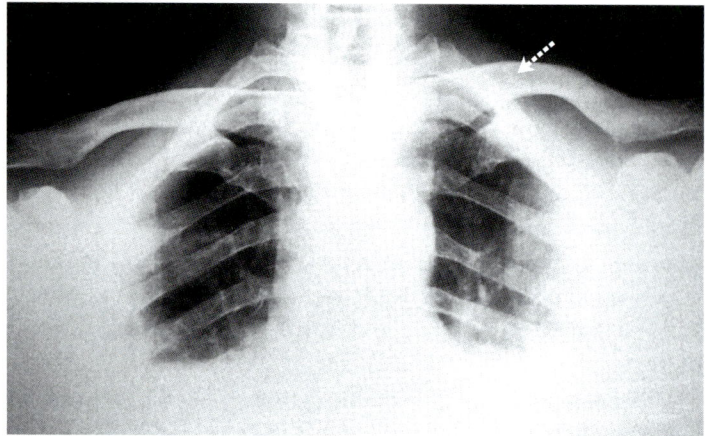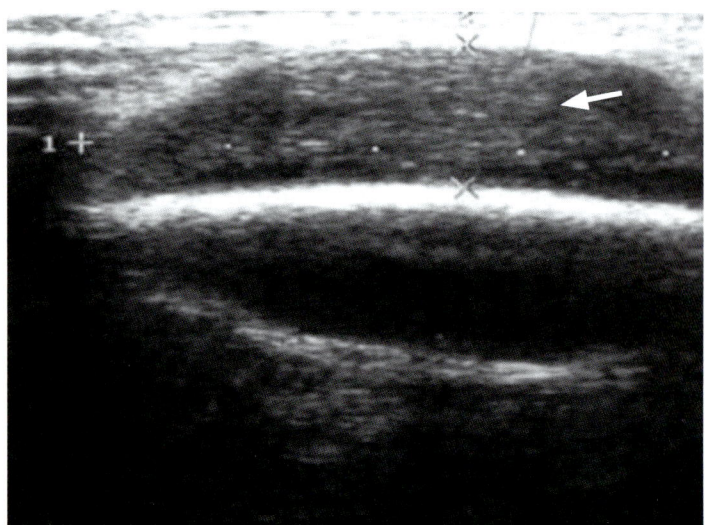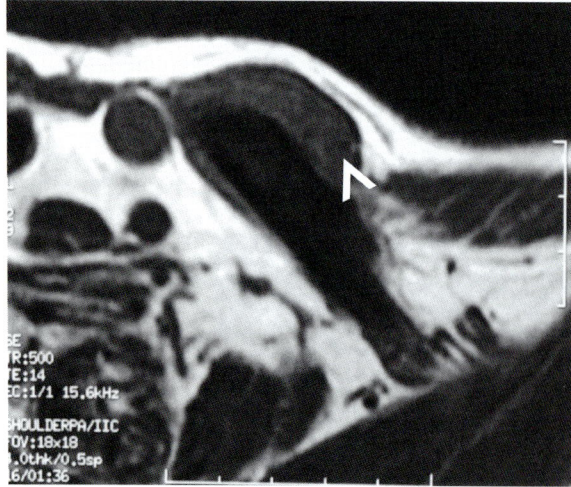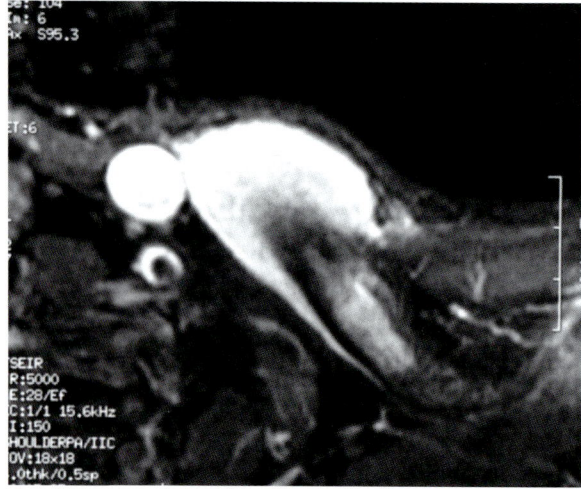

A 75-year-old man was admitted to the hospital with a 1-month history of a firm soft-tissue mass in the left clavicular region. Physical examination revealed a palpable mass in the middle-third of the left clavicle. The superficial lymph nodes were not enlarged. The complete hemogram, biochemical tests, and levels of tumor markers were normal.

Comments

Primary lymphoma of bone is an uncommon tumor, accounting for 3–4% of all malignant bone tumors. Lymphoma is considered primary in bone only when a complete systematic workup reveals no evidence of extraosseous involvement. Distinguishing primary bone lymphoma from other bone tumors is important as the former has a better response to therapy and a better prognosis. Patients treated for primary bone lymphoma have a much better 5 year survival rate (50%). The disease may occur at any age (peak 35–45 years) and is more common in males, with a sex ratio (1.4:1). Primary lymphoma of bone predominantly involves the appendicular skeleton in the region of the diaphysis or metaphysis.

The radiographic appearance of the disease is variable and nonspecific; a wide spectrum of patterns might be depicted, from nearly normal-appearing bone to a focal lytic lesion or a diffusely mixed permeative or blastic appearance process with cortical destruction.

MRI demonstrates bone marrow involvement. On T1-weighted images, diffuse infiltration is demonstrated as an area of low signal intensity. On T2-weighted images, the lesion is hyperintense compared to muscle. On STIR, the foci of lymphomatous infiltration exhibit high signal intensity.

The prognosis for patients with extraosseous soft-tissue masses is worse.

The differential diagnosis must include other primary bone tumors: Ewing's sarcoma, metastatic carcinoma, plasmacytoma, and osteomyelitis.

Imaging Findings

The radiological findings on plain film might be subtle; lordotic projection of the thorax shows a slight sclerotic area (dotted arrow) in the middle-third of the left clavicle without periosteal reaction (Fig. 6.9.1).

Ultrasound study (Fig. 6.9.2) reveals a hypoechogenic soft-tissue mass surrounding the clavicle (*arrow*).

Axial T1-weighted MR image (Fig. 6.9.3) shows abnormal low signal intensity within the bone marrow of the clavicle and the soft-tissue extension surrounding the bone (*open arrowhead*).

Axial STIR MR image (Fig. 6.9.4) demonstrates the homogeneous high signal intensity of the tumor.

Case 10
■
Enchondroma

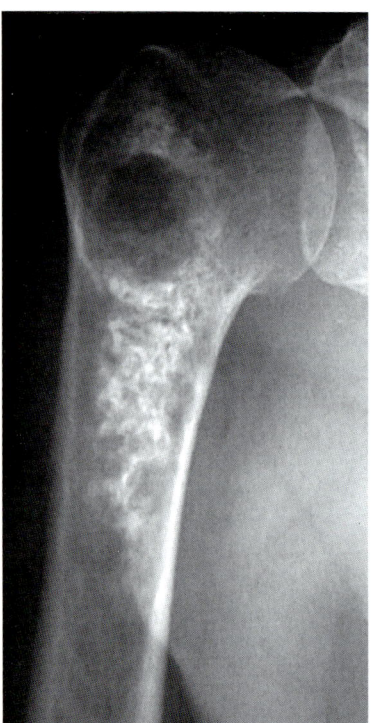

Fig. 6.10.1

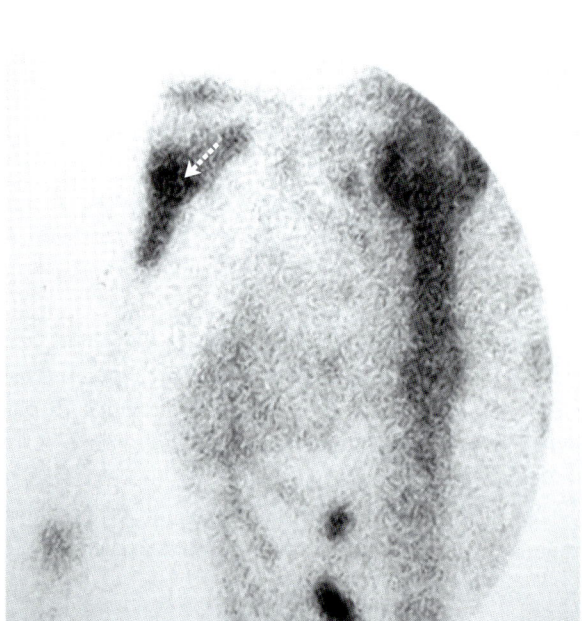

Fig. 6.10.2

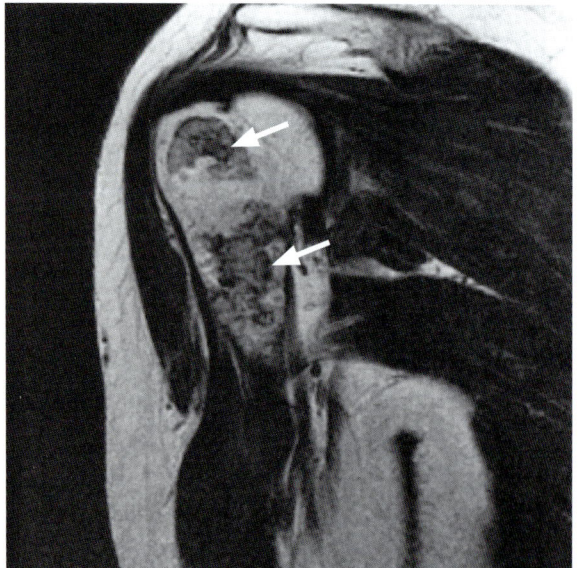

Fig. 6.10.3

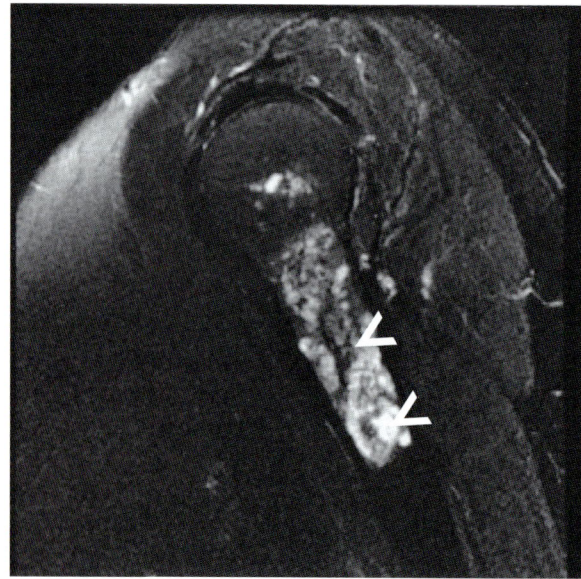

Fig. 6.10.4

52-year-old woman with incidental finding on plain film obtained after trauma.

Enchondroma is a common chondroid musculoskeletal neoplasm representing 3–17% of primary bone tumors. It may be solitary or multiple (enchondromatosis – Ollier's disease). Enchondroma is the result of the continued growth of residual benign cartilaginous remains that are displaced from the growth plate. The neoplasm is usually discovered in the third or fourth decade of life with the same frequency in men and woman. Malignant transformation is exceptional.

Between 40–65% of solitary enchondromas occur in the hand, although long tubular bones are affected in 25% of cases, more frequently in the bones of the upper extremity. Enchondromas are usually located in the metaphysis of a long tubular bone or in the diaphysis of a short tubular bone.

Cartilaginous tumors are typically recognized on radiographs as a lytic lesion with mineralized cartilage matrix within and lobulated contour, but CT is the best modality to detect mineralization characteristic of a chondroid neoplasm, showing the typical rings and arcs pattern. Scintigraphic bone scans show slightly increased activity. On MRI, enchondroma appears as a well-circumscribed lobulated lesion of low signal intensity on T1-weighted images, intermediate intensity on T2-weighted images, and high signal on T2-weighted fat-suppression sequences. Calcified foci have low signal intensity on all sequences.

Low-grade chondrosarcoma may be indistinguishable from enchondroma; however, in most cases, chondrosarcoma has certain imaging features that are indicative of its aggressive behavior. Cortical breakthrough, soft-tissue mass, and deep endosteal scalloping of the cortex are three features that are described more frequently in chondrosarcoma.

On plain radiography, the classic pattern of calcifications, described as rings and arcs, is pathognomonic for enchondroma (Fig. 6.10.1). Bone scintigraphy shows only mild uptake (dotted *arrow*) in the right humerus (Fig. 6.10.2). Oblique coronal T2-weighted MR image (Fig. 6.10.3) shows intermediate signal intensity from entrapment of residual normal fatty marrow with a cluster of numerous tiny low signal intensity foci (arrows) representing mineralized matrix (Fig. 6.10.3)

Oblique sagittal T2-weighted fat-suppression MR image (Fig. 6.10.4) reveals calcified foci as areas of low signal intensity, and hyperintense areas with lobulated margins correspond to chondroid tumor (*open arrowheads*). Enchondroma spares the cortex and there is no soft-tissue extension or other signs of an aggressive lesion.

Further Readings

Books

Arthritis: in Black and White. Brower AC, Flemming DJ (1997) Saunders (W.B.). ISBN-13: 9780721651521

Diagnosis of Bone and Joint Disorders. Vol 1–5. Resnik D (2002) Saunders (W.B.). ISBN-13: 9780721689210

Fundamentals of Skeletal Radiology. Helms CA (2005) Saunders (W.B.). ISBN-13: 9780721605708

Imaging of Soft Tissue Tumors. 3rd ed. De Schepper AM (2005) Springer, Berlin. ISBN-13: 9783540248095

Magnetic Resonance Imaging in Orthopaedics and Sports Medicine. Stoller DW (2006) Lippincott Williams & Wilkins. ISBN-13: 9780781773577

Musculoskeletal MRI. Kaplan PA, Helms CA, Dussault R, Anderson MW, Major NM (2001) Saunders (W.B.). ISBN-13: 9780721690278

Musculoskeletal Imaging: The Requisites (Requisites in Radiology). 3rd ed. Manaster BJ, May DA, Disler DG (2006) Mosby. ISBN-13: 9780323043618

Orthopedic Radiology: A Practical Approach. 3rd ed. Greenspan A (2000) Lippincott Williams & Wilkins. ISBN-13: 9780781715898

Spinal Imaging: Diagnostic Imaging of the Spine and Spinal Cord. Van Goethem JW, Hauwe L, Parizel PM (2007) Springer, Berlin. ISBN-13: 9783540213444

Ultrasound of the Musculoskeletal System. Bianchi S, Martinoli C (2007) Springer, Berlin. ISBN-13: 9783540422679

Web Sites

http://bonetumor.org/tumors/pages/page174.html

http://chorus.rad.mcw.edu/index/6.html (Chorus: collaborative hypertext of radiology>musculoskeletal system)

http://emedicine.com/radio/MUSCULOSKELETAL.htm

http://gentili.net/ (The Musculoskeletal Radiologist Guide to the Internet. A. Gentili, MD, A.P. Lai, MD. UCLA and WLA VAMC. Los Angeles, California)

http://indyrad.iupui.edu/public/ddaven/main.htm (Skeletal Radiology Tutorial. Department of Radiology. Indiana University Medical Center)

http://med-ed.virginia.edu/courses/rad/ext/ (Introduction to radiology > skeletal trauma radiology)

http://orthop.washington.edu/

http://rad.washington.edu/mskbook (Approaches to Differential Diagnosis in Musculoskeletal Imaging by Richardson ML)

http://radiographics.rsnajnls.org/cgi/collection/skeletal_radiology

https://skeletalrad.org/Default.aspx (American Society of Skeletal Radiology)

Articles

Adams ME, Saifuddin A. Characterisation of intra-articular soft tissue tumours and tumour-like lesions. Eur Radiol 2007; 17(4):950–958

Baur A, Reiser MF. Diffusion-weighted imaging of the musculoskeletal system in humans. Skeletal Radiol 2000; 29(10):555–562

Beaman FD, Kransdorf MJ, Andrews TR, Murphey MD, Arcara LK, Keeling JH. Superficial soft-tissue masses: analysis, diagnosis, and differential considerations. Radiographics 2007;27(2):509–523

Beck M, Kalhor M, Leunig M, Ganz R. Hip morphology influences the pattern of damage to the acetabular cartilage: femoroacetabular impingement as a cause of early osteoarthritis of the hip. J Bone Joint Surg Br 2005; 87(7):1012–1018

Beltran J, Bencardino J, Mellado J, Rosenberg ZS, Irish RD. MR arthrography of the shoulder: variants and pitfalls. Radiographics 1997; 17(6):1403–1412

Bergin D, Morrison WB, Carrino JA, Nallamshetty SN, Bartolozzi AR. Anterior cruciate ligament ganglia and mucoid degeneration: coexistence and clinical correlation. AJR Am J Roentgenol 2004; 182(5):1283–1287

Bianchi S, Martinoli C, Abdelwahab IF. Ultrasound of tendon tears. Part 1: general considerations and upper extremity. Skeletal Radiol 2005; 34(9):500–512

Bianchi S, Poletti PA, Martinoli C, Abdelwahab IF. Ultrasound appearance of tendon tears. Part 2: lower extremity and myotendinous tears. Skeletal Radiol 2006; 35(2):63–77

Blumenkrantz G, Lindsey CT, Dunn TC, et al. A pilot, two-year longitudinal study of the interrelationship between trabecular bone and articular cartilage in the osteoarthritic knee. Osteoarthritis Cartilage 2004; 12(12):997–1005

Brown WE, Potter HG, Marx RG, Wickiewicz TL, Warren RF. Magnetic resonance imaging appearance of cartilage repair in the knee. Clin Orthop Relat Res 2004; (422):214–223

Byun WM, Shin SO, Chang Y, Lee SJ, Finsterbusch J, Frahm J. Diffusion-weighted MR imaging of metastatic disease of the spine: assessment of response to therapy. AJNR Am J Neuroradiol 2002; 23(6):906–912

Cerezal L, Del PF, Abascal F, Garcia-Valtuille R, Pereda T, Canga A. Imaging findings in ulnar-sided wrist impaction syndromes. Radiographics 2002; 22(1):105–121

Cheng EY, Thongtrangan I, Laorr A, Saleh KJ. Spontaneous resolution of osteonecrosis of the femoral head. J Bone Joint Surg Am 2004; 86-A(12):2594–2599

Clavero JA, Alomar X, Monill JM, et al. MR imaging of ligament and tendon injuries of the fingers. Radiographics 2002; 22(2):237–256

Davies AM, Vanel D. Follow-up of musculoskeletal tumors. I. Local recurrence. Eur Radiol 1998; 8(5):791–799

Davies AM, Hall AD, Strouhal PD, Evans N, Grimer RJ. The MR imaging appearances and natural history of seromas following excision of soft tissue tumours. Eur Radiol 2004; 14(7):1196–1202

Davies M, Cassar-Pullicino VN, Davies AM, McCall IW, Tyrrell PN. The diagnostic accuracy of MR imaging in osteoid osteoma. Skeletal Radiol 2002; 31(10):559–569

Dehdashti F, Siegel BA, Griffeth LK, et al. Benign versus malignant intraosseous lesions: discrimination by means of PET with 2-[F-18]fluoro-2-deoxy-D-glucose. Radiology 1996; 200(1):243–247

Drape JL, Guerini H, Duffaut-Andreux C. Musculoskeletal radiology. J Radiol 2004; 85(7–8):973–978

Duc SR, Mengiardi B, Pfirrmann CW, Jost B, Hodler J, Zanetti M. Diagnostic performance of MR arthrography after rotator cuff repair. AJR Am J Roentgenol 2006; 186(1):237–241

Dupuy DE, Hangen DH, Zachazewski JE, Boland AL, Palmer W. Kinematic CT of the patellofemoral joint. AJR Am J Roentgenol 1997; 169(1):211–215

Elfering A, Semmer N, Birkhofer D, Zanetti M, Hodler J, Boos N. Risk factors for lumbar disc degeneration: a 5-year prospective MRI study in asymptomatic individuals. Spine 2002; 27(2):125–134

Elias DA, White LM, Fithian DC. Acute lateral patellar dislocation at MR imaging: injury patterns of medial patellar soft-tissue restraints and osteochondral injuries of the inferomedial patella. Radiology 2002; 225(3):736–743

Erickson SJ. High-resolution imaging of the musculoskeletal system. Radiology 1997; 205(3):593–618

Fayad LM, Johnson P, Fishman EK. Multidetector CT of musculoskeletal disease in the pediatric patient: principles, techniques, and clinical applications. Radiographics 2005; 25(3):603–618

Feldman F, Staron R, Zwass A, Rubin S, Haramati N. MR imaging: its role in detecting occult fractures. Skeletal Radiol 1994; 23(6):439–444

Garcia R, Kim EE, Wong FC, Korkmaz M, Wong WH, Yang DJ, et al. Comparison of fluorine-18-FDG PET and technetium-99m-MIBI SPECT in evaluation of musculoskeletal sarcomas. J Nucl Med 1996; 37(9):1476–1479

Geijer M, El-Khoury GY. MDCT in the evaluation of skeletal trauma: principles, protocols, and clinical applications. Emerg Radiol 2006; 13(1):7–18

Gil HC, Levine SM, Zoga AC. MRI findings in the subchondral bone marrow: a discussion of conditions including transient osteoporosis, transient bone marrow edema syndrome, SONK, and shifting bone marrow edema of the knee. Semin Musculoskelet Radiol 2006; 10(3):177–186

Gilbert FJ, Grant AM, Gillan MG, et al. Low back pain: influence of early MR imaging or CT on treatment and outcome – multicenter randomized trial. Radiology 2004; 231(2):343–351

Gillan MG, Gilbert FJ, Andrew JE, et al. Influence of imaging on clinical decision making in the treatment of lower back pain. Radiology 2001; 220(2):393–399

Glaves J. The use of radiological guidelines to achieve a sustained reduction in the number of radiographic examinations of the cervical spine, lumbar spine and knees performed for GPs. Clin Radiol 2005; 60(8):914–920

Gottlieb RH. Imaging for whom: patient or physician? AJR Am J Roentgenol 2005; 185(6):1399–1403

Haig AJ, Geisser ME, Tong HC, et al. Electromyographic and magnetic resonance imaging to predict lumbar stenosis, low-back pain, and no back symptoms. J Bone Joint Surg Am 2007; 89(2):358–366

Hernigou P, Poignard A, Nogier A, Manicom O. Fate of very small asymptomatic stage-I osteonecrotic lesions of the hip. J Bone Joint Surg Am 2004; 86-A(12):2589–2593

Hodler J, Resnick D. Current status of imaging of articular cartilage. Skeletal Radiol 1996; 25(8):703–709

Jacobson JA. Musculoskeletal ultrasound and MRI: which do I choose? Semin Musculoskelet Radiol 2005; 9(2):135–149

Jee WH, McCauley TR, Kim JM, et al. Meniscal tear configurations: categorization with MR imaging. AJR Am J Roentgenol 2003; 180(1):93–97

Kirwan JR. Conceptual issues in scoring radiographic progression in rheumatoid arthritis. J Rheumatol 1999; 26(3):720–725

Kiuru MJ, Pihlajamaki HK, Hietanen HJ, Ahovuo JA. MR imaging, bone scintigraphy, and radiography in bone stress injuries of the pelvis and the lower extremity. Acta Radiol 2002; 43(2):207–212

Kjaer P, Leboeuf-Yde C, Korsholm L, Sorensen JS, Bendix T. Magnetic resonance imaging and low back pain in adults: a diagnostic imaging study of 40-year-old men and women. Spine 2005; 30(10):1173–1180

Kobayashi Y, Kimura M, Higuchi H, Terauchi M, Shirakura K, Takagishi K. Juxta-articular bone marrow signal changes on magnetic resonance imaging following arthroscopic meniscectomy. Arthroscopy 2002; 18(3):238–245

Koulouris G, Connell D. Hamstring muscle complex: an imaging review. Radiographics 2005; 25(3):571–586

Kransdorf MJ. Benign soft-tissue tumors in a large referral population: distribution of specific diagnoses by age, sex, and location. AJR Am J Roentgenol 1995; 164(2):395–402

Kransdorf MJ. Malignant soft-tissue tumors in a large referral population: distribution of diagnoses by age, sex, and location. AJR Am J Roentgenol 1995; 164(1):129–134

Lang P, Honda G, Roberts T, Vahlensieck M, Johnston JO, Rosenau W, et al. Musculoskeletal neoplasm: perineoplastic edema versus tumor on dynamic postcontrast MR images with spatial mapping of instantaneous enhancement rates. Radiology 1995; 197(3):831–839

Leunig M, Beck M, Kalhor M, Kim YJ, Werlen S, Ganz R. Fibrocystic changes at anterosuperior femoral neck: prevalence in hips with femoroacetabular impingement. Radiology 2005; 236(1):237–246

Llauger J, Palmer J, Roson N, Bague S, Camins A, Cremades R. Nonseptic monoarthritis: imaging features with clinical and histopathologic correlation. Radiographics 2000; 20 Spec No:S263–S278

Low G, Raby N. Can follow-up radiography for acute scaphoid fracture still be considered a valid investigation? Clin Radiol 2005; 60(10):1106–1110

Ma LD, Frassica FJ, McCarthy EF, Bluemke DA, Zerhouni EA. Benign and malignant musculoskeletal masses: MR imaging differentiation with rim-to-center differential enhancement ratios. Radiology 1997; 202(3):739–744

Mackenzie R, Dixon AK, Keene GS, Hollingworth W, Lomas DJ, Villar RN. Magnetic resonance imaging of the knee: assessment of effectiveness. Clin Radiol 1996; 51(4):245–250

Malizos KN, Zibis AH, Dailiana Z, Hantes M, Karachalios T, Karantanas AH. MR imaging findings in transient osteoporosis of the hip. Eur J Radiol 2004; 50(3):238–244

Matava MJ, Eck K, Totty W, Wright RW, Shively RA. Magnetic resonance imaging as a tool to predict meniscal reparability. Am J Sports Med 1999; 27(4):436–443

McQueen FM, Stewart N, Crabbe J, Robinson E, Yeoman S, Tan PL, et al. Magnetic resonance imaging of the wrist in early rheumatoid arthritis reveals a high prevalence of erosions at four months after symptom onset. Ann Rheum Dis 1998 Jun;57(6):350–6

Milette PC, Fontaine S, Lepanto L, Dery R, Breton G. Clinical impact of contrast-enhanced MR imaging reports in patients with previous lumbar disk surgery. AJR Am J Roentgenol 1996; 167(1):217–223

Milette PC. Reporting lumbar disk abnormalities: at last, consensus! AJNR Am J Neuroradiol 2001; 22(3):428–429

Mitra D, Cassar-Pullicino VN, McCall IW. Longitudinal study of vertebral type-1 end-plate changes on MR of the lumbar spine. Eur Radiol 2004; 14(9):1574–1581

Modic MT. Degenerative disc disease and back pain. Magn Reson Imaging Clin N Am 1999; 7(3):481–491, viii

Modic MT, Obuchowski NA, Ross JS, et al. Acute low back pain and radiculopathy: MR imaging findings and their prognostic role and effect on outcome. Radiology 2005; 237(2):597–604

Mohana-Borges AV, Chung CB, Resnick D. Superior labral anteroposterior tear: classification and diagnosis on MRI and MR arthrography. AJR Am J Roentgenol 2003; 181(6):1449–1462

Moore SL, Teirstein A, Golimbu C. MRI of sarcoidosis patients with musculoskeletal symptoms. AJR Am J Roentgenol 2005; 185(1):154–159

Morag Y, Jacobson JA, Shields G, et al. MR arthrography of rotator interval, long head of the biceps brachii, and biceps pulley of the shoulder. Radiology 2005; 235(1):21–30

Muller R, Hildebrand T, Ruegsegger P. Non-invasive bone biopsy: a new method to analyse and display the three-dimensional structure of trabecular bone. Phys Med Biol 1994; 39(1):145–164

Munter FM, Wasserman BA, Wu HM, Yousem DM. Serial MR Imaging of Annular Tears in Lumbar Intervertebral Disks. AJNR Am J Neuroradiol 2002; 23(7):1105–1109

Murphey MD, Robbin MR, McRae GA, Flemming DJ, Temple HT, Kransdorf MJ. The many faces of osteosarcoma. Radiographics 1997; 17(5):1205–1231

Murphey MD, Smith WS, Smith SE, Kransdorf MJ, Temple HT. From the archives of the AFIP. Imaging of musculoskeletal neurogenic tumors: radiologic-pathologic correlation. Radiographics 1999; 19(5):1253–1280

Murphey MD, Carroll JF, Flemming DJ, Pope TL, Gannon FH, Kransdorf MJ. From the archives of the AFIP: benign musculoskeletal lipomatous lesions. Radiographics 2004; 24(5):1433–1466

Narvaez JA, Narvaez J, Ortega R, Aguilera C, Sanchez A, Andia E. Painful heel: MR imaging findings. Radiographics 2000; 20(2):333–352

Neyman EG, Corl FS, Fishman EK. 3D-CT evaluation of metallic implants: principles, techniques, and applications. Crit Rev Comput Tomogr 2002; 43(6):419–452

Nikken JJ, Oei EH, Ginai AZ, et al. Acute peripheral joint injury: cost and effectiveness of low-field-strength MR imaging – results of randomized controlled trial. Radiology 2005; 236(3):958–967

Pfirrmann CW, Theumann NH, Chung CB, Botte MJ, Trudell DJ, Resnick D. What happens to the triangular fibrocartilage complex during pronation and supination of the forearm? Analysis of its morphology and diagnostic assessment with MR arthrography. Skeletal Radiol 2001; 30(12):677–685

Pfirrmann CW, Mengiardi B, Dora C, Kalberer F, Zanetti M, Hodler J. Cam and pincer femoroacetabular impingement: characteristic MR arthrographic findings in 50 patients. Radiology 2006; 240(3):778–785

Potter HG, Weinstein M, Allen AA, Wickiewicz TL, Helfet DL. Magnetic resonance imaging of the multiple-ligament injured knee. J Orthop Trauma 2002; 16(5):330–339

Ramnath RR, Kattapuram SV. MR appearance of SONK-like subchondral abnormalities in the adult knee: SONK redefined. Skeletal Radiol 2004; 33(10):575–581

Recht MP, Goodwin DW, Winalski CS, White LM. MRI of articular cartilage: revisiting current status and future directions. AJR Am J Roentgenol 2005; 185(4):899–914

Resnick D, Niwayama G, Guerra J Jr, Vint V, Usselman J. Spinal vacuum phenomena: anatomical study and review. Radiology 1981; 139(2):341–348

Robertson DD, Walker PS, Granholm JW, et al. Design of custom hip stem prostheses using three-dimensional CT modeling. J Comput Assist Tomogr 1987; 11(5):804–809

Roposch A, Wright JG. Increased diagnostic information and understanding disease: uncertainty in the diagnosis of developmental hip dysplasia. Radiology 2007; 242(2):355–359

Rosenberg AE. Malignant fibrous histiocytoma: past, present, and future. Skeletal Radiol 2003; 32(11):613–618

Rosenthal DI, Hornicek FJ, Wolfe MW, Jennings LC, Gebhardt MC, Mankin HJ. Percutaneous radiofrequency coagulation of osteoid osteoma compared with operative treatment. J Bone Joint Surg Am 1998; 80(6):815–821

Rupp S, Seil R, Jochum P, Kohn D. Popliteal cysts in adults. Prevalence, associated intraarticular lesions, and results after arthroscopic treatment. Am J Sports Med 2002; 30(1):112–115

Sabharwal S, Zhao C, McKeon J, Melaghari T, Blacksin M, Wenekor C. Reliability analysis for radiographic measurement of limb length discrepancy: full-length standing anteroposterior radiograph versus scanogram. J Pediatr Orthop 2007; 27(1):46–50

Sanders TG, Medynski MA, Feller JF, Lawhorn KW. Bone contusion patterns of the knee at MR imaging: footprint of the mechanism of injury. Radiographics 2000; 20 Spec No:S135–S151

Santiago RC, Gimenez CR, McCarthy K. Imaging of osteomyelitis and musculoskeletal soft tissue infections: current concepts. Rheum Dis Clin North Am 2003; 29(1):89–109

Schweitzer ME, Morrison WB. MR imaging of the diabetic foot. Radiol Clin North Am 2004; 42(1):61–71, vi

Shapeero LG, Vanel D, Verstraete KL, Bloem JL. Fast magnetic resonance imaging with contrast for soft tissue sarcoma viability. Clin Orthop Relat Res 2002; (397):212–227

Shepard MF, Hunter DM, Davies MR, Shapiro MS, Seeger LL. The clinical significance of anterior horn meniscal tears diagnosed on magnetic resonance images. Am J Sports Med 2002; 30(2):189–192

Sims WF, Jacobson KE. The posteromedial corner of the knee: medial-sided injury patterns revisited. Am J Sports Med 2004; 32(2):337–345

Teefey SA, Rubin DA, Middleton WD, Hildebolt CF, Leibold RA, Yamaguchi K. Detection and quantification of rotator cuff tears. Comparison of ultrasonographic, magnetic resonance imaging, and arthroscopic findings in seventy-one consecutive cases. J Bone Joint Surg Am 2004; 86-A(4):708–716

Thain LM, Adler RS. Sonography of the rotator cuff and biceps tendon: technique, normal anatomy, and pathology. J Clin Ultrasound 1999; 27(8):446–458

Theumann NH, Pfirrmann CW, Chung CB, Antonio GE, Trudell DJ, Resnick D. Ligamentous and tendinous anatomy of the intermetacarpal and common carpometacarpal joints: evaluation with MR imaging and MR arthrography. J Comput Assist Tomogr 2002; 26(1):145–152

Theumann NH, Etechami G, Duvoisin B, et al. Association between extrinsic and intrinsic carpal ligament injuries at MR arthrography and carpal instability at radiography: initial observations. Radiology 2006; 238(3):950–957

Vande Berg BC, Malghem J, Lecouvet FE, Maldague B. Magnetic resonance imaging of normal bone marrow. Eur Radiol 1998; 8(8):1327–1334

Vanel D, Shapeero LG, Tardivon A, Western A, Guinebretiere JM. Dynamic contrast-enhanced MRI with subtraction of aggressive soft tissue tumors after resection. Skeletal Radiol 1998; 27(9):505–510

Verstraete KL, Van der Woude HJ, Hogendoorn PC, DeDeene Y, Kunnen M, Bloem JL. Dynamic contrast-enhanced MR imaging of musculoskeletal tumors: basic principles and clinical applications. J Magn Reson Imaging 1996; 6(2):311–321

Vilanova JC, Woertler K, Narvaez JA, et al. Soft-tissue tumors update: MR imaging features according to the WHO classification. Eur Radiol 2007; 17(1):125–138

Vincken PW, Ter Braak BP, van Erkell AR, et al. Effectiveness of MR imaging in selection of patients for arthroscopy of the knee. Radiology 2002; 223(3):739–746

Waldschmidt JG, Rilling RJ, Kajdacsy-Balla AA, Boynton MD, Erickson SJ. In vitro and in vivo MR imaging of hyaline cartilage: zonal anatomy, imaging pitfalls, and pathologic conditions. Radiographics 1997; 17(6):1387–1402

Younger AS, Sawatzky B, Dryden P. Radiographic assessment of adult flatfoot. Foot Ankle Int 2005; 26(10):820–825

Zanetti M, Bruder E, Romero J, Hodler J. Bone marrow edema pattern in osteoarthritic knees: correlation between MR imaging and histologic findings. Radiology 2000; 215(3):835–840

F. Bravo-Rodriguez and Rocio Diaz-Aguilera

Introduction

Neuroradiology is the branch of radiology dealing with both diagnostic and interventional aspects of the central nervous system (CNS) and head and neck.

The introduction of computed tomography (CT) in 1972 and magnetic resonance imaging (MRI) in 1981 have contributed greatly to this highly specialized radiological subspecialty.

Moreover, radiologists working in the interventional branch of neuroradiology must acquire specialized manual and surgical skills in addition to extensive knowledge of anatomy, physiology, pathology, and diagnostic techniques required of all neuroradiologists.

Thus, neuroradiology comprises two closely related disciplines which are, at the same time, clearly different from each other. On the one hand, diagnostic neuroradiology based on noninvasive imaging modalities and, on the other hand, interventional neuroradiology, based on digital subtraction angiography (DSA), which permits the treatment of many neurological conditions by means of endovascular approaches.

Neuroradiology is widely connected to many specialities such as neurology, neurosurgery, otolaryngology, oral and maxillofacial surgery, among others, and neuroradiologists work in close contact with specialists in these fields, enabling faster and more accurate diagnoses through imaging modalities such as conventional X-ray, ultrasound, CT, and/or MRI. Moreover, interventional neuroradiologists contribute to the management of numerous neurological conditions through minimally invasive procedures such as extracranial or intracranial stenting in cases of arterial stenoses, endovascular treatment of intracranial aneurysms, embolization of head and neck tumors, etc.

The current scope of this radiological discipline is extensive and its future is promising. The advent of functional MR imaging, diffusion-weighted imaging, and perfusion-weighted imaging, have replaced the mere anatomical view of classic neuroradiology with a wider perspective that includes cerebral pathophysiology. Furthermore, recent research into endovascular stem cell implantation opens a new and fascinating field with regard to the treatment of strokes and degenerative diseases.

Case 1
■
Meningioma

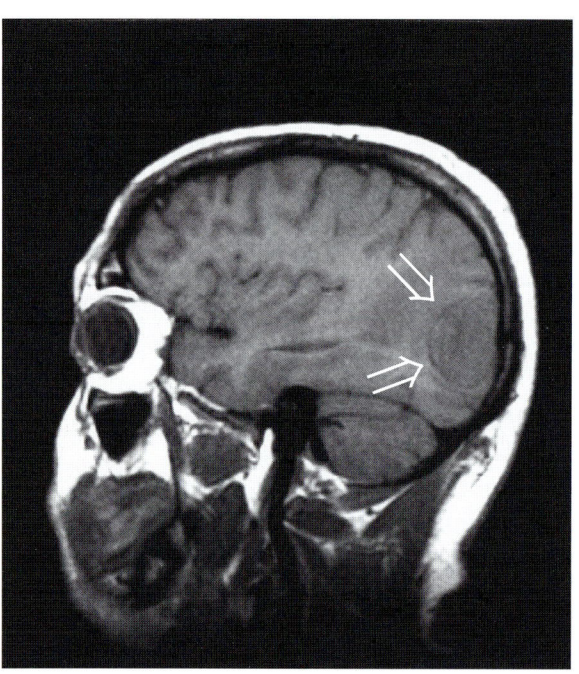

Fig. 7.1.1

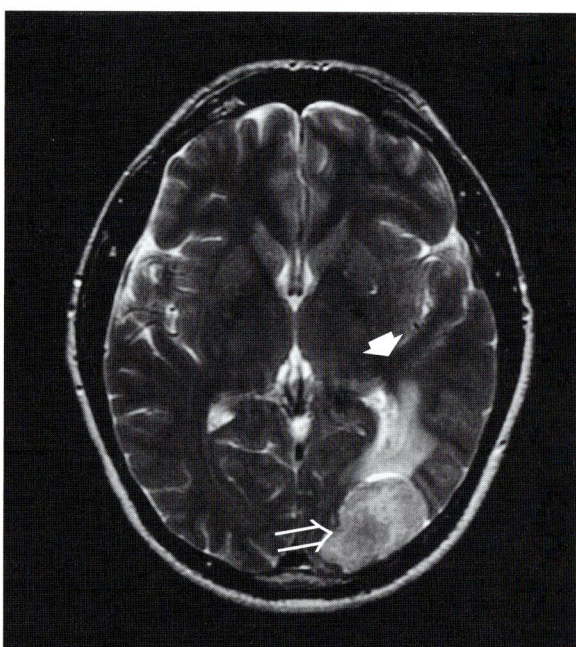

Fig. 7.1.2

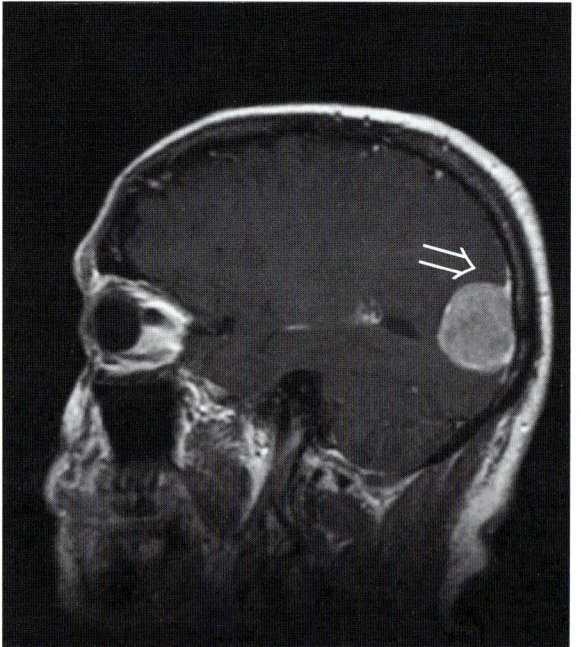

Fig. 7.1.3

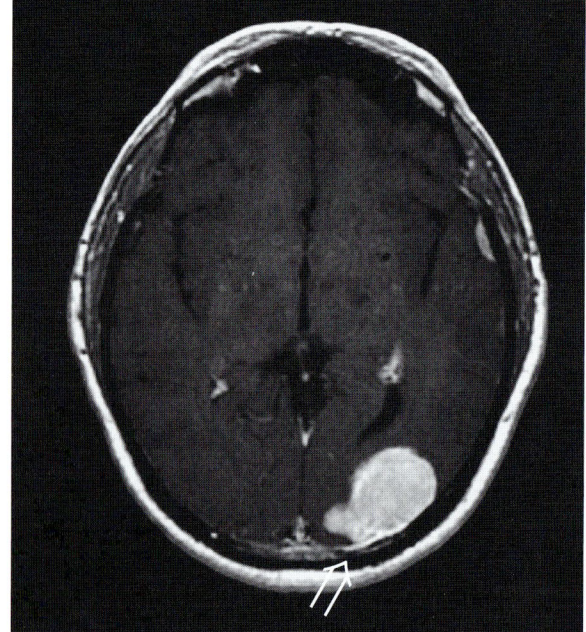

Fig. 7.1.4

A 43-year-old man with no relevant past medical history was admitted to the emergency room with a 10 minute seizure. The patient presented a slight decrease in cognitive function in the postcritical period. The clinical examination was otherwise unremarkable. Brain MRI showed several extraaxial lesions consistent with multiple meningiomas.

Comments

Meningiomas are tumors that arise from arachnoid cap cells, which reside in the arachnoid layer covering the surface of the brain. They account for 13–20% of all primary intracranial tumors in adulthood. There is a female predilection (1.5:1 to 3:1) and the mean age of presentation is over 50 years. Meningiomas are multiple in 5–40% of cases, and multiple lesions are more frequent in patients suffering from neurofibromatosis-2 (NF-2), an inheritable disorder with an autosomal dominant mode of transmission secondary to a mutation of a gene located on chromosome 22.

Meningiomas are supratentorial in up to 90% of cases. The most common locations are the parasagittal region (25%), convexity (20%), and sphenoid ridge (15%). Clinical manifestations depend on location. Symptoms of a meningioma in the convexity or parasagittal region are seizures, focal neurological deficits, or headaches; sphenoid meningiomas can cause visual problems or facial numbness. Complete surgical resection is the treatment of choice.

Imaging Findings

On CT scans, meningiomas are usually dural-based tumors that are slightly hyperattenuating in up to 70% of cases. They enhance homogeneously and intensely after the injection of iodinated contrast material. In nearly 25% of cases, calcifications are present. Hyperostosis of the adjacent bone can be seen in some cases.

On T1-weighted images (Fig. 7.1.1), most meningiomas have similar signal intensity to cortical gray matter. Meningiomas present as extraaxial masses with a broad dural attachment and a thin hypointense rim/cleft (*open arrow*) between the tumor and the brain, corresponding to cerebrospinal fluid.

On T2-weighted images (Fig. 7.1.2), meningiomas may have different appearances. In general, the tumor is hypointense to gray matter if calcium or fibrotic components are present (*open arrow*). Meningiomas can show extensive perilesional edema (*solid arrow*).

After the injection of gadolinium, these tumors show intense and homogeneous enhancement. In a majority of cases, enhancing of the tissue that surrounds the dural attachment is seen; this radiological finding is known as the dural tail (Figs. 7.1.3 and 7.1.4, *open arrows*).

Digital subtraction angiography – not shown – showed meningeal arteries penetrating into the tumor through its dural attachment, with inside branches with a characteristic radial distribution. Homogeneous sharp tumor staining was seen in early and late phases.

Although complete surgical resection is the treatment of choice for benign meningiomas, preoperative embolization to reduce the blood supply to the tumor may be useful.

Case 2
■ Multiple Sclerosis

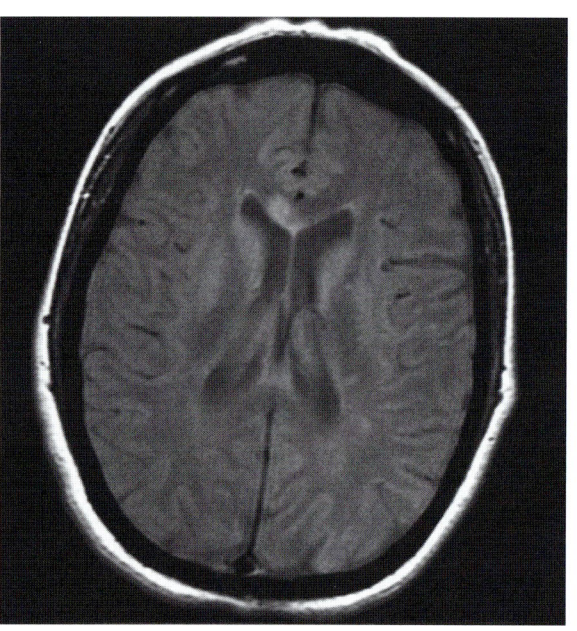

Fig. 7.2.1

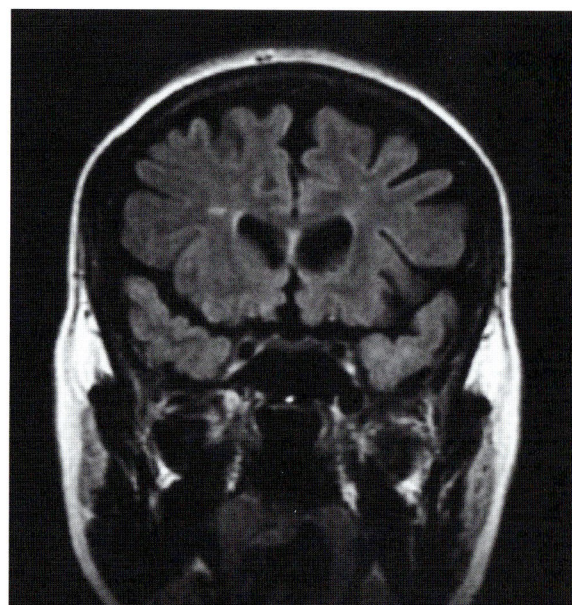

Fig. 7.2.2

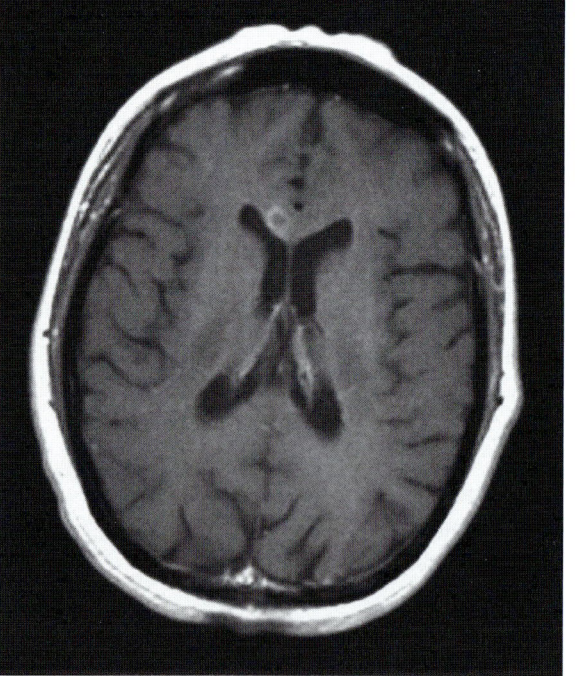

Fig. 7.2.3

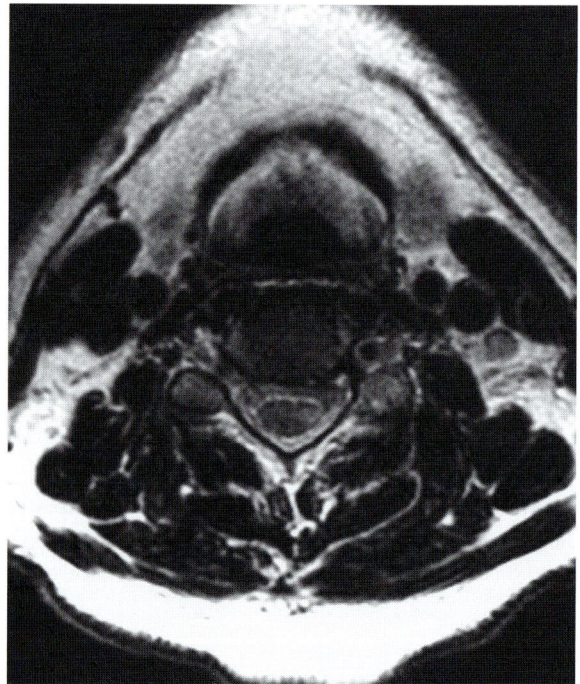

Fig. 7.2.4

A 40-year-old woman with sudden left-limb monoparesis and hyporeflexia. Cerebral MRI showed lesions consistent with multiple sclerosis.

Multiple sclerosis (MS) is an inflammatory, demyelinating disease of the central nervous system (CNS). It is considered an autoimmune disease. MS most commonly afflicts young people between the ages of 20 and 30 years, but any age group can be affected. It has a prevalence of nearly 100 cases per 100,000 inhabitants. MS affects females more than males (2:1).

Optic neuritis (ON) or other isolated neurological symptoms are the usual initial presentation. The disease can present in different forms, such as primary progressive, relapsing remitting, or relapsing progressive. MS diagnosis is mainly based on the clinical symptoms. Visual evoked potential testing and laboratory studies are useful as well; oligoclonal bands of IgG are demonstrated in cerebrospinal fluid samples in approximately 85% of patients with MS. With the advent of MRI, the ability to confirm the diagnosis of MS has improved dramatically. On MRI, MS lesions are detected in up to 95% of patients. Newer MRI techniques promise to yield important information regarding MS heterogeneity, prognosis, and treatment effects.

Currently, the Barkhof MRI criteria are applied to establish the diagnosis in patients with clinically isolated syndromes suggestive of MS.

Spatial progress criteria
9 T2-weighted images lesions or 1 enhancing lesion
1 or more infratentorial lesions
1 or more juxtacortical lesions
3 or more periventricular lesions

Time progress criteria
1 new enhancing lesion 3 months after an acute attack
New lesions on T2-weighted images or new enhancing lesions 6 months after a first episode of symptoms suggestive of MS

No highly effective treatment is currently available to counteract acute MS attacks after their onset. The most widely used therapy is high-dose intravenous steroids. This medication may help expedite the timing of recovery but will not affect the actual degree of recovery. To prevent relapses or disease progression, immunomodulatory drugs (e.g., interferon) are used with different results.

MRI characteristically shows lesions of high T2, PD and FLAIR signal intensity of variable location in the white matter of the brain, brain stem, optic nerves, or spinal cord. In typical cases, the lesions tend to occur in periventricular areas (Fig. 7.2.1) and may affect in the corpus callosum. They have an ovoid shape with their largest axis oriented perpendicular to the ventricular surface (Fig. 7.2.2); they typically involve only the white matter and usually present peripheral enhancement after gadolinium administration (Fig. 7.2.3).

Spinal cord lesions are detected in 75% of cases. They usually appear in the cervical spine and present a vertical orientation (Fig. 7.2.4).

Case 3
Cerebral Abscess

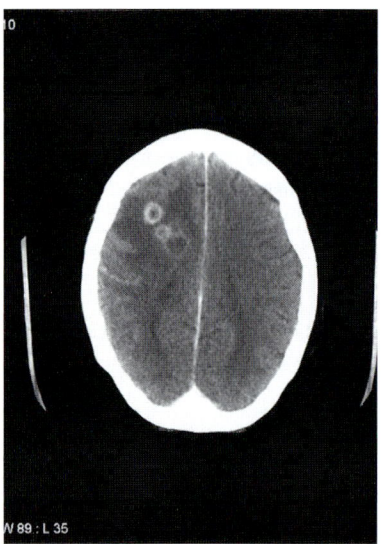

Fig. 7.3.1

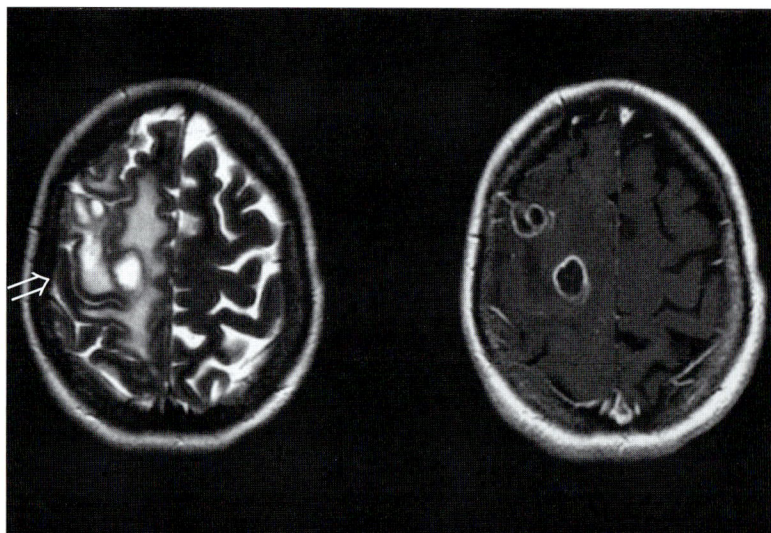

Fig. 7.3.2

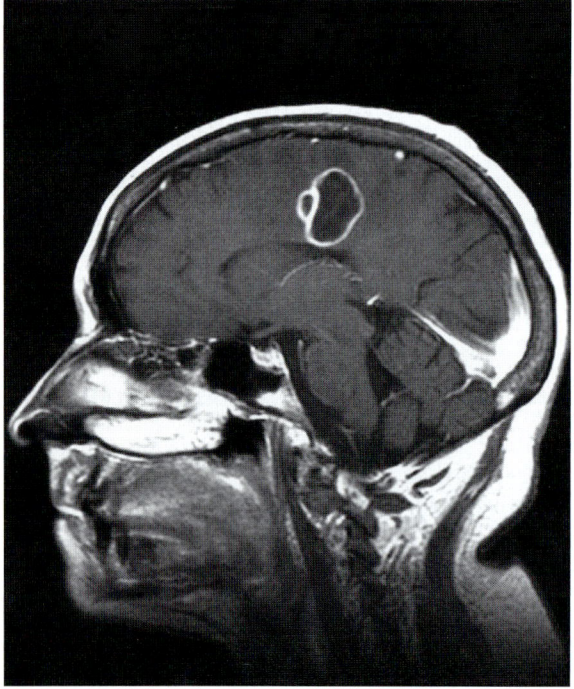

Fig. 7.3.3

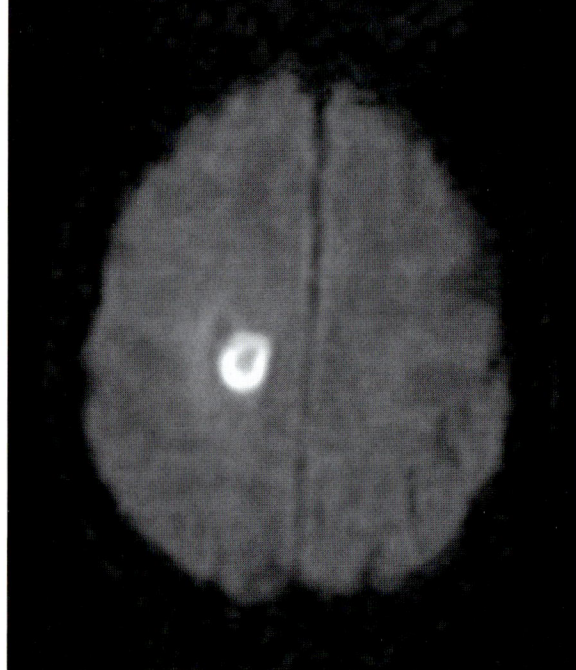

Fig. 7.3.4

A 32-year-old woman presented with a 24 hour history of progressive holocranial headache and left hemiparesis. She had a recent history of upper tooth arcade phlegmon. On physical examination, severe left hemiparesis and facial palsy were found. Blood cultures revealed Staphylococcus hyicus. She was treated with cefotaxime and metronidazole. Unenhanced and contrast-enhanced CT scans showed right frontal lobe abscesses.

Comments

Brain abscess is a focal infectious process. Most commonly, microorganisms reach the CNS from a contiguous focus of infection, such as otitis media, mastoiditis, infection of the paranasal sinuses, or dental infection. Hematogenous spread from an extracranial site is also possible. The origin of the infection remains unknown in up to 10–40% of cases. Brain abscesses typically undergo four stages in their development: early cerebritis, late cerebritis, early capsule formation, and late capsule formation.

Brain abscesses are more common between the ages of 20 and 40 years and have a male predilection. They generally occur in the frontal and temporal lobes.

Clinical symptoms of cerebral abscess depend on the size and location of the space occupied and on the overall reaction of the brain to the presence of the organism. The most common symptom is headache, typically progressive and treatment-resistant. Other symptoms are fever, focal neurologic deficits, and decreased level of consciousness.

In adults, most brain abscesses are produced by gram-negative organisms in cases of hematogenous spread. In children, gram-positive bacteria from ENT entities are the most common microorganisms involved.

The treatment of choice is abscess drainage through aspiration of infectious material. Surgery is considered in cases of established abscesses. In early stages, intravenous antibiotic medication can be used. The current mortality rate is less than 10%.

Imaging Findings

CT manifestations of an intracranial abscess depend on the stage of abscess formation. During early cerebritis, unenhanced CT scans may demonstrate only poorly delineated hypodense areas surrounded by vasogenic edema. After contrast administration, an ill-defined and faint enhancing area within the edematous region can be seen. When an abscess capsule is present, an irregular enhancing rim surrounding a central low-attenuating area is shown (Fig. 7.3.1). Sometimes, satellite abscesses can be demonstrated.

On MRI, cerebritis appears as hypointense areas on T1-weighted images that are hyperintense on T2-weighted images, proton density-weighted and FLAIR images. After gadolinium administration, these areas present a similar pattern of enhancement to that of CT-scans. In advanced stages, the necrotic core is hyperintense on PD- and T2-weighted images and is surrounded by a variable degree of perilesional edema (Fig. 7.2.2, *open arrow*). The capsule enhances intensely following gadolinium administration (Figs. 7.2.2 and 7.3.3). On diffusion-weighted imaging (Fig. 7.3.4), abscesses present a strongly hyperintense signal; this MR sequence is of great value in differentiating brain abscesses from other entities with necrotic components, such as neoplasms and metastases, which appear hypointense.

Case 4
■
Acute Head Trauma

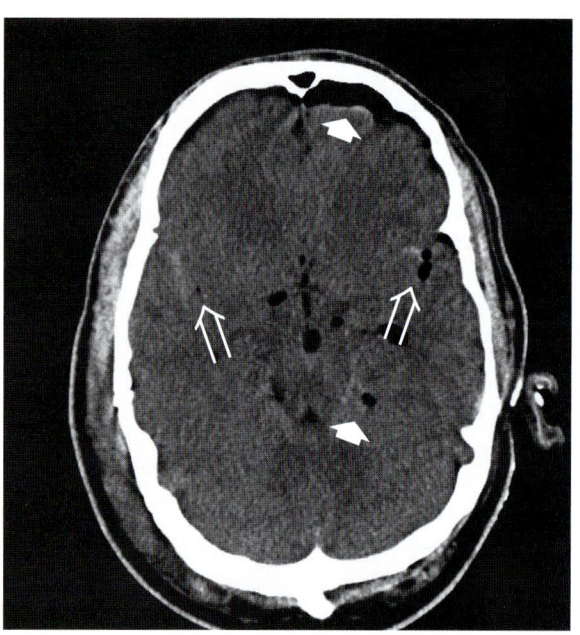

Fig. 7.4.1

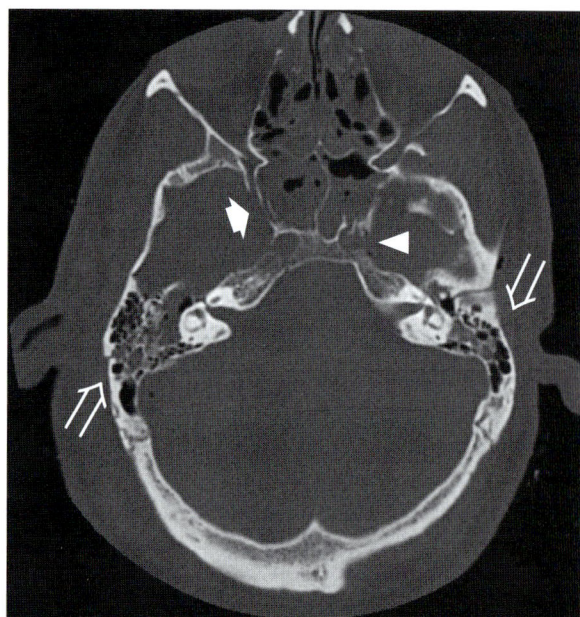

Fig. 7.4.2

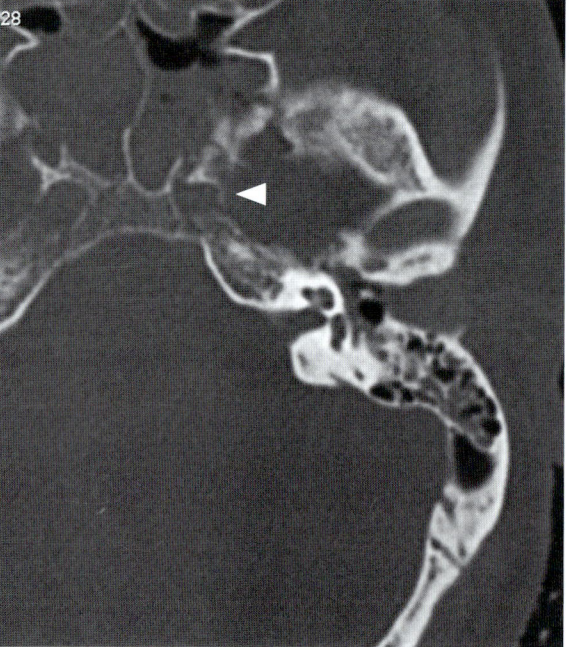

Fig. 7.4.3

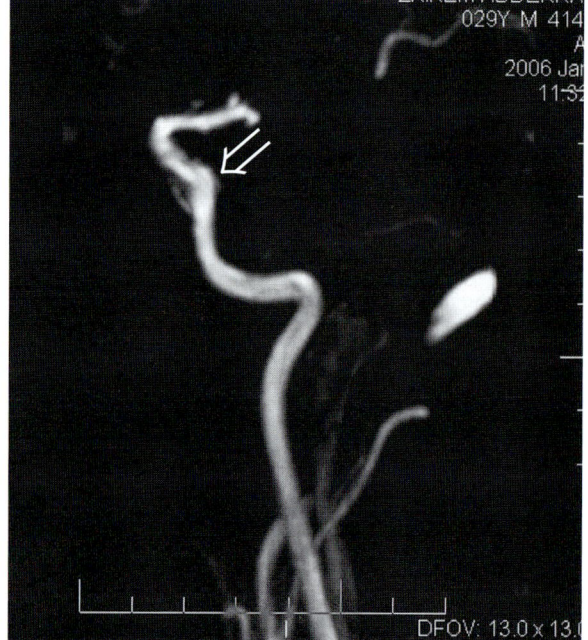

Fig. 7.4.4

A 30-year-old man was admitted to the emergency room with head trauma after a motor vehicle accident. He was alert and oriented but slightly agitated. On examination, bilateral otorrhea and probable left Horner's syndrome were found.

An urgent unenhanced CT of brain and skull base was performed. Diffusion-weighted MR imaging and extracranial MR angiography were carried out next.

Comments

Approximately 15% of head trauma patients die and another 15% present chronic impairment.

Primary and secondary injuries occur in head trauma. The primary injury occurs at the time of impact, either by a direct injury to the brain parenchyma or by an indirect injury to the long white matter tracts caused by acceleration-deceleration forces. Specific types of primary injury include scalp injury, skull fracture, cerebral contusion, subarachnoid hemorrhage, epidural hematoma, subdural hematoma, penetrating injuries, and diffuse axonal injury.

The secondary injury consists of systemic and intracranial events that occur in response to the primary injury and further contribute to neuronal damage and cell death. Secondary injuries include brain herniation, cerebral edema, ischemia, cerebral death, extracranial and intracranial vessel dissection, and carotid-cavernous fistula.

CT scanning is the imaging modality of choice in cases of severe head trauma. CT is widely available and has excellent sensitivity for the detection of hemorrhage and osseous involvement. Moreover, only a few minutes are required to perform the entire examination.

MRI is carried out when diffuse axonal injury is suspected because this entity may not be detected on CT.

CT and MR angiography may be useful to study intracranial or extracranial vessels in cases of suspected dissection. Digital subtraction angiography is performed in doubtful cases or for therapeutic purposes.

Imaging Findings

CT scan (Fig. 7.4.1) showing post-traumatic subarachnoid hemorrhage with blood within the Sylvian fissures (*open arrows*). Air bubbles consistent with pneumoencephalus are seen in the ventricular system and subarachnoid space (*solid arrows*).

CT scan of the skull base (Figs. 7.4.2 and 7.4.3) demonstrates several fractures affecting the petrous temporal bone (*open arrows*), paranasal sinuses (*solid arrow*), and left carotid channel (*arrowhead*).

MR angiography (Fig. 7.4.4) shows irregularity and enlargement of the cavernous segment of the left internal carotid artery consistent with post-traumatic pseudoaneurysm (*open arrow*).

Case 5

■
Stroke

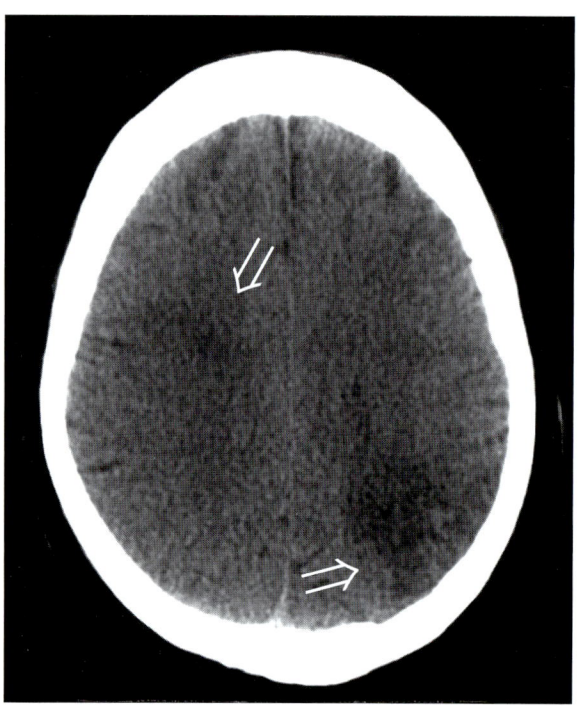

Fig. 7.5.1

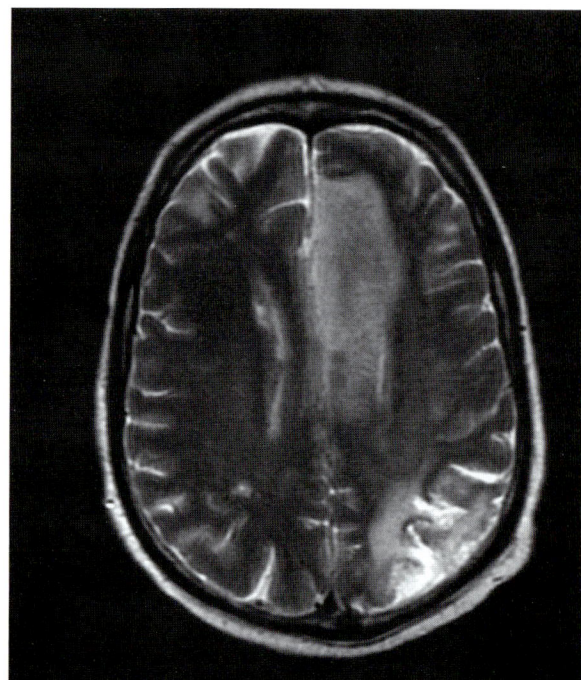

Fig. 7.5.2

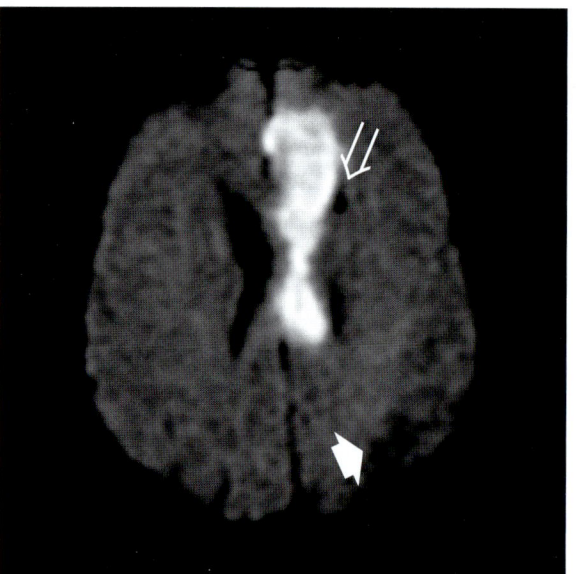

Fig. 7.5.3

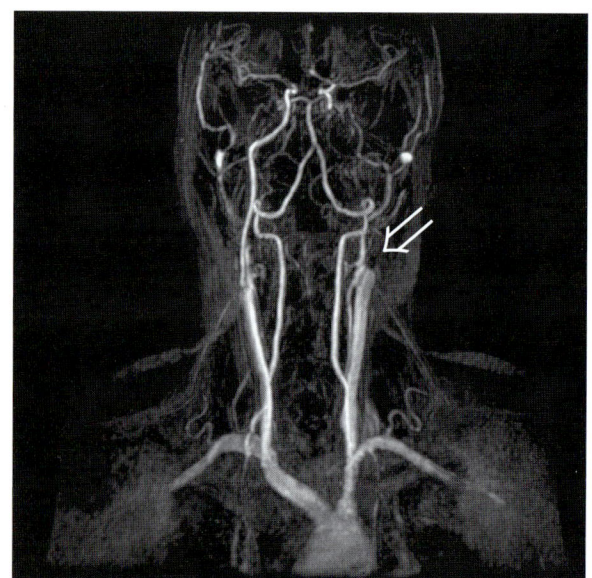

Fig. 7.5.4

A 57-year-old man presented with sudden aphasia and right hemiparesis. An urgent CT scan was performed and showed two old lesions. Brain MRI and MR angiography 24 hours later showed left anterior cerebral artery ischemic infarction.

Stroke is the third cause of death in the world and the first cause of disability, according to the WHO. Ischemic strokes represent nearly 80% of cases. At the macroscopic level, ischemic strokes most often are caused by extracranial embolism from the heart or extracranial arteries or intracranial thrombosis secondary to arterial stenosis or atherosclerosis; however, ischemic strokes may also be caused by a decrease in cerebral blood flow. At the cellular level, any process that disrupts blood flow to a portion of the brain unleashes an ischemic cascade, leading to the death of neurons and cerebral infarction. Clinically, the patient presents with an acute neurologic deficit which can be reversible (acute ischemic attack) or definitive (stroke).

Unenhanced CT has traditionally been considered the imaging method of choice. CT is fast and widely available; it is also very useful in distinguishing ischemic from hemorrhagic infarction. Unfortunately, CT scans are normal early after the onset of symptoms in up to 50% of patients.

The advent of new MRI sequences, especially diffusion-weighted MRI (DWI-MRI) with a higher sensitivity than standard unenhanced head CT in detecting infarcts early after symptom onset, has represented a huge advance in stroke diagnosis.

Recent multimodal CT and MR evaluations demonstrate not only the core area of infarction but also the surrounding area of oligemia (ischemic penumbra). On the other hand, CT and MR angiographies allow the evaluation of cerebral vessels showing possible vascular stenosis or occlusion.

Therapeutic procedures aim to open the occluded vessel as soon as possible because the duration of ischemia is the most important factor affecting prognosis – remember the catch phrase: "time is brain". Intravenous thrombolytic therapy is indicated within three hours of symptoms onset. This time window may be extended to 6 hours if fibrinolytic medication is administered intraarterially, or even longer if mechanical endovascular methods for clot retrieval are performed. Hopefully, multimodal techniques and new fibrinolytic agents will enable the therapeutic window to be extended beyond 3 or 6 hours.

CT scan (Fig. 7.5.1) demonstrates the presence of two old lesions (*open arrows*). No acute lesion is detected. T2-weighted image (Fig. 7.5.2) showing several hyperintense lesions located in the frontal parasagittal region and left posterior parietal region. On DWI-MRI (Fig. 7.5.3.), the frontal parasagittal lesion presents high signal intensity (acute lesion) (*open arrow*) in contrast with the hypointense parietal lesion (old lesion) (*arrow*).

Extracranial MR angiography (Fig. 7.5.4) shows left internal carotid artery occlusion (*open arrow*).

Case 6
■
Subarachnoid Hemorrhage

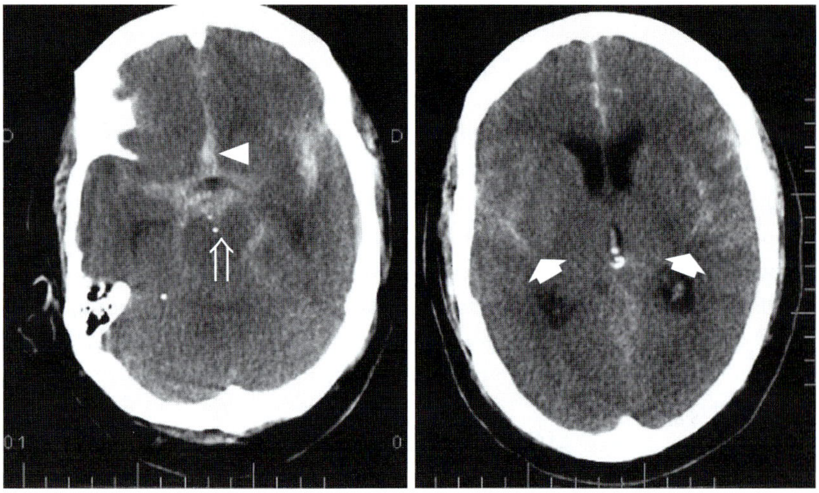

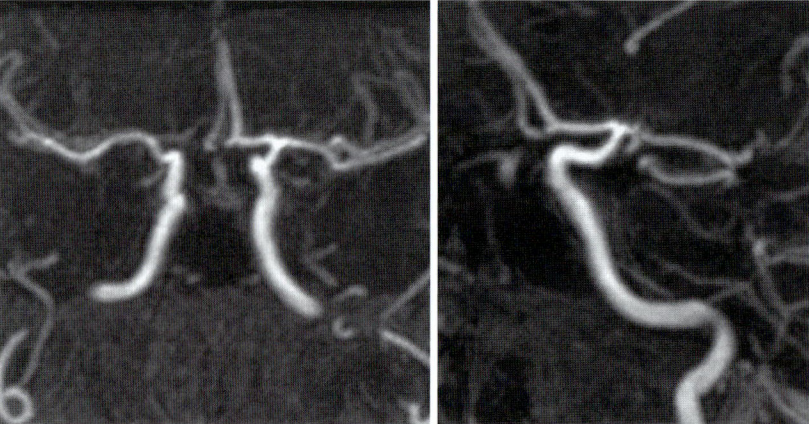

Fig. 7.6.1

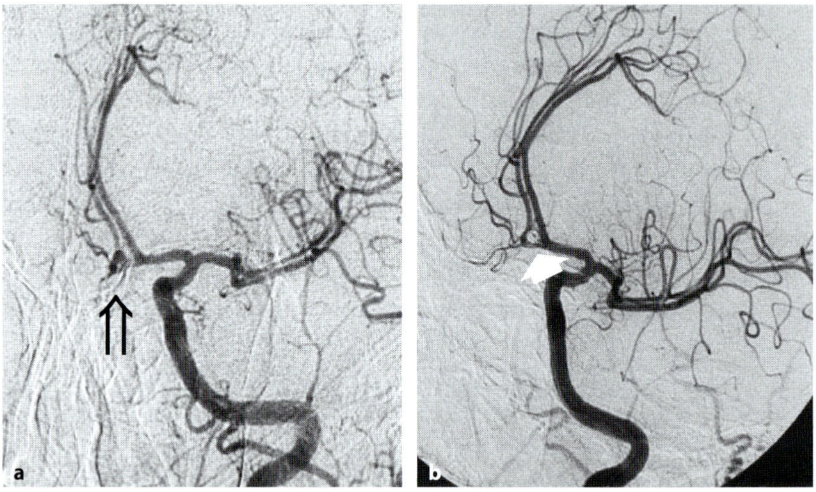

Fig. 7.6.2a,b

Fig. 7.6.3

A 47-year-old male was admitted to the emergency room with sudden occipital headache, vomiting, and progressive loss of consciousness. CT showed a subarachnoid hemorrhage. The patient was transferred to the intensive care unit and digital subtraction angiography (DSA) carried out 12 hours after the onset of symptoms revealed an anterior communicating artery aneurysm. In the same procedure, the aneurysm was completely occluded with GDC coils. A contrast-enhanced MRA performed 6 months after embolization for surveillance showed total occlusion of the aneurysm.

Comments

Subarachnoid hemorrhage (SAH), which implies the presence of blood within the subarachnoid space, could be traumatic or nontraumatic. The common medical use of the term SAH refers to the nontraumatic type, usually from rupture of an intracranial berry aneurysm (in 85% of cases), which accounts for 5% of strokes. The incidence is 6–8 events per 100,000 person years, being higher in women than in men.

The most common presentation is an unusually severe headache that starts suddenly. Other possible features are vomiting, focal deficits, and/or loss of consciousness.

The mortality rate is as high as 25 to 50%.

If SAH is suspected, unenhanced CT scan is the first-line imaging modality because the characteristically hyperdense appearance of extravasated blood in the basal cisterns and sulci is virtually pathognomonic. Additionally, the pattern of hemorrhage often suggests the location of any underlying aneurysm (sentinel clot). CT scanning presents a high sensitivity (93–100%) when it is performed within the first 24 hours.

Nevertheless, the method of choice to detect an intracranial aneurysm is DSA, which allows a better assessment of the architecture of the aneurysm in order to decide on the most appropriate therapeutic procedure, endovascular embolization (the current treatment of choice) or surgery.

On the other hand, as DSA is an invasive technique, other less invasive methods, such as CT-angiography or MR-angiography, should be considered during follow-up.

Imaging Findings

Unenhanced CT-scan showing SAH (Fig. 7.6.1) with blood in perimesencephalic cisterns (*open arrow*), SYLVIAN fissures (*arrows*), and sulci. Notice the sentinel clot in the anterior interhemispheric fissure (*arrowhead*).

DSA (Fig. 7.6.2a) reveals a 2 mm anterior communicating artery aneurysm (*open arrow*). DSA after coiling with GDC showing complete occlusion of the aneurysm (*arrow*) (Fig. 7.6.2b).

Gadolinium-enhanced MRA, MIP reconstruction, obtained 6 months after treatment (Fig. 7.6.3). No recurrence of the aneurysm is seen. Notice the magnetic susceptibility artifact secondary to the coils in the aneurysm. Magnetic susceptibility artifacts can be a limitation in the MRA follow-up of intracranial aneurysms.

Case 7
■
Cerebral Venous Thrombosis

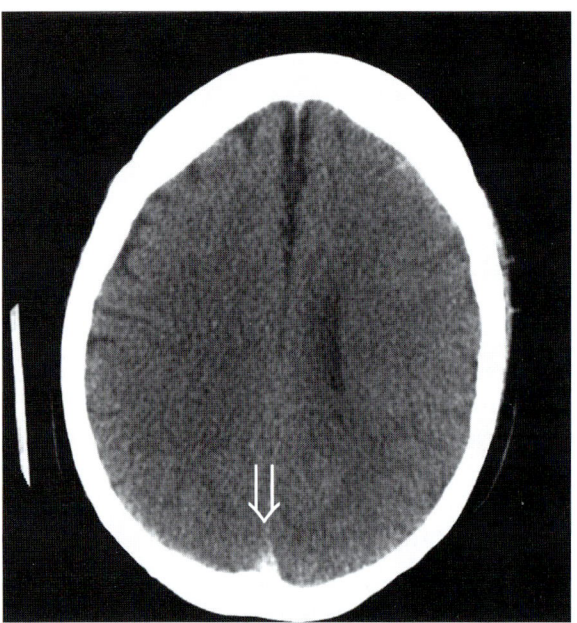

Fig. 7.7.1

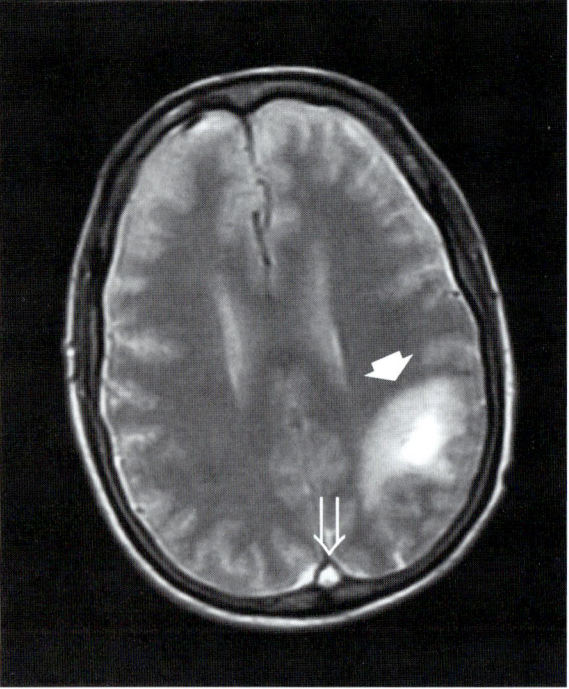

Fig. 7.7.3

Fig. 7.7.2

Fig. 7.7.4

A 24-year-old woman presented with headache and confusion followed by upper left limb paresthesia, incoordination, and motor dysphasia.

Cerebral venous thrombosis was suspected after an urgent CT scan. The diagnosis was confirmed by MRI and MR venography.

Cerebral venous thrombosis (CVT) represents 1% of all acute strokes. This entity consists of venous occlusion that may affect dural sinuses (venous dural thrombosis), cortical veins (cortical thrombosis), the internal cerebral veins, Galen veins, or sinus rectus (deep cerebral venous thrombosis). CVT is more common in women than men and has no age predilection. Over one hundred causative conditions have been described in CVT. In general, any condition that produces hypercoagulability or decreased cerebral blood flow may predispose to CVT, for instance, dehydratation, coagulopathies, pregnancy, oral contraceptives, infections, or malignancies. However, no cause is identified in approximately 25% of cases.

The most common presentation is progressive headache with nausea and vomiting. Focal neurologic deficits can occur as well.

The venous occlusion produces edema in the adjacent cerebral parenchyma. Venous thrombosis may progress to infarction, characteristically cortical and hemorrhagic. Prognosis is variable depending on the extension of thrombosis and the patient's clinical condition at admission.

Anticoagulation is the treatment of choice for CVT. Endovascular thrombolytic therapy is reserved for cases with unfavorable evolution despite anticoagulation.

Unenhanced CT may show a hyperattenuating sinus (*open arrow*) (Fig. 7.7.1) or a hyperdense cortical vein, known as the "cord sign". Cortical infarctions appear as hypodense cortical areas or hyperdense zones if hemorrhage is present. After contrast administration, the "empty delta sign", which corresponds to the filling defect of the clot inside the sinus, can be seen.

T1- and proton-density-weighted MR images show a lack of normal flow in the involved vessels and an increased signal within the thrombosed vein on all pulse sequences (*open arrows*) (Figs. 7.7.2 and 7.7.3). Edema or hemorrhage can be detected as well (*solid arrows*). After gadolinium administration , the empty delta sign can be seen.

MR venography may be useful for determining the extension of thrombosis. MR venography (Fig. 7.7.4) demonstrates enlargement of the affected sinus and filling defects (*open arrows*) secondary to the presence of thrombi.

Digital subtraction angiography (DSA) is not necessary in the majority of cases and is used only when the diagnosis is not clear.

Case 8
■
Cavernous Angioma

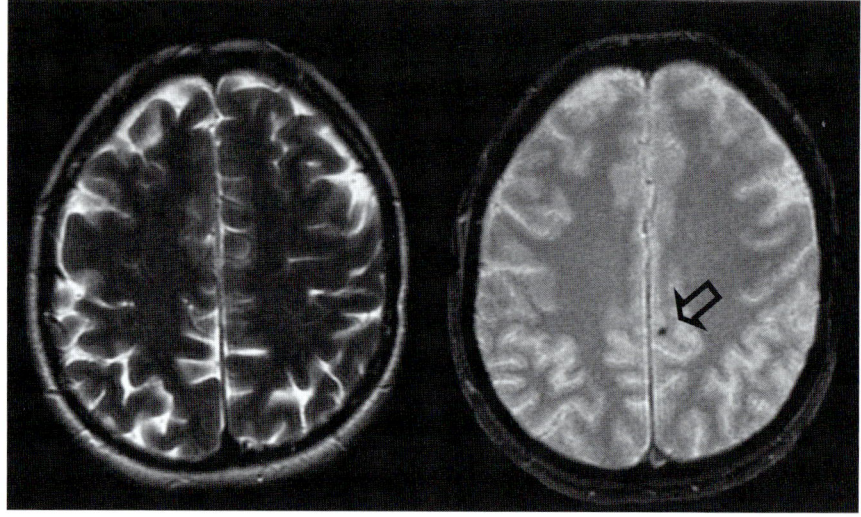

Fig. 7.8.1

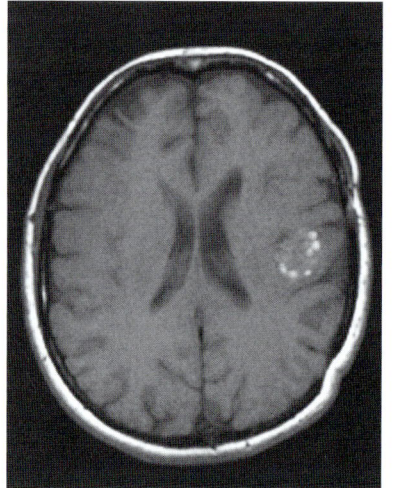

Fig. 7.8.2

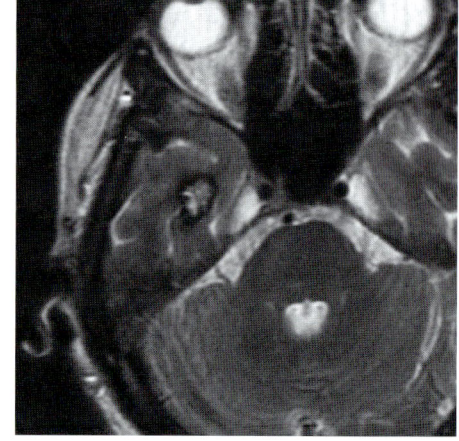

Fig. 7.8.3

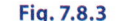

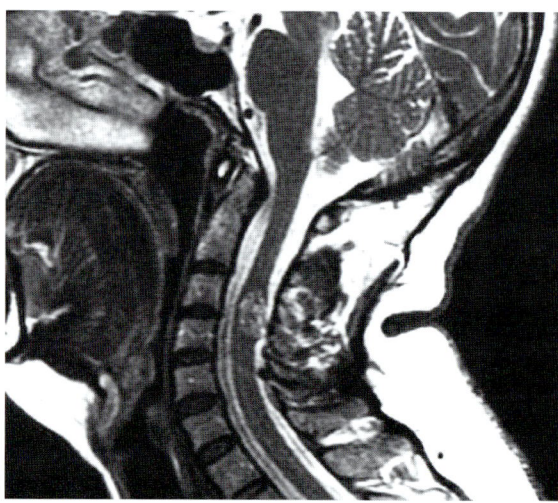

Fig. 7.8.4

A 35-year-old woman with a prior medical history of seizures and surgical resection of a cavernoma 10 years prior was being treated with carbamazepine and presented with isolated seizures. Brain and spine MRI were performed for surveillance of multiple cavernomatosis.

Comments

Cavernous malformations (cavernomas, cavernous angiomas, or hemangiomas,...) consist of well-circumscribed sinusoidal vascular channels containing blood in various stages of evolution. They represent approximately 1% of intracranial vascular lesions and 15% of cerebrovascular malformations. With the advent of MRI, cavernomas have become the most commonly identified vascular malformations in the brain. Cavernous angiomas vary from several millimeters to several centimeters in diameter although they are usually <3 cm in size. Multiple lesions are seen in approximately 10–30% of spontaneous cases. A familial form of the disorder exists and is inherited as an autosomal dominant trait with variable expression. Multiple lesions are more common in the familial form, occurring in as many as 80% of patients. About 80–90% of lesions are supratentorial and only 5% of cavernomas are seen in the spinal cord of adult patients. There is no gender predilection.

Cavernous angiomas are considered to be a congenital entity although de novo lesions may occur in patients with previous radiation exposure or in familial form cases. In early studies of major autopsy reports, the calculated prevalence was 0.3–0.9%. Cavernomas can occur at any age, but they are most likely to become clinically apparent in patients aged 20–40 years. Common clinical symptoms are seizures secondary to cortical lesions, focal neurologic deficits secondary to deep cerebral white matter and pons lesions, and headache as a result of intralesional hemorrhage.

The treatment of choice is surgical removal. Resection is indicated even in cases affecting the pons, due to the increased risk of subsequent and progressive neurologic disability in cases of rehemorrhage.

Imaging Findings

The sensitivity of CT for these lesions is 70–80%. Cavernous angiomas are typically hyperdense and present calcifications in 30% of cases. Lesions show a mottled pattern of enhancement after contrast administration. When surrounding edema is present, it is indicative of a recent bleed.

MRI is the imaging modality of choice. Gradient-echo imaging, with its increased sensitivity to susceptibility artifacts, is useful in the detection of smaller and concomitant lesions, which may not be detected with SE and FSE sequences (Fig. 7.8.1, *open arrow*). Cavernous angiomas present as a typical "popcorn-like" lesion with a large amount of hemosiderin surrounding a core of hemorrhage in different stages of evolution. The central area appears hyperintense on T1-weighted images (Fig. 7.8.2) and the hemosiderin rim is hypointense on gradient-refocused and FSE T2-weighted images (Figs. 7.8.3 and 7.8.4).

In general, cavernomas are considered angiographically occult because of the extremely low flow of blood through these lesions.

Case 9
■
Epidermoid Cyst

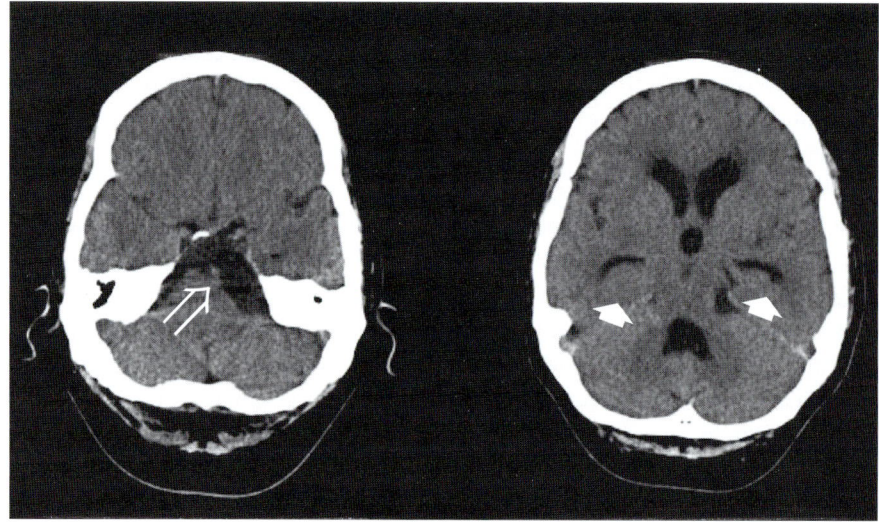

Fig. 7.9.1

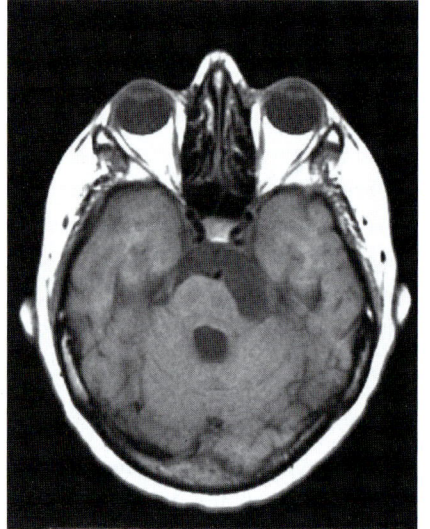

Fig. 7.9.2

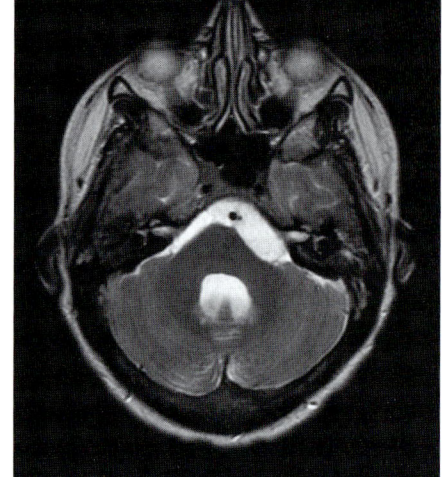

Fig. 7.9.3

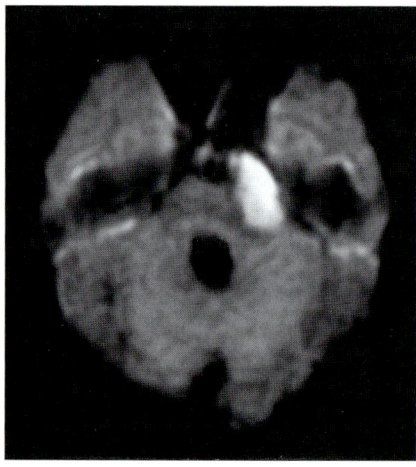

Fig. 7.9.4

A 32-year-old woman was admitted to the emergency room with a 24 hour history of diplopia, left hypoacusia, tinnitus, and vertigo. The patient had a prior medical history of headache and occasional vomiting for 5 years.

On physical examination, bilateral papilledema, diplopia, and hypoalgesia of the left maxillary nerve (V2) and cornea were found.

A CT scan showed hydrocephalus and the presence of an extraaxial lesion located in the posterior fossa, consistent with epidermoid cyst. MRI confirmed the suspected diagnosis.

Comments

Epidermoid cysts are benign congenital lesions of ectodermal origin secondary to epithelial inclusion during neural tube closure between the third and fifth weeks of embryonic life. They represent approximately 0.2–1.8% of all primary intracranial tumors. Epidermoid cysts occur most commonly in the cerebellopontine angle (40–50% of cases) and fourth ventricle. They tend to be well-circumscribed, smooth or lobulated, encapsulated lesions with a characteristic glistening, pearl-like sheen. The tumor presents as a slowly enlarging lesion that tends to adapt to the subarachnoid space, which is why patients are usually not symptomatic until age 30–40. Clinical features depend on the location of the lesion. Headache and cranial-nerve neuropathy are the most common symptoms. The differential diagnosis includes arachnoid cysts which appear isointense to CSF in all MRI pulse sequences, including diffusion-weighted images.

The treatment of choice is microsurgery. Total excision of the tumor is not always possible and there is a high rate of recurrences in these cases.

Imaging Findings

CT scan (Fig. 7.9.1) demonstrates an extraaxial hypodense lesion located in the left cerebellopontine angle (CPA) and prepontine cistern. The tumor envelops the basilar artery (*open arrow*) and causes a mild mass effect over the pons. A superior slice shows dilatation of the third and fourth ventricles as well as of the frontal and temporal horns (*solid arrows*).

MRI demonstrates a lesion in the left CPA which extends anteriorly to the prepontine cistern and superiorly to suprasellar and chiasmatic regions and ambiens cistern. Note that the signal intensity of the lesion is slightly different from that of CSF on T1- and T2-weighted images (Figs. 7.9.2 and 7.9.3). As epidermoid cysts have markedly restricted diffusion, they show high signal intensity on diffusion-weighted images (Fig. 7.9.4). This feature is useful in the distinction between arachnoid cysts, which are hypointense on DWI, and epidermoid cysts.

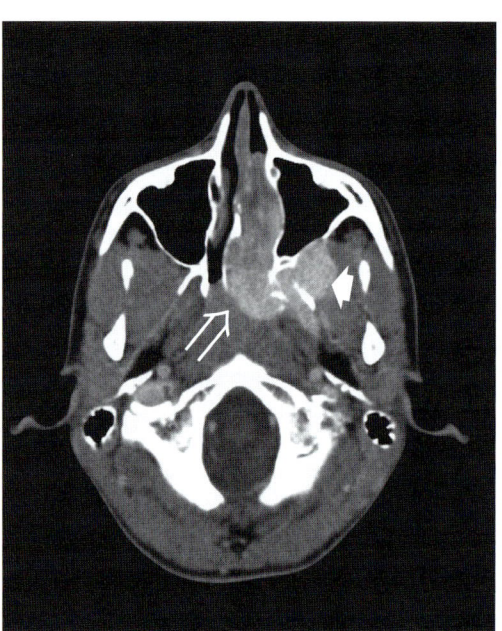

Fig. 7.10.1

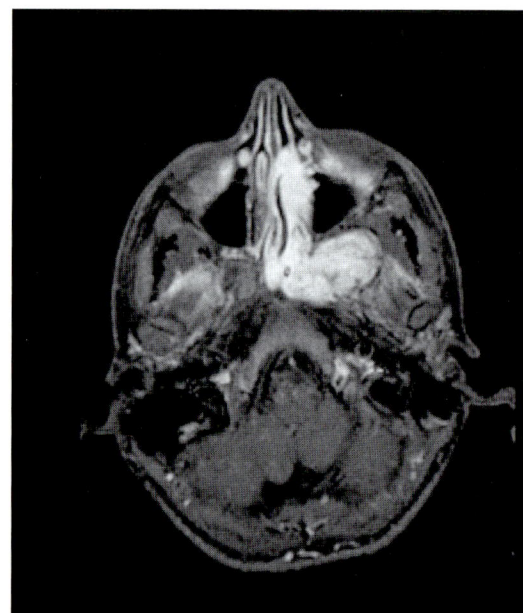

Fig. 7.10.2

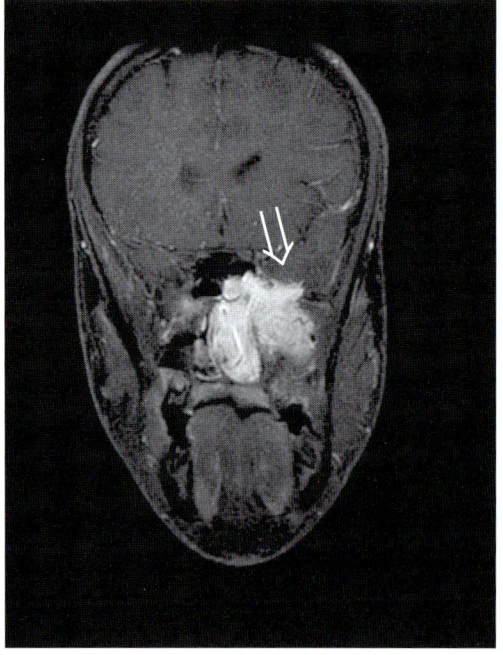

Fig. 7.10.3

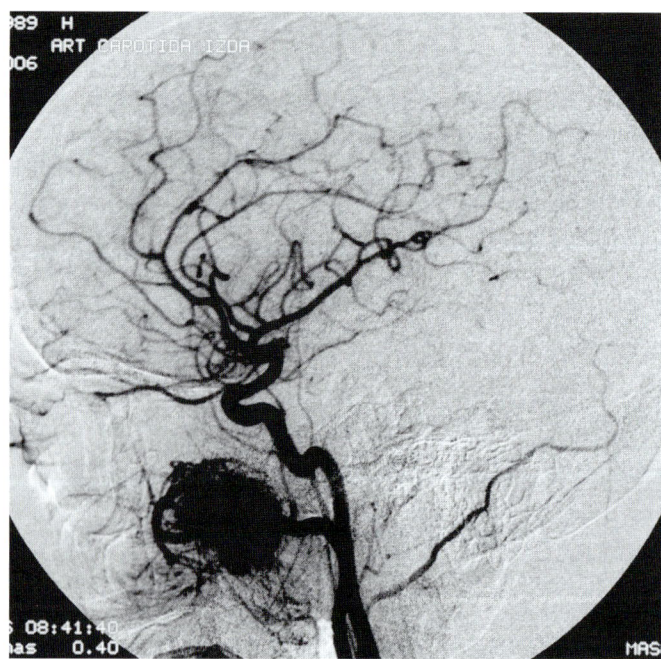

Fig. 7.10.4

A 14-year-old male presented with nasal stuffiness, continuous rhinorrhea and occasional epistaxis. On the endoscopic examination a polypoid lesion was found arising from the nasopharynx and filling the left posterior nasal cavity.

Comments

Nasopharyngeal angiofibroma is a benign vascular tumor that occurs in the nasopharynx of prepubertal and adolescent males. The most frequent symptoms are unilateral nasal obstruction and spontaneous epistaxis. The lesion typically arises in the sphenopalatine foramen and it often acts in a malignant manner by eroding into the surrounding sinuses, orbit, or cranial vault. This tumor is highly vascularized, with its main blood supply coming from the internal maxillary artery, although the ascending pharyngeal or vidian arteries may also feed the lesion.

Treatment is usually preoperative embolization to reduce blood loss followed by surgical resection (preferably endoscopic). Radiation therapy is a treatment option reserved for patients with incomplete resection, intracranial disease, or recurrent cases.

Imaging Findings

CT scan after contrast administration (Fig. 7.10.1) showing an enhancing mass in the left posterior nasal cavity extending into the cavum (*open arrow*). The lesion extends laterally through the pterygomaxillary fissure into the infratemporal fossa (*solid arrow*) and erodes the posterior wall of the maxillary sinus. Note the aggressiveness of the tumor, which produces erosion of the greater wing of the sphenoid and left side of the clivus.

Axial and coronal T1-weighted MR images after gadolinium administration and fat saturation (Figs. 7.10.2 and 7.10.3) demonstrate intense enhancement of the lesion. The borders are clearly depicted. A nodule is seen protruding into the middle fossa dura (*open arrow*); no cerebral involvement is detected.

DSA (Fig. 7.10.4) before embolization. The lesion is fed by branches of the internal maxillary artery (*open arrow*).

Acknowledgements

The authors wish to thank F. Delgado, A. Cano, M.J. Ramos, and R. Oteros of the Neuroradiology Unit of Reina Sofía Universitary Hospital in Córdoba, Spain for their contribution to the preparation of this chapter.

Further Readings

Books

Clinical Neuroanatomy. 6th ed. Snell RS (2006) Lippincott Williams & Wilkins. ISBN-13: 9780781759939

Diagnostic Cerebral Angiography. 2nd ed. Osborn AG (1999) Lippincott Williams & Wilkins. ISBN-13: 9780397584048

Diagnostic Imaging: Brain. Osborn AG (2004) Elsevier-Amirsys. ISBN-13: 9780721629056

Diagnostic Imaging: Head and Neck. Harnsberger R (2004) Elsevier-Amirsys. ISBN-13: 9780721628905

Diagnostic Imaging: Spine. Ross J, Brant-Zawadzki M, Chen MZ, Moore KR (2005) Elsevier-Amirsys. ISBN-13: 9780721628806

Head and Neck Imaging. Som PM, Curtin HD (2003) Elsevier-Mosby. ISBN-13: 9780323009423

Magnetic Resonance Imaging of the Brain and Spine. 3rd ed. Atlas SW (2001) Lippincott Williams & Wilkins. ISBN-13: 9780781720366

Neurorradiología diagnóstica y terapéutica. Mercader JM, Viñuela F (2004) Elsevier-Masson. ISBN: 9788445813300

Neuroradiology. 2nd ed. Grossman RI, Yousem DM (2003) Elsevier-Mosby. ISBN-13: 9780323005081

Pediatric Neuroimaging 4th ed. Barkovich AJ (2005) Lippincott Williams & Wilkins. ISBN-13: 9780781757669

Web Links

http://ashnr.org
http://asnr.org/
http://esnr.org/00.asp
http://neuroguide.com/
http://neurorad.ucsf.edu/index.html
http://radiographics.rsnajnls.org/cgi/collection/neuroradiology
http://silan.org/Spanish/society.html
http://springerlink.com/content/100446/
http://stroke-university.com/
http://wfns.org/

Articles

Abe O, Aoki S, Shirouzu I, Kunimatsu A, Hayashi N, Masumoto T, Mori H, Yamada H, Watanabe M, Masutani Y, Ohtomo K. MR imaging of ischemic penumbra. Eur J Radiol 2003; 46(1):67–78

Anslow P. Cranial bacterial infection. Eur Radiol 2004; 14 Suppl 3:E145–154

Barkovich AJ. MR imaging of the neonatal brain. Neuroimaging Clin N Am 2006; 16(1):117–135

Bode MK, Ruohonen J, Nieminen MT, Pyhtinen J. Potential of diffusion imaging in brain tumors: a review. Acta Radiol 2006; 47(6):585–594

Bonneville F, Sourour N, Biondi A. Intracranial aneurysms: an overview. Neuroimaging Clin N Am 2006; 16(3):371–382

Bonneville JF, Bonneville F, Cattin F. Magnetic resonance imaging of pituitary adenomas. Eur Radiol 2005; 15(3):543–548. Epub 2004 Dec 31

Brisman JL, Song JK, Newell DW. Cerebral aneurysms. N Engl J Med 2006; 355(9):928–939

Bravo-Rodriguez Fde A, Delgado Acosta F, Cano Sánchez A, Bautista Rodriguez MD. Trombosis venosa cerebral. Tratamiento mediante fibrinolisis local con alteplasa. Radiología 2002; 44(1):23–26

Bravo-Rodriguez Fde A, Espejo Herrero JJ, Bautista Rodriguez MD, Delgado Acosta F. Spontaneous dissection of vertebral arteries. Med Clin (Barc) 2004; 122(8):317–318

Burtscher IM, Holtas S. Proton magnetic resonance spectroscopy in brain tumours: clinical applications. Neuroradiology 2001; 43(5):345–352

Castillo M. Imaging of the upper cranial nerves I, III–VIII, and the cavernous sinuses. Neuroimaging Clin N Am 2004; 14(4):579–593

Caruso PA, Rincon S, Weber AL. Lesions of the maxilla: crossroads of the head and neck. Neuroimaging Clin N Am 2003; 13(3):411–426

Cha S. Update on brain tumor imaging: from anatomy to physiology. AJNR Am J Neuroradiol 2006; 27(3):475–487

Charil A, Yousry TA, Rovaris M, Barkhof F, De Stefano N, Fazekas F, Miller DH, Montalban X, Simon JH, Polman C, Filippi M. MRI and the diagnosis of multiple sclerosis: expanding the concept of "no better explanation". Lancet Neurol 2006; 5(10):841–852

Charles-Edwards EM, deSouza NM. Diffusion-weighted magnetic resonance imaging and its application to cancer. Cancer Imaging 2006; 6:135–143

Cognard C, Gobin YP, Pierot L, Bailly AL, Houdart E, Casasco A, Chiras J, Merland JJ. Cerebral dural arteriovenous fistulas: clinical and angiographic correlation with a revised classification of venous drainage. Radiology 1995; 194(3):671–680

Connor SE, Flis C, Langdon JD. Vascular masses of the head and neck. Clin Radiol 2005; 60(8):856–868

Cruz Junior LC, Sorensen AG. Diffusion tensor magnetic resonance imaging of brain tumors. Neurosurg Clin N Am 2005; 16(1):115–134

DeAngelis LM. Brain tumors. N Engl J Med 2001; 344(2):114–123

Delgado F, Bravo-Rodríguez FA, Bautista MD, Chirosa MA, Molina T, Martos JM, Canis M. Carotid pseudoaneurysms secondary to dissection: endovascular management with bare stent-graft. Cerebrovasc Dis 2005; 19(2):136–138

Diaz-Aguilera R, Martos-Becerra JM, Bravo-Rodriguez F, Ramos-Gomez MJ, Vinals-Torras M. Transient lesion in the corpus callosum associated with the use of antiepileptic drugs. Rev Neurol 2005; 41(4):254–255

Di Costanzo A, Scarabino T, Trojsi F, Giannatempo GM, Popolizio T, Catapano D, Bonavita S, Maggialetti N, Tosetti M, Salvolini U, d'Angelo VA, Tedeschi G. Multiparametric 3T MR approach to the assessment of cerebral gliomas: tumor extent and malignancy. Neuroradiology 2006; 48(9):622–631. Epub 2006 Jun 3

Drevelegas A. Extra-axial brain tumors. Eur Radiol 2005; 15(3):453–467

Essig M. MultiHance in brain perfusion. Eur Radiol 2004; 14 Suppl 7:O10–15

Esteban JM, Cervera V. Perfusion CT and angio CT in the assessment of acute stroke. Neuroradiology 2004; 46(9):705–715

Fiebach JB, Schellinger PD, Geletneky K, Wilde P, Meyer M, Hacke W, Sartor K. MRI in acute subarachnoid haemorrhage; findings with a standardised stroke protocol. Neuroradiology 2004; 46(1):44–48

Flis CM, Connor SE. Imaging of head and neck venous malformations. Eur Radiol 2005; 15(10):2185–2193. Epub 2005 Jul 8

Forsting M, Weber J. MR perfusion imaging: a tool for more than stroke. Eur Radiol 2004; 14 Suppl 5:M2–7

Fox AJ. Carotid endarterectomy trials. Neuroimaging Clin N Am 1996; 6(4):931–938

Gao PY, Osborn AG, Smirniotopoulos JG, Harris CP. Radiologic-pathologic correlation. Epidermoid tumor of the cerebellopontine angle. AJNR Am J Neuroradiol 1992; 13(3):863–872

Ge Y. Multiple sclerosis: the role of MR imaging. AJNR Am J Neuroradiol 2006; 27(6):1165–1176

Gil-Peralta A, Mayol A, Marcos JR, Gonzalez A, Ruano J, Boza F, Duran F. Percutaneous transluminal angioplasty of the symptomatic atherosclerotic carotid arteries. Results, complications, and follow-up. Stroke 1996; 27(12):2271–2273

Glenn OA, Barkovich J. Magnetic resonance imaging of the fetal brain and spine: an increasingly important tool in prenatal diagnosis: part 2. AJNR Am J Neuroradiol 2006; 27(9):1807–1814

Glenn OA, Barkovich AJ. Magnetic resonance imaging of the fetal brain and spine: an increasingly important tool in prenatal diagnosis, part 1. AJNR Am J Neuroradiol 2006; 27(8):1604–1611

Gonzalez A, Mayol A, Martinez E, Gonzalez-Marcos JR, Gil-Peralta A. Mechanical thrombectomy with snare in patients with acute ischemic stroke. Neuroradiology 2007; 49(4):365–372

Guglielmi G, Viñuela F, Dion J, Duckwiler G. Electrothrombosis of saccular aneurysms via endovascular approach. Part 2: Preliminary clinical experience.J Neurosurg 1991; 75(1):8–14

Hillis AE, Wityk RJ, Beauchamp NJ, Ulatowski JA, Jacobs MA, Barker PB. Perfusion-weighted MRI as a marker of response to treatment in acute and subacute stroke. Neuroradiology 2004; 46(1):31–39

Higashida RT, Meyers PM. Intracranial angioplasty and stenting for cerebral atherosclerosis: new treatments for stroke are needed! Neuroradiology 2006; 48(6):367–372

Higashida RT, Furlan AJ, Roberts H, Tomsick T, Connors B, Barr J, Dillon W, Warach S, Broderick J, Tilley B, Sacks D; Technology Assessment Committee of the American Society of Interventional and Therapeutic Neuroradiology; Technology Assessment Committee of the Society of Interventional Radiology. Trial design and reporting standards for intra-arterial cerebral thrombolysis for acute ischemic stroke. Stroke 2003; 34(8):e109–137

Hutter A, Schwetye KE, Bierhals AJ, McKinstry RC. Brain neoplasms: epidemiology, diagnosis, and prospects for cost-effective imaging. Neuroimaging Clin N Am 2003; 13(2):237–250

Jellison BJ, Field AS, Medow J, Lazar M, Salamat MS, Alexander AL. Diffusion tensor imaging of cerebral white matter: a pictorial review of physics, fiber tract anatomy, and tumor imaging patterns. AJNR Am J Neuroradiol 2004; 25(3):356–369

Jensen ME, Dion JE. Percutaneous vertebroplasty in the treatment of osteoporotic compression fractures. Neuroimaging Clin N Am 2000; 10(3):547–568

Kai Y, Hamada J, Morioka M, Yano S, Todaka T, Ushio Y. Appropriate interval between embolization and surgery in patients with meningioma. AJNR Am J Neuroradiol 2002; 23(1):139–142

Kane I, Sandercock P, Wardlaw J. Magnetic resonance perfusion diffusion mismatch and thrombolysis in acute ischaemic stroke: a systematic review of the evidence to date. J Neurol Neurosurg Psychiatry 2007; 78(5):485–491. Epub 2006 Oct 20

Kim LJ, Spetzler RF. Classification and surgical management of spinal arteriovenous lesions: arteriovenous fistulae and arteriovenous malformations. Neurosurgery 2006; 59(5 Suppl 3):S195–201

Korteweg T, Tintore M, Uitdehaag B, Rovira A, Frederiksen J, Miller D, Fernando K, Filippi M, Agosta F, Rocca M, Fazekas F, Enzinger C, Matthews P, Parry A, Polman C, Montalban X, Barkhof F. MRI criteria for dissemination in space in patients with clinically isolated syndromes: a multicentre follow-up study. Lancet Neurol 2006; 5(3):221–227

Lasjaunias PL, Chng SM, Sachet M, Alvarez H, Rodesch G, Garcia-Monaco R. The management of vein of Galen aneurysmal malformations. Neurosurgery 2006; 59(5 Suppl 3):S184–194

Lai R, Rosenblum MK, DeAngelis LM. Primary CNS lymphoma: a whole-brain disease? Neurology 2002; 59(10):1557–1562

Law M, Yang S, Wang H, Babb JS, Johnson G, Cha S, Knopp EA, Zagzag D. Glioma grading: sensitivity, specificity, and predictive values of perfusion MR imaging and proton MR spectroscopic imaging compared with conventional MR imaging. AJNR Am J Neuroradiol 2003; 24(10):1989–1998

Law M. MR spectroscopy of brain tumors. Top Magn Reson Imaging 2004; 15(5).291–313

Leira R, Davalos A, Silva Y, Gil-Peralta A, Tejada J, Garcia M, Castillo J; Stroke Project, Cerebrovascular Diseases Group of the Spanish Neurological Society. Early neurologic deterioration in intracerebral hemorrhage: predictors and associated factors. Neurology 2004; 63(3):461–467

Majos C, Alonso J, Aguilera C, Serrallonga M, Coll S, Acebes JJ, Arus C, Gili J. Utility of proton MR spectroscopy in the diagnosis of radiologically atypical intracranial meningiomas. Neuroradiology 2003; 45(3):129–136. Epub 2003 Feb 19

Mathis JM, Barr JD, Jungreis CA, Yonas H, Sekhar LN, Vincent D, Pentheny SL, Horton JA. Temporary balloon test occlusion of the internal carotid artery: experience in 500 cases. AJNR Am J Neuroradiol 1995; 16(4):749–754

Mezzapesa DM, Petruzzellis M, Lucivero V, Prontera M, Tinelli A, Sancilio M, Carella A, Federico F. Multimodal MR examination in acute ischemic stroke. Neuroradiology 2006; 48(4):238–246

Mitra D, Herwadkar A, Soh C, Gholkar A. Follow-up of intracranial aneurysms treated with matrix detachable coils: a single-center experience. AJNR Am J Neuroradiol 2007; 28(2):362–367

Molyneux AJ. Ruptured intracranial aneurysms – clinical aspects of subarachnoid hemorrhage management and the International Subarachnoid Aneurysm Trial. Neuroimaging Clin N Am 2006; 16(3):391–396

Molyneux A, Kerr R, Stratton I, Sandercock P, Clarke M, Shrimpton J, Holman R; International Subarachnoid Aneurysm Trial (ISAT) Collaborative Group. International Subarachnoid Aneurysm Trial (ISAT) of neurosurgical clipping versus endovascular coiling in 2143 patients with ruptured intracranial aneurysms: a randomised trial. Lancet 2002; 360(9342):1267–1274

Munoz del Castillo F, Jurado Ramos A, Bravo-Rodriguez F, Delgado Acosta F, Lopez Villarejo P. Endoscopic surgery of nasopharyngeal angiofibroma. Acta Otorrinolaringol Esp 2004; 55(8):369–375

Murphy KJ, Deramons H. Percutaneous vertebroplasty in benign and malignant disease. Neuroimaging Clin N Am 2000; 10(3):535–545

Murray TJ. Diagnosis and treatment of multiple sclerosis. BMJ 2006; 332(7540):525–527

Osborn AG, Preece MT. Intracranial cysts: radiologic-pathologic correlation and imaging approach. Radiology 2006; 239(3):650–664

Parizel PM, Van Goethem JW, Ozsarlak O, Maes M, Phillips CD. New developments in the neuroradiological diagnosis of craniocerebral trauma. Eur Radiol 2005; 15(3):569–581

Pinero P, Gonzalez A, Mayol A, Martinez E, Gonzalez-Marcos JR, Boza F, Cayuela A, Gil-Peralta A. Silent ischemia after neuroprotected percutaneous carotid stenting: a diffusion-weighted MRI study. AJNR Am J Neuroradiol 2006; 27(6):1338–1345

Poussaint TY, Rodriguez D. Advanced neuroimaging of pediatric brain tumors: MR diffusion, MR perfusion, and MR spectroscopy. Neuroimaging Clin N Am 2006; 16(1):169–192

Provenzale JM, Mukundan S, Barboriak DP. Diffusion-weighted and perfusion MR imaging for brain tumor characterization and assessment of treatment response. Radiology 2006; 239(3):632–649

Reijneveld JC, van der Grond J, Ramos LM, Bromberg JE, Taphoorn MJ. Proton MRS imaging in the follow-up of patients with suspected low-grade gliomas. Neuroradiology 2005; 47(12):887–891. Epub 2005 Aug 20

Rivera PP, Willinsky RA, Porter PJ. Intracranial cavernous malformations. Neuroimaging Clin N Am 2003; 13(1):27–40

Rovira A, Grive E, Rovira A, Alvarez-Sabin J. Distribution territories and causative mechanisms of ischemic stroke. Eur Radiol 2005; 15(3):416–426

Rovira A, Orellana P, Alvarez-Sabin J, Arenillas JF, Aymerich X, Grive E, Molina C, Rovira-Gols A. Hyperacute ischemic stroke: middle cerebral artery susceptibility sign at echo-planar gradient-echo MR imaging. Radiology 2004; 232(2):466–473

Rovira A, Pericot I, Alonso J, Rio J, Grive E, Montalban X. Serial diffusion-weighted MR imaging and proton MR spectroscopy of acute large demyelinating brain lesions: case report. AJNR Am J Neuroradiol 2002; 23(6):989–994

Rovira A, Rovira-Gols A, Pedraza S, Grive E, Molina C, Alvarez-Sabin J. Diffusion-weighted MR imaging in the acute phase of transient ischemic attacks. AJNR Am J Neuroradiol 2002; 23(1):77–83

Rovira A, Pedraza S, Molina C, Capellades J, Grive E, Rovira A, Montaner J. Diffusion-weighted magnetic resonance in the diagnosis of acute subcortical infarcts. Rev Neurol 2000; 30(10):914–919

Sanchez-Arjona MB, Sanz-Fernandez G, Franco-Macias E, Gil-Peralta A. Cerebral hemodynamic changes after carotid angioplasty and stenting. AJNR Am J Neuroradiol 2007; 28(4):640–644

Schaefer PW, Copen WA, Lev MH, Gonzalez RG. Diffusion-weighted imaging in acute stroke. Neuroimaging Clin N Am 2005; 15(3):503–530

Schellinger PD, Fiebach JB, Hacke W. Imaging-based decision making in thrombolytic therapy for ischemic stroke: present status. Stroke 2003; 34(2):575–583

Schievink WI. Spontaneous dissection of the carotid and vertebral arteries. N Engl J Med 2001; 344(12):898–906

Shetty SK, Lev MH. CT perfusion in acute stroke. Neuroimaging Clin N Am 2005; 15(3):481–501

Smith WS. Safety of mechanical thrombectomy and intravenous tissue plasminogen activator in acute ischemic stroke. Results of the multi Mechanical Embolus Removal in Cerebral Ischemia (MERCI) trial, part I. AJNR Am J Neuroradiol 2006; 27(6): 1177–1182

Srinivasan A, Goyal M, Al Azri F, Lum C. State-of-the-art imaging of acute stroke. Radiographics 2006; 26 Suppl 1:S75–95

Spetzler RF, Martin NA. A proposed grading system for arteriovenous malformations. J Neurosurg 1986; 65(4):476–483

Stadnik TW, Demaerel P, Luypaert RR, Chaskis C, Van Rompaey KL, Michotte A, Osteaux MJ. Imaging tutorial: differential diagnosis of bright lesions on diffusion-weighted MR images. Radiographics 2003; 23(1):e7

Sundgren PC, Dong Q, Gomez-Hassan D, Mukherji SK, Maly P, Welsh R. Diffusion tensor imaging of the brain: review of clinical applications. Neuroradiology 2004; 46(5):339–350

Tharin S, Golby A. Functional brain mapping and its applications to neurosurgery. Neurosurgery 2007; 60(4 Suppl 2):185–201

Thurnher MM, Castillo M. Imaging in acute stroke. Eur Radiol 2005; 15(3): 408–415

Urtasun F, Biondi A, Casaco A, Houdart E, Caputo N, Aymard A, Merland JJ. Cerebral dural arteriovenous fistulas: percutaneous transvenous embolization. Radiology 1996; 199(1):209–217

Valavanis A. The role of angiography in the evaluation of cerebral vascular malformations. Neuroimaging Clin N Am 1996; 6(3):679–704 van Gijn J, Kerr RS, Rinkel GJ. Subarachnoid haemorrhage. Lancet 2007; 369(9558):306–318

Vates GE, Chang S, Lamborn KR, Prados M, Berger MS. Gliomatosis cerebri: a review of 22 cases. Neurosurgery 2003; 53(2):261–271

Vattipally VR, Bronen RA. MR imaging of epilepsy: strategies for successful interpretation. Neuroimaging Clin N Am 2004; 14(3):349–372

Vinuela F, Duckwiler G, Mawad M. Guglielmi detachable coil embolization of acute intracraneial aneurysm: perioperative anatomical and clinical outcome in 403 patients. J Neurosurg 1997; 86(3):475–482

Weber AL, Caruso P, Sabates NR. The optic nerve: radiologic, clinical, and pathologic evaluation. Neuroimaging Clin N Am 2005; 15(1):175–201

Wetzel S, Bongartz G. MR angiography: supra-aortic vessels. Eur Radiol 1999; 9(7):1277–1284

White PM, Wardlaw JM, Lindsay KW, Sloss S, Patel DK, Teasdale EM. The non-invasive detection of intracranial aneurysms: are neuroradiologists any better than other observers? Eur Radiol 2003; 13(2):389–396

Wiebers DO. Unruptured intracranial aneurysms: natural history and clinical management. Update on the international study of unruptured intracranial aneurysms. Neuroimaging Clin N Am 2006; 16(3):383–390

Wilms G, Demaerel P, Sunaert S. Intra-axial brain tumours. Eur Radiol 2005; 15(3):468–484

Wintermark M. Brain perfusion-CT in acute stroke patients. Eur Radiol 2005; 15 Suppl 4:D28–31

Witte RJ, Lane JI, Driscoll CL, Lundy LB, Bernstein MA, Kotsenas AL, Kocharian A. Pediatric and adult cochlear implantation. Radiographics 2003; 23(5):1185–1200

Wittenberg KH, Adkins MC. MR imaging of nontraumatic brachial plexopathies: frequency and spectrum of findings. Radiographics 2000; 20(4):1023–1032

Yuh WT, Christoforidis GA, Koch RM, Sammet S, Schmalbrock P, Yang M, Knopp MV. Clinical magnetic resonance imaging of brain tumors at ultrahigh field: a state-of-the-art review. Top Magn Reson Imaging 2006; 17(2):53–61

Young RJ, Sills AK, Brem S, Knopp EA. Neuroimaging of metastatic brain disease. Neurosurgery 2005; 57(5 Suppl): S10–23

Nuclear Medicine

8

Juan Antonio Vallejo Casas and Angel C. Rebollo Aguirre
Luisa M. Mena Bares (Contributor)

Introduction

Nuclear medicine is the medical specialty that uses radioactive isotopes, nuclear radiation, electromagnetic changes of the nuclear components, and biophysical techniques to prevent, diagnose, and treat medical conditions.

In a nuclear medicine test, small amounts of radiopharmaceuticals are introduced into the body by injection, swallowing, or inhalation. Radiopharmaceuticals are substances that are attracted to specific organs and provide information about both their structure and function. The amount of radiopharmaceutical used is carefully selected to ensure an accurate test while providing the least amount of radiation exposure to the patient. A special camera (PET, SPECT or gamma camera) is used to detect the radiopharmaceutical in the target organ or tissue and shows images of the area in question.

The capability of nuclear medicine to determine the presence of disease is based on biophysiological changes rather than anatomical ones.

Widespread clinical use of nuclear medicine began in the early 1950s, with the application of radioiodine to patients suffering from thyroid disease. In the 1960s and the years that followed, the growth of nuclear medicine was phenomenal. In the 1970s most organs of the body could be visualized. In 1971 the American Medical Association officially recognized nuclear medicine as a distinct medical specialty.

As more is learned about the fundamental processes of diseases and new radiopharmaceuticals and analytical tools are developed, PET and CT/PET scanning will prove to be invaluable tools in the diagnosis and management of some of the most critical diseases challenging modern medicine. The development of new therapeutic agents, especially those related to radioimmunotherapy of many oncological conditions, will give nuclear medicine a prominent role in the management and treatment of oncological patients.

Case 1
■
Brain Death

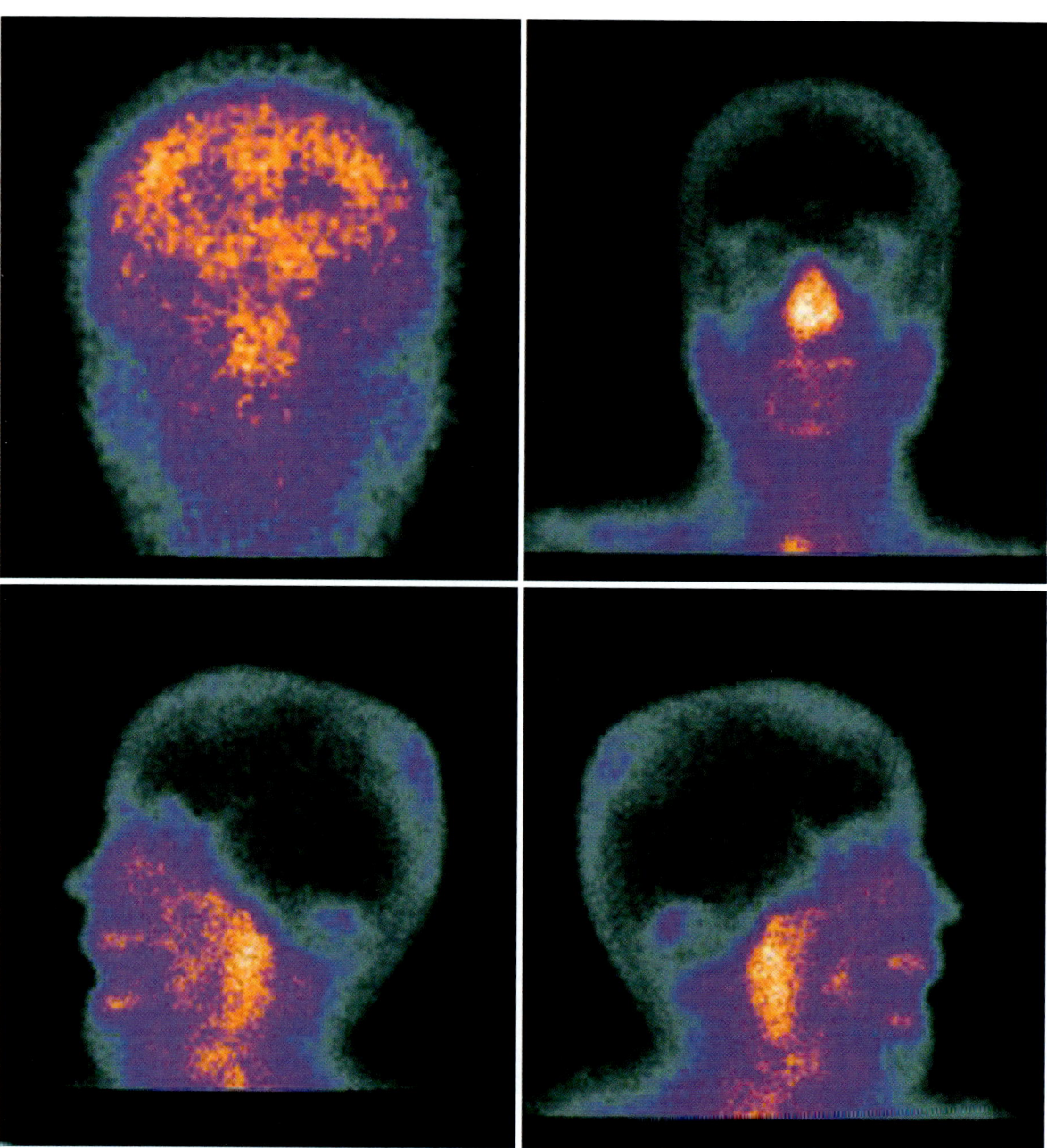

Fig. 8.1.1

A 53-year-old woman suffered occipital trauma and presented with loss of consciousness. The initial clinical examination showed areactive mydriasis with Glasgow score 3; 48 hours after admission the patient was in deep coma and ^{99m}Tc-HMPAO cerebral perfusion scintigraphy was performed to confirm the diagnosis of cerebral death.

Comments

The term "brain death" is used to signify the irreversible loss of function of the entire brain and, by general consensus, is accepted as a criterion for human death. The determination of brain death has gained importance in modern health care to prevent futile attempts to sustain ventilation and blood circulation artificially for prolonged periods and to ensure the potential availability of organs for transplantation.

Although physicians generally agree that a patient can be declared brain dead when the loss of brain function is total and irreversible, different approaches have been taken to define what constitutes brain-death. A thorough clinical examination is essential to the diagnosis. The role of confirmatory tests differ among countries but they are generally indicated when a specific part of the clinical examination cannot be performed or is deemed unreliable. Under certain circumstances, confirmatory tests can be used to shorten the period of clinical observation.

Cerebral scintigraphy is a safe, reliable and widely available alternative that can be performed rapidly and can be interpreted in a straightforward manner. It is not affected by metabolic aberrations or pharmacologic intoxicants. Electrical interference and the presence of skull defects or scalp trauma do not preclude its performance either. The radiopharmaceuticals used in scintigraphy (Tc-99m hexamethylpropyleneamine oxime) have no deleterious effects on potential donor organs.

Tc-99m HMPAO cerebral scintigraphy is highly sensitive and appears to be 100% specific.

Imaging Findings

After the intravenous administration of Tc-99m HMPAO in an alive patient, the first pass radionuclide cerebral angiogram shows flow in the common carotids as well as within the regions supplied by the external carotid arteries and by the middle cerebral arteries. The anterior static view (Fig. 8.1.1) shows the location of the radiopharmaceutical within the cerebral hemispheres.

In brain death, the anterior and middle cerebral artery complexes are not visualized in the first pass. Subsequent planar images (anterior, left and right lateral) show no radiopharmaceutical within the cerebral cortices, basal ganglia, or cerebellar hemispheres. The presence of early, increased activity in the nasopharyngeal region at radionuclide blood flow scanning, dubbed the "hot nose sign", is supportive of but not diagnostic of brain death.

Case 2
■
Gastrointestinal Bleeding

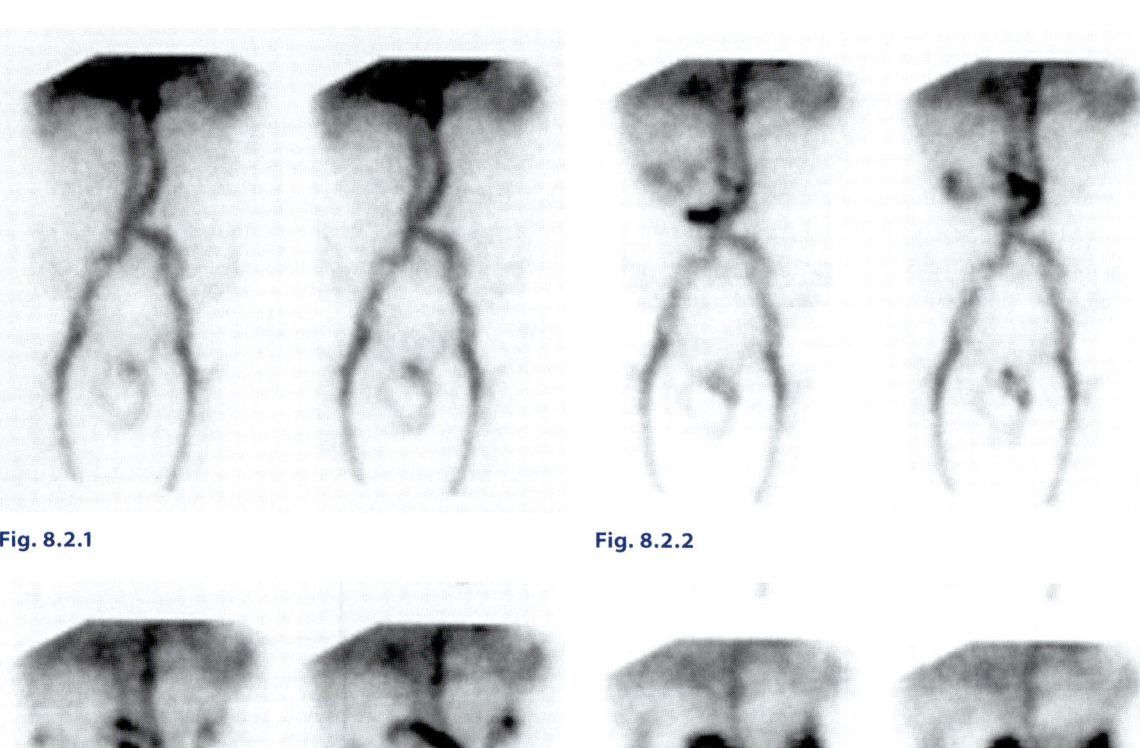

Fig. 8.2.1

Fig. 8.2.2

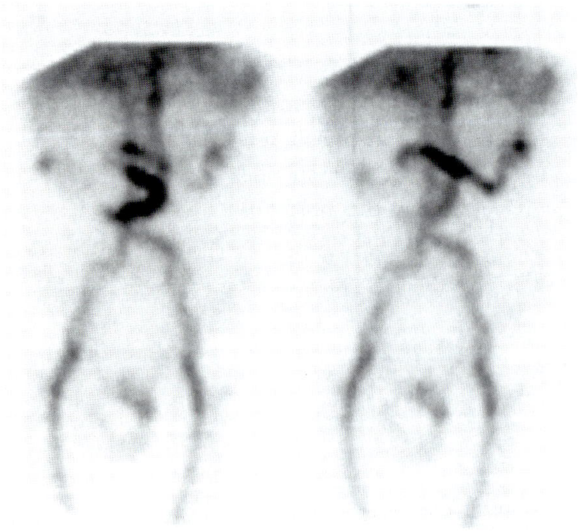

Fig. 8.2.3

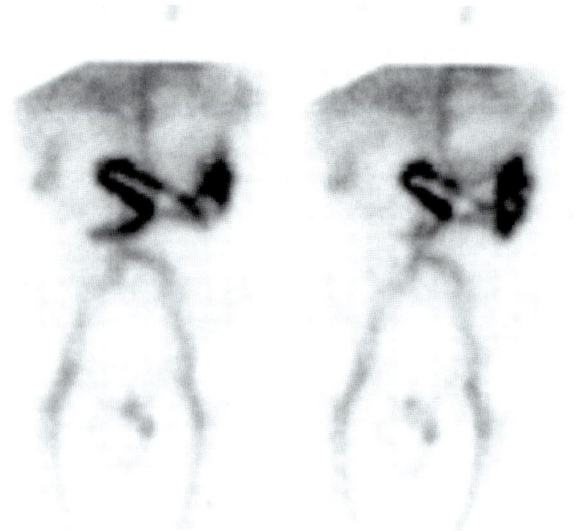

Fig. 8.2.4

A 53-year-old man was referred with suspicion of GI bleeding and negative upper GI endoscopy. At colonoscopy, blood in the bowel precluded the visualization of eventual lesions. Non-colonic diverticulosis or inflammatory bowel disease were suspected.

The patient was hemodynamically unstable, with paleness and severe hypotension, and required blood transfusion. He was referred to the nuclear medicine department to determine the location and extent of GI bleeding. During the isotopic study, the patient had a new episode of hemodynamic instability and a second blood transfusion was performed.

Successful management of patients with acute gastrointestinal (GI) bleeding often depends on accurate location of the bleeding site. In suspected lower GI bleeding, nuclear medicine imaging techniques are the methods of choice because they are highly sensitive.

Isotopic studies, especially 99mTc-labeled red blood cells, may detect bleeding rates as low as 0.05 to 0.1 ml/min, while angiography will only demonstrate bleeding rates greater than 0.5 ml/min. ^{99m}Tc-sulphur colloid techniques are also used for this purpose.

The labeled red blood cell technique has the advantage of a longer potential period during which bleeding may be visualized. Moreover, the patient's clinical needs can be taken care of and blood transfusions can be performed during the study.

The procedure for red blood cell labeling is easy, fast, safe, and inexpensive.

The bleeding site will be visualized as a focal area of abnormal radiopharmaceutical accumulation. Acute GI bleeding is diagnosed when the radiopharmaceutical moves in an antegrade or retrograde direction within the bowel lumen.

A negative isotopic study for GI bleeding indicates no active bleeding and no other imaging modalities are usually needed

Figure 8.2.1 shows the major abdominal structures and the liver and spleen blood pools

Figure 8.2.2 shows a focus of activity in the middle abdominal area, deriving from blood extravasated from a small bowel bleeding site. We can see the movement of the activity in the lumen.

Figures 8.2.3 and 8.2.4 (60 and 90 minutes after injection) show a new bleeding episode in the same location and antegrade activity progression within the small bowel lumen.

The diagnosis of active small bowel bleeding at the point shown was confirmed surgically.

Case 3
■ Inflammatory Bowel Disease

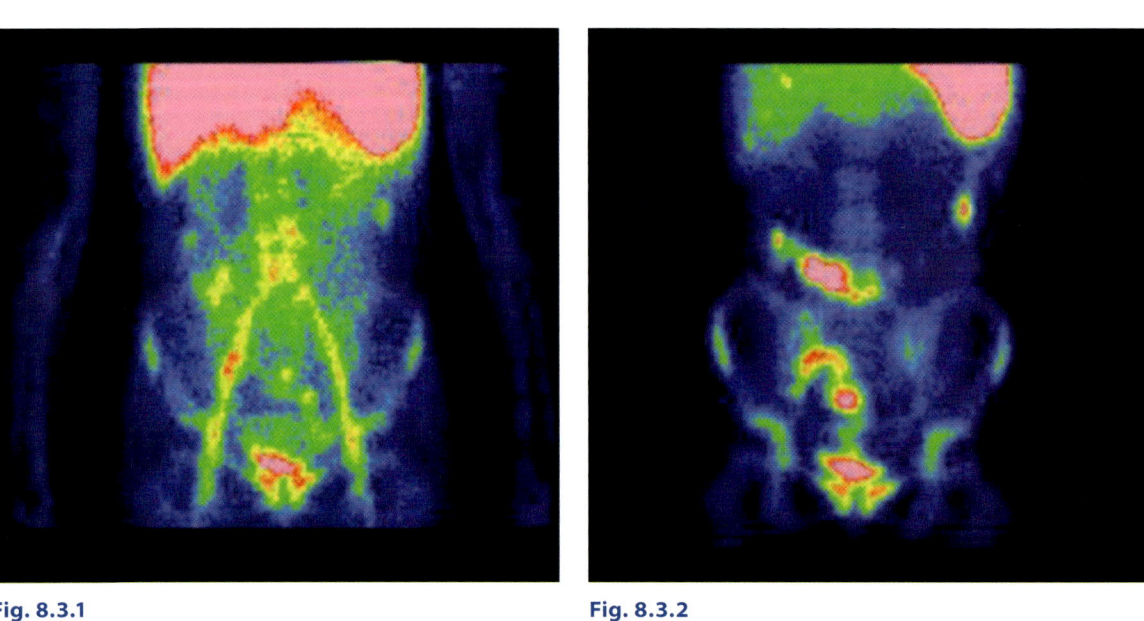

Fig. 8.3.1

Fig. 8.3.2

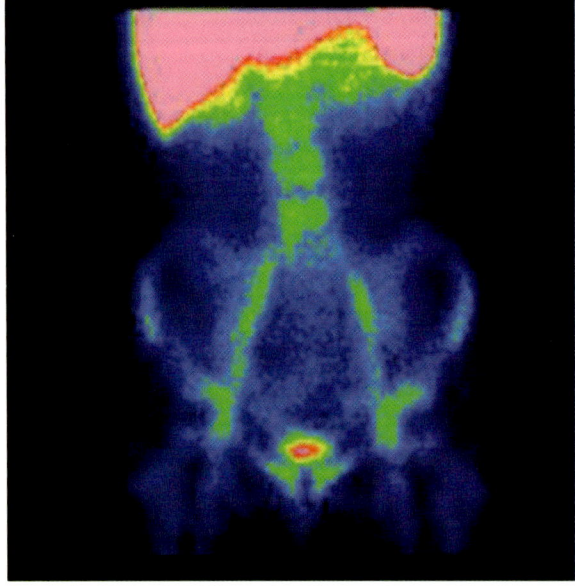

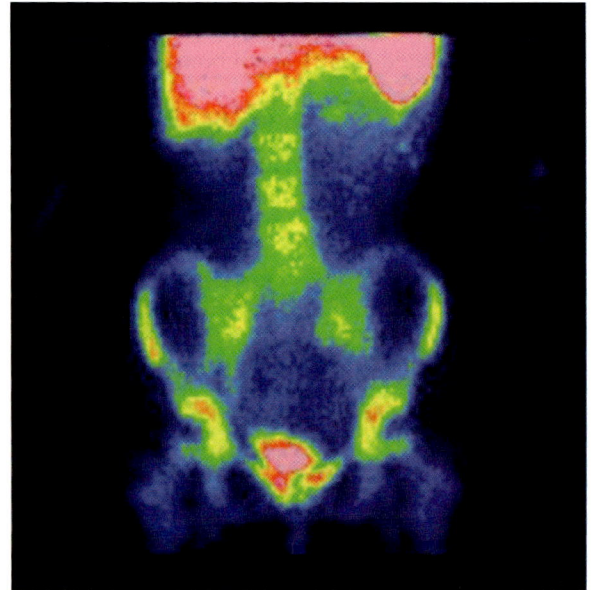

Fig. 8.3.3

Fig. 8.3.4

A 10-year-old girl presented with abdominal distress. The patient had a recent history of acute pain episodes, loss of appetite, weight loss, and mucous diarrhea. Biochemical parameters were indicative of inflammatory activity.

Comments

99mTc-hexamethylpropyleneamine oxime (HMPAO)-labeled autologous leukocyte imaging is the first-line investigation to detect inflammatory bowel disease.

Management of ulcerative colitis and Crohn's disease depends on the knowledge of the site, extent, and activity of inflammation, as well as on the presence of complications. Leukocyte-labeled scintigraphy can provide information about the location, extent, and severity of inflammatory disease.

The labeled-leukocyte procedures are carried out "in vitro", after blood extraction, sample anticoagulation, and application of centrifugation gradients to separate white blood cells. After a short incubation with the radiopharmaceutical ^{99m}Tc-HMPAO, the labeled leukocytes are re-injected. Quality control before re-injection is obligatory.

Images are obtained at 30 minutes (early set) and 150 minutes (late set) after injection. The findings are generally easy to interpret.

Imaging Findings

Figures 8.3.1 and 8.3.2 were obtained in the acute episode and show inflammatory activity in the ileum, cecum, and transverse colon, with greater intensity than the normal reference (activity of bone marrow in the iliac spine). For increased clinical accuracy, both the early and late image sets must show pathological uptake. If only the late images are abnormal, there is a risk of false-positive results.

After this study, infliximab was infused and the patient underwent a new leukocyte-labeled scan (Figs. 8.3.3 and 8.3.4) to evaluate the response; this study showed normal uptake in bone marrow, liver, and spleen, without bowel uptake.

Case 4
■
Movement Disorders

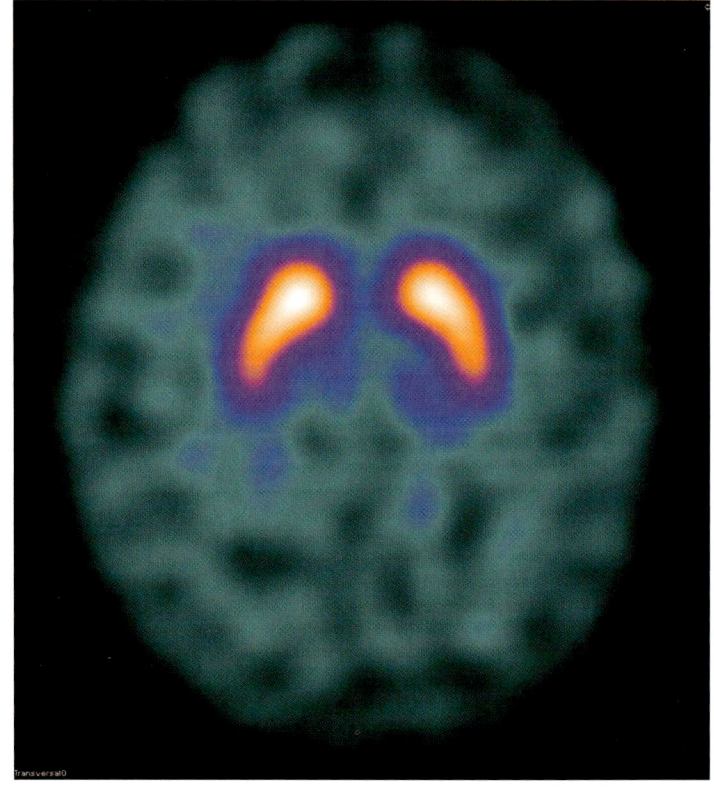

Fig. 8.4.1

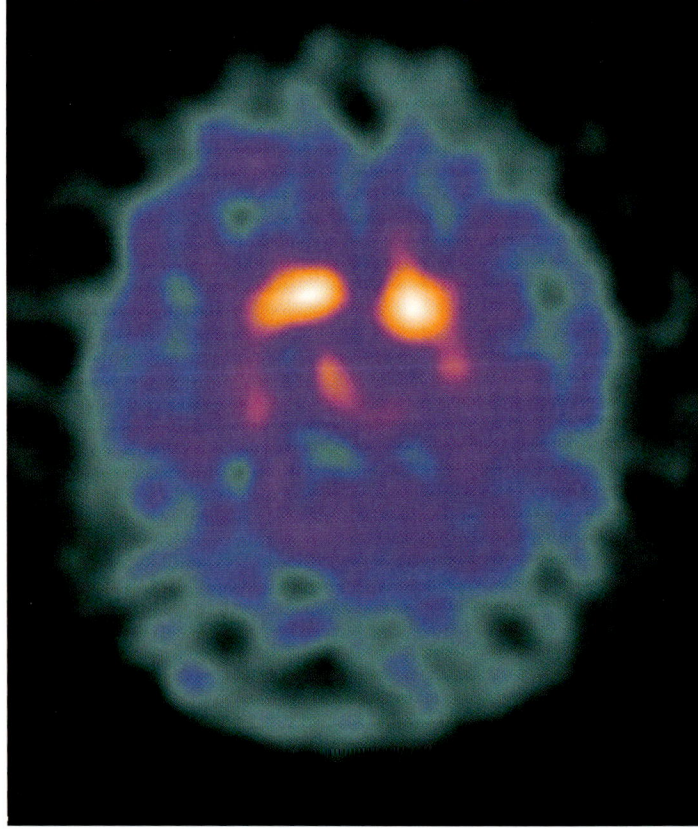

Fig. 8.4.2

A 78-year-old woman complained of tremor affecting both upper limbs, more pronounced on the left, and mild depression symptoms. Possible Parkinson's disease or drug-induced parkinsonism were potential diagnoses.

Functional imaging provides a sensitive means of detecting and characterizing brain changes in movement disorders.

Symptoms typically include tremor, rigidity, and bradykinesia. The principal physiopathological feature is the degeneration of nigrostriatal dopaminergic neurons. The number of presynaptic striatal dopaminergic neurons is greatly reduced in Parkinson's disease. Together with progressive supranuclear palsy and multi-system atrophy, this results in a reduction of dopamine transport.

SPECT imaging with 123-I-Ioflupane (DaTSCAN®, General Electric Healthcare) has proven to be both sensitive and specific in the detection of dopaminergic dysfunction in these patients. Ioflupane can differentiate essential tremor from Parkinson's disease and related syndromes.

Cases that may benefit from Ioflupane study include atypical presentation, early onset of tremor, and patients on medication with potential parkinsonian effects.

Figure 8.4.1 shows the normal appearance, with normal bilateral striatal uptake (largely symmetrical activity in the putamen and caudate nuclei).

Figure 8.4.2 image is a tomographic image of this patient, showing significantly reduced putamen uptake bilaterally, with activity confined to the caudate nuclei.

These findings demonstrate severe damage to nigrostriatal dopaminergic pathways, diagnostic of Parkinson's disease.

123-I-Ioflupane had a significant impact on the clinical management of this patient, making it possible to establish the correct treatment.

Case 5
■
Obstructive Uropathy

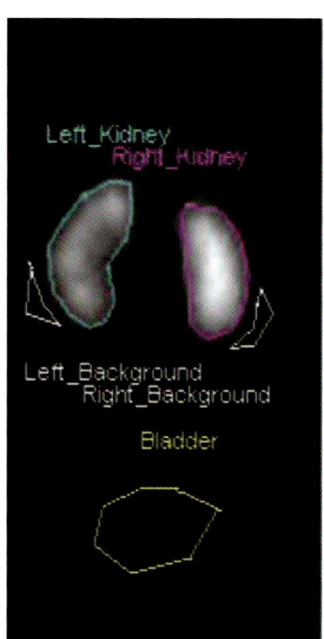

Fig. 8.5.1

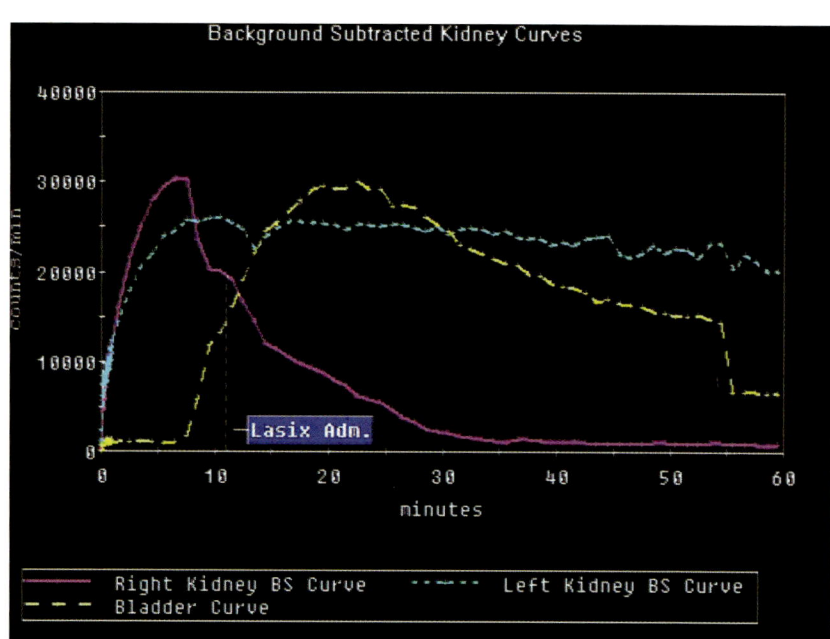

Fig. 8.5.2

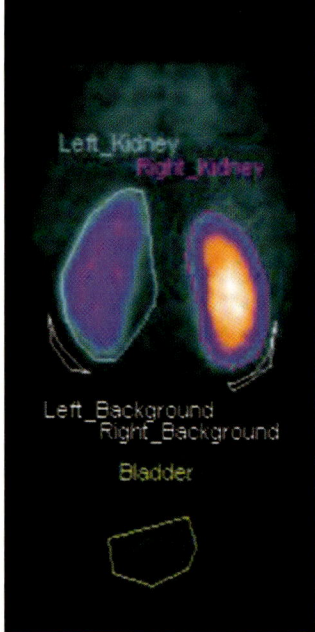

Fig. 8.5.3

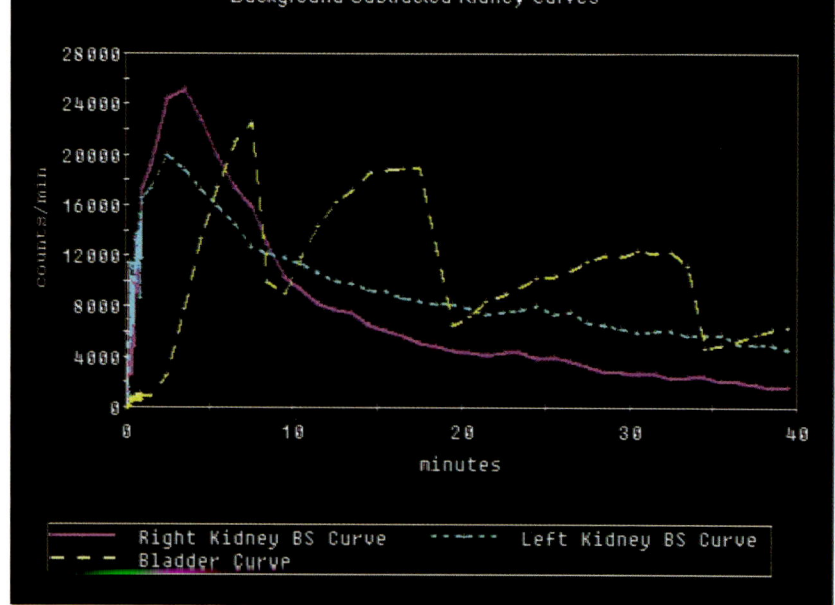

Fig. 8.5.4

A 3-year-old girl with a history of urinary tract infection was referred to the nuclear medicine department after left hydronephrosis was detected at ultrasonography. Pathological findings at kidney scan necessitated surgery.

Follow-up ultrasonography four months after surgery showed persistent dilatation of the pelvis.

Comments

Different radiotracers are used to assess renal function. ^{99m}Tc- mercaptoacetyltriglycine (MAG3) is currently the most widely used in children; it is secreted by renal tubules and has much greater extraction efficiency than glomerular-filtered agents.

After intravenous injection, the images are obtained in the posterior projection, with the child supine. Serial images are acquired over a determinate period. If urinary obstruction is suspected, furosemide is administered. There is no current consensus about the best time for diuretic injection. Some protocols call for injection 15 minutes before radiotracer injection; however, the classical protocol injects the diuretic 20 minutes after injection.

Computer-generated time-activity curves are obtained from areas drawn over the kidneys (background corrected). In normal patients, this curve shows rapid and intense tracer concentration, with time to the peak lower than 5 minutes. After the peak, the activity declines faster (to less than 50% of the peak value at 20 minutes). We can also the compare the function of one kidney compared to the other quantitatively.

Hydronephrosis is one of the most frequent indications for renograms in children. Renograms can differentiate between an unobstructed dilated renal pelvis and a true obstructed renal pelvis. In obstructive hydronephrosis, the half-washout time point on the curve is greater than 20 minutes. However, the diagnosis must be made taking the entire radionuclide study into consideration: the morphology and size of the kidneys, intensity of renal uptake, cortical transit time, and appearance of tracer in the collecting systems are all important.

Imaging Findings

Figure 8.5.1 shows the difference in the parenchymal uptake between the two kidneys, with an enlarged left kidney and low intensity in the MAG3 activity.

On the renogram curve (Fig. 8.5.2), the morphology of the right kidney (*pink line*) is normal; the left kidney (*blue line*) is dilated and obstructed and does not respond to the injection of the diuretic.

Ultrasonography after surgery – not shown – showed persistent hydronephrosis. The ^{99m}Tc-MAG3 renogram (Fig. 8.5.3) shows the difference in uptake between the two kidneys; however, the left kidney curve (*blue line*) has normalized compared with the previous study.

In spite of the persistence of abnormal morphological features, the functional study shows the resolution of obstructive uropathy (Fig. 8.5.4).

Case 6
■
Thromboembolic Pulmonary Disease

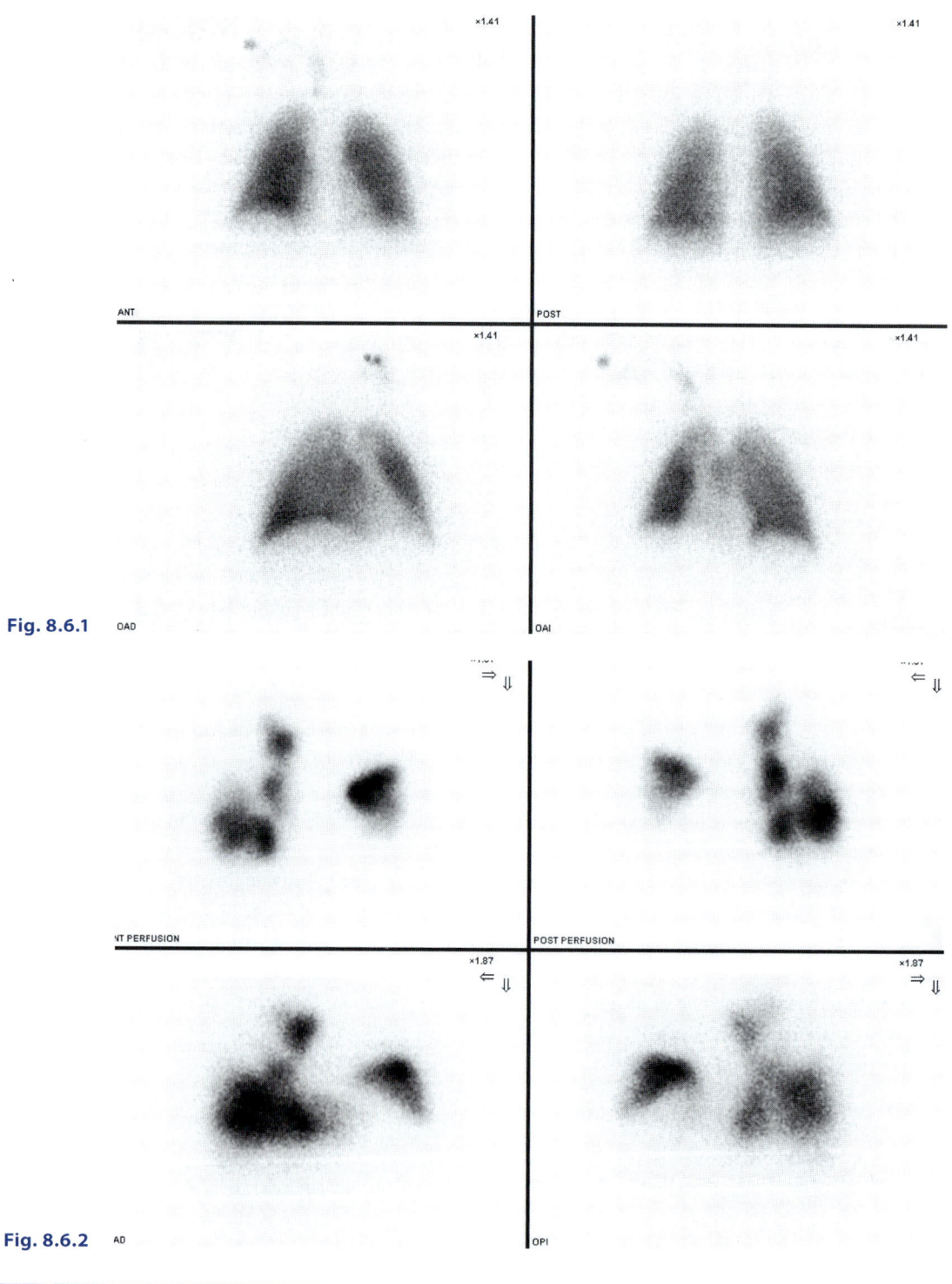

Fig. 8.6.1

Fig. 8.6.2

A 65-year-old man presented at the emergency department with dyspnea and lateral chest pain of sudden onset. Clinical examination showed no alterations at auscultation or in leg perfusion. Arterial blood gasometry showed hypoxemia with hypocapnia. The chest X-ray was unremarkable .

The patient was referred to the nuclear medicine department for ventilation-perfusion scintigraphy to evaluate clinical suspicion of pulmonary thromboembolic disease.

Comments

Pulmonary thromboembolic disease is a potentially life-threatening condition. The major difficulty in its diagnosis is suspecting it in the first place. The vast majority of pulmonary emboli originate in the lower extremities. Leg trauma and prolonged immobilization can be predisposing factors.

The clinical signs and symptoms of pulmonary thromboembolism are nonspecific. The classic triad of chest paint, thrombophlebitis, and hemoptysis only occurs in one third of the patients. Moreover, pulmonary embolism may be asymptomatic.

Pulmonary angiography is the most specify modality for the diagnosis; however, this technique is invasive and is not appropriate for screening.

Scintigraphic studies for pulmonary thromboembolism involve simultaneous imaging of pulmonary ventilation and blood flow. The principle findings for the diagnosis are normal ventilation remains with abnormal pulmonary perfusion, the so-called mismatched defect.

Ventilation imaging can use radioactive inert gases (expensive and limited availability) or radiolabeled aerosols (widely used). Aerosol administration requires patient cooperation to coordinate breathing.

The perfusion lung scan is performed after the ventilation study. The perfusion scan involves the intravenous injection of microparticles of human protein (human serum albumin) labeled with technetium-99m. The distribution of lung radioactivity is proportional to the pulmonary blood flow.

Imaging Findings

Figure 8.6.1 shows a ^{99m}Tc-Technegas ventilation study. Multiple views must be acquired to evaluate each patient. In this study, we can observe uniform distribution of aerosols to both lungs, without ventilatory defects.

The perfusion scan reveals multiple mismatched perfusion defects in both lungs, indicating a high probability of pulmonary thromboembolic disease (Fig. 8.6.2).

In this clinical scenario, a high probability ventilation/perfusion scan indicates a probability of pulmonary embolism of over 90%.

Case 7
■
Coronary Disease

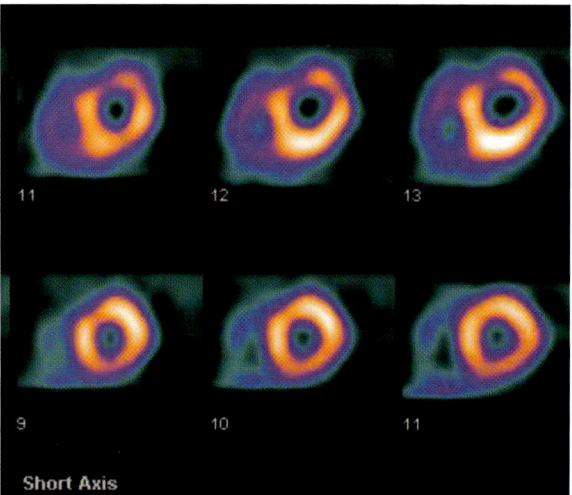

Fig. 8.7.1

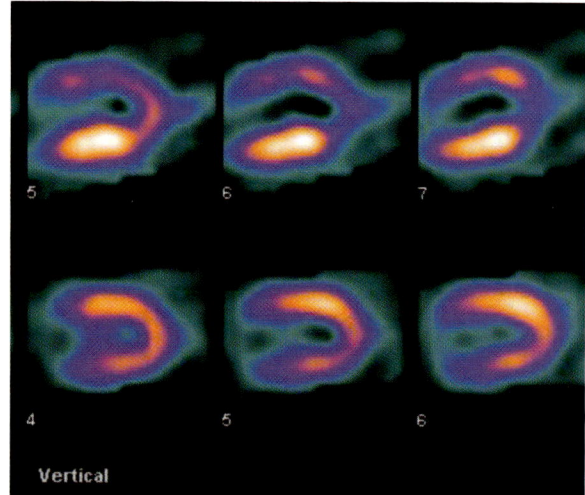

Fig. 8.7.2

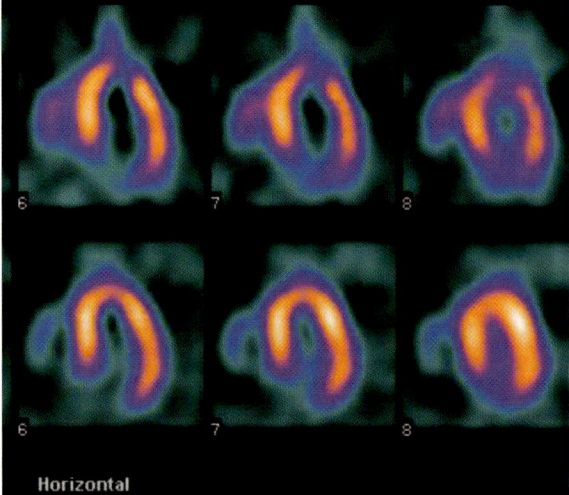

Fig. 8.7.3

Fig. 8.7.4

A 60-year-old man consulted for oppressive chest pain, not directly related with physical exercise. The patient related a tendency to tire easily and occasional dyspnea.

He was heavy smoker and had various episodes of angina, which had become more frequent in the two months prior to consultation. The EKG showed ST depression.

Coronary disease was suspected and he was referred to the nuclear medicine department to assess myocardial blood flow.

Coronary artery disease is a common clinical problem. Many patients present with atypical symptoms, making diagnostic investigation necessary in patients with acute or chronic chest pain.

Several ^{99m}Tc derivatives have been developed for myocardial perfusion studies and have replaced the classical use of 201-Tl. The initial myocardial uptake is linearly related to regional blood flow, without appreciable redistribution.

To compare resting and stress myocardial perfusion, two injections must be given, generally on separate days. The most important use of this technique is to demonstrate myocardial ischemia and detect viable myocardium. Myocardial perfusion imaging is a powerful tool for risk stratification and to formulate management strategies for a wide variety of patients.

The "stress" procedure can be carried out using exercise testing or by pharmacologically induced coronary hyperemia (adenosine or dobutamine). At present we can also analyze wall motion, using EKG-gated acquisition with good correlation between regional wall motion studies and echocardiography.

Areas of decreased or absent perfusion in the stress images that are less severe or normal on the rest images may be due to ischemia. A constant perfusion defect is usually due to myocardial infarction.

SPECT images were obtained 45 minutes after intravenous administration of ^{99m}Tc-tetrofosmin (MYOVIEW®) during the stress test. This study shows an area of decreased perfusion in the anterior wall and in the apex, with contractile alteration in the same region.

Two days later, the rest study was performed. In this case, the myocardial wall showed normal perfusion in all territories.

This myocardinal risk area is shown in the short, vertical, and horizontal axes in the stress study (Figs. 8.7.1–8.7.3 upper row)

The polar map (Fig. 8.7.4) shows an extensive severe reversible defect.

These findings were diagnostic of coronary disease and the patient was referred for coronary angiography. Cardiac catheterization showed severe obstruction of the left anterior descending artery due to atherosclerotic plaques and angioplasty was carried out.

Case 8
Parathyroid Adenoma

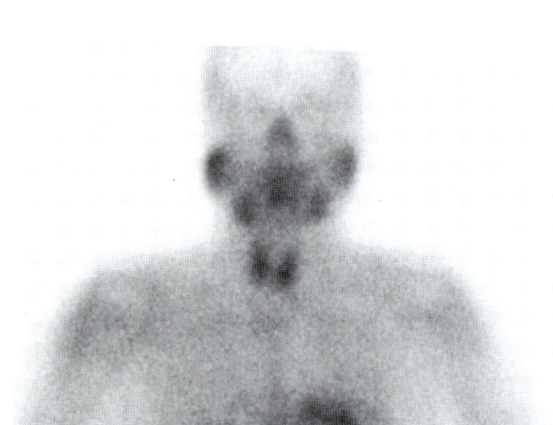

Fig. 8.8.1

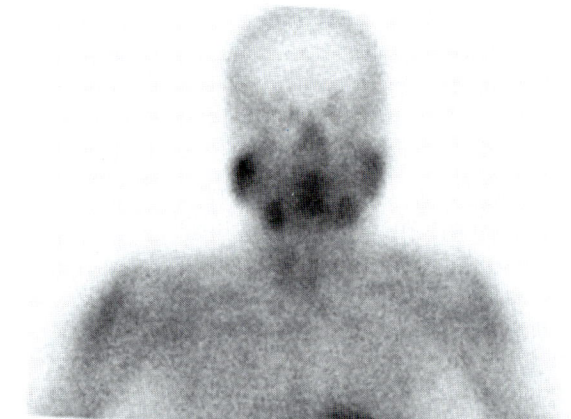

Fig. 8.8.2

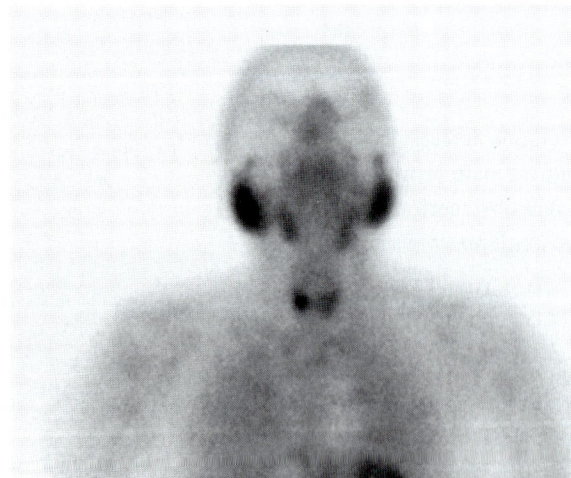

Fig. 8.8.3

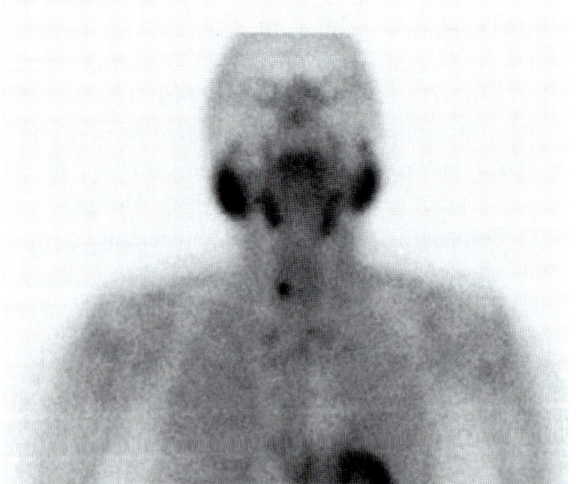

Fig. 8.8.4

An asymptomatic 47-year-old woman presented biochemical evidence of elevated parathyroid hormone levels.

Her neck was normal at physical examination. Neck ultrasound was inconclusive and she was referred for radionuclide examination.

Primary hyperparathyroidism is caused by hyper-functioning parathyroid glands. It is characterized by secretion of more parathyroid hormone than is necessary to maintain normal serum calcium levels. Most patients with hyperparathyroidism are asymptomatic at presentation.

Although it has certain limitations due to the small size of parathyroid glands, in the hands of an experienced operator, ultrasound of the neck is a useful technique for parathyroid abnormalities. CT and MRI effectively demonstrate the location of the parathyroids or their enlargement.

Scintigraphic methods for the study of the parathyroid glands include tallium-201/technetium-99m subtraction and the isonitrile compounds (^{99m}Tc-sestamibi). Both of these procedures have shown a high degree of reliability in clinical use. Parathyroid scintigraphy should only be performed when there is biochemical evidence of hyperparathyroidism.

After the intravenous injection of radiotracer (^{99m}Tc-sestamibi in our institution), early images (obtained at 15 minutes) are compared with delayed images (at 2 hours). Sestamibi "washes out" more rapidly from thyroid (the early image normally depicts the thyroid morphology) than from the parathyroid tissue. The difference in retention may be due to increased number of mitochondria in the cells of an adenoma.

Figure 8.8.1 shows the normal appearance of early acquisition, with normal uptake of ^{99m}Tc-sestamibi in the thyroid gland, as well as in the salivary glands and the myocardium. The delayed image (Fig. 8.8.2) shows normal washout in the thyroid tissue and in non-pathological parathyroid tissue.

On the early acquisition (Fig. 8.8.3), increased uptake in the right lower pole of the thyroid is evident. On the delayed image (Fig. 8.8.4), the thyroid uptake has washed out and the right inferior parathyroid adenoma is clearly visualized.

Case 9

Pulmonary Solitary Node. Pet-CT Evaluation

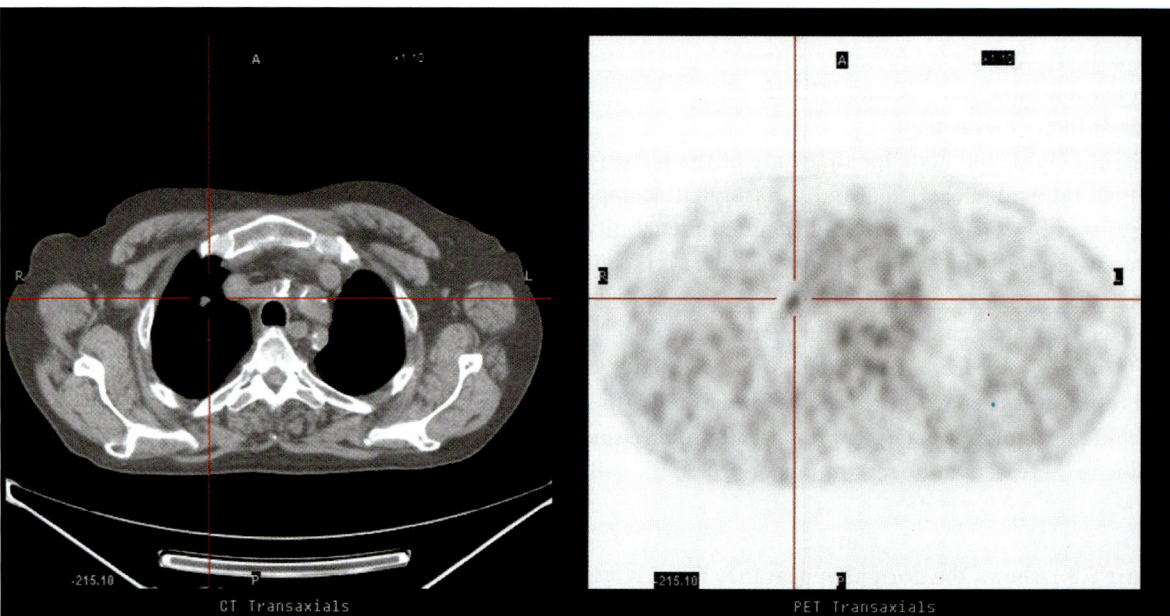

Fig. 8.9.1

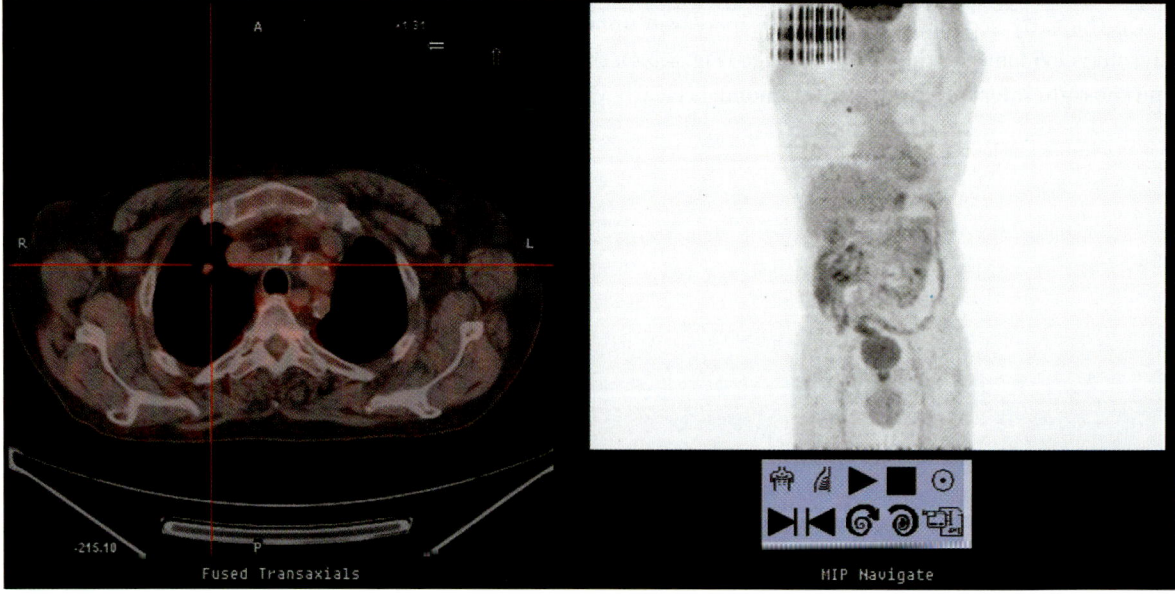

Fig. 8.9.2

A 68-year-old man with a noncalcified solitary pulmonary nodule with lobulated margins and measuring 1×0.9 cms observed at CT was referred to the nuclear medicine department to evaluate the malignant or benign nature of this finding.

A solitary pulmonary nodule is defined as single rounded lesion not associated with any other lung lesions, without lymphadenopathy. Over 40% of solitary pulmonary nodules are malignant in the majority of reported series.

The sensitivity and specificity of 18-FDG PET is high. Any degree of FDG uptake must initially be considered suspicious for malignancy (although benign lesions can also exhibit variable degrees of FDG uptake).

A negative PET scan indicates that a nodule has a high probability of being benign, but a small number of nodules without glycolytic activity in PET will be malignant and follow-up is needed.

Nodules smaller than 1cm are best evaluated using dynamic contrast-enhanced CT.

Dual point PET images (at 1 and 3 hours post-injection) and evaluation of changes in the standardized uptake value (SUV) improve accuracy. Malignant lesions show increased FDG uptake on late images whereas benign lesions have the same or inferior index in the second scan. This is especially useful in SUVs around 2.5 I.

Axial CT shows the solitary pulmonary nodule in the right upper lobe (Fig. 8.9.1).

Figure 8.9.2. Axial PET image shows focal moderately increased glycolytic activity in this area, with an SUV of 7.2 (malignity range).

Axial PET-CT image (Fig. 8.9.3) shows a hypermetabolic solitary pulmonary nodule in the right upper lobe.

The lesion was considered malignant, the patient was referred for resection and histological study confirmed the malignancy of the lesion.

We express our gratitude to Jose R. Infante de la Torre (Badajoz Hospital) for providing the images.

Case 10

Lymphoma. Pet-CT Evaluation

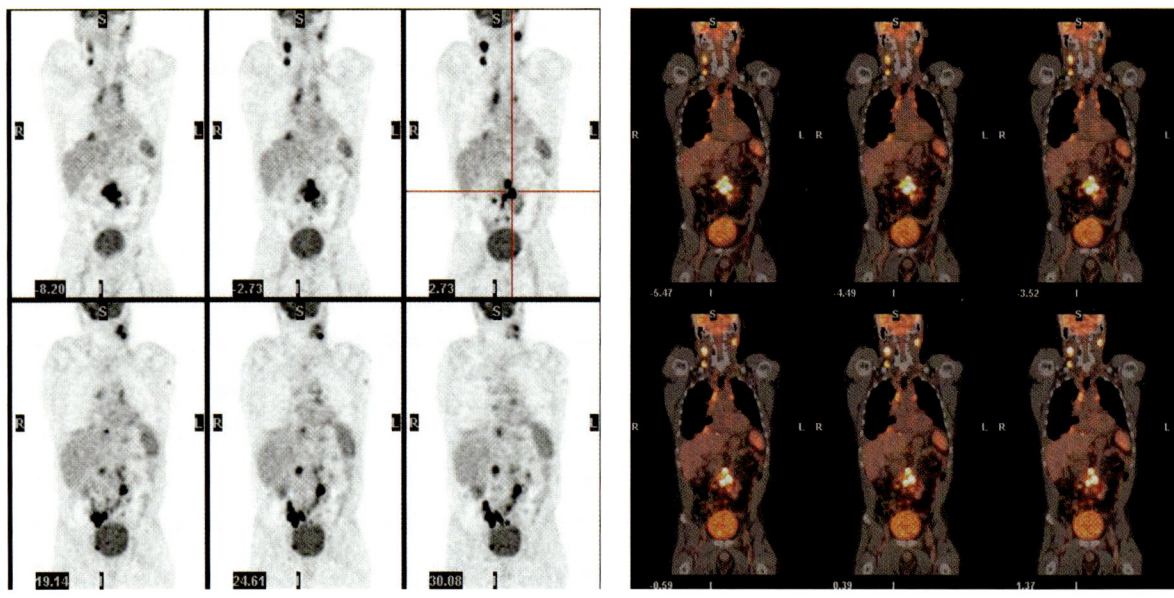

Fig. 8.10.1   Fig. 8.10.2

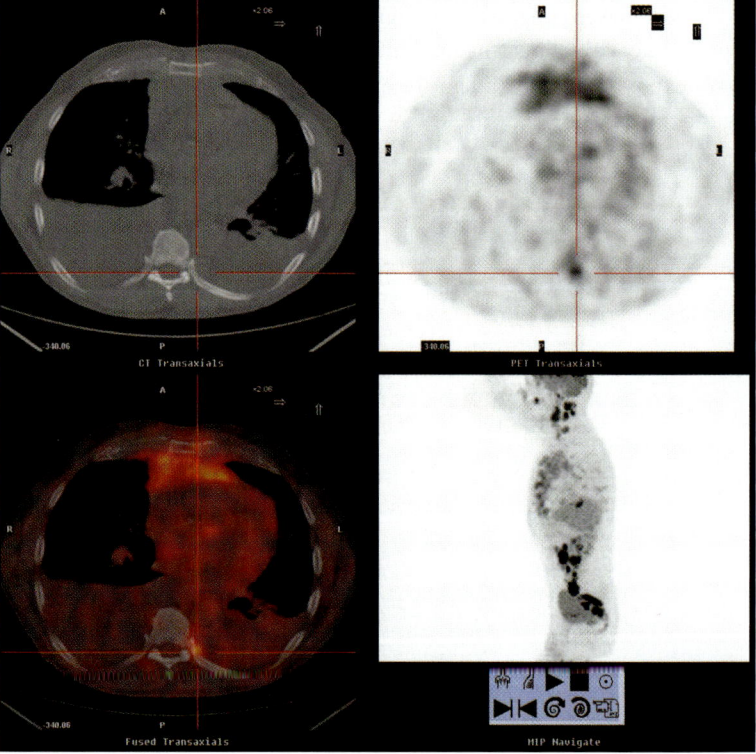

Fig. 8.10.3

A 40-year-old man with a nodular non-Hodgkin's lymphoma was referred for staging before the first therapeutic approach.

The main purpose of combining PET and CT systems in a single device is to determine the anatomical site of metabolic PET tracer uptake.

The typical PET-CT study begins with a CT scout to define the scan area, followed by helical CT scan, and finally PET images. The CT images are used for attenuation correction of the PET data.

Fluorodeoxyglucose-18F (FDG) is the most commonly used radiotracer in PET. It has demonstrated wide utility in a variety of indications, including oncology, cardiology, and brain diseases.

The primary attribute of PET imaging is the great contrast resolution compared with anatomical imaging techniques. PET can detect early disease before anatomical changes become evident. It usually has a greater contrast-to-noise ratio of abnormal/normal areas. The disadvantages are its sensitivity for small lesions, which increases the possibility of false positives due to inflammatory, infectious, or other benign etiologies. PET-CT has remedied the problem of anatomical localization with PET images alone and has also increased the accuracy of technique. The only disadvantages of PET-CT relative to PET alone are artifacts.

The standardized uptake value (SUV) is a semiquantitative measurement of activity in the region of interest , which is normalized for surface area and weight and injected dose. We can use the SUV as tool to compare different studies in the same patient (evaluation of the response to treatment, or clinical situation); however, the SUV must be used with caution for decisions regarding cutoffs. There is little evidence that SUV values are superior to visual interpretation in reaching the correct diagnosis.

18-FDG study shows extensive lymphoma. Coronal PET scan (Fig. 8.10.1) shows uptake in cervical, mediastinal, axillary, retroperitoneal, and sacral nodes. PET-CT images (Fig. 8.10.2) are more sensitive for both nodal and extranodal disease (sensitivity 94%).

Figure 8.10.3 demonstrates the procedure to locate a paravertebral node suspicious for malignancy. Note the usefulness of PET-CT in determining the anatomic localization of the focally increased uptake.

In this group of patients, baseline pre-treatment PET-CT scans are very useful for staging. PET-CT is also useful in the evaluation of the response to therapy (lack of response suggests that the treatment regimen should be changed) and in the detection of relapse.

We express our gratitude to Jose R. Infante de la Torre (Badajoz Hospital) for providing the images.

Further Readings

Books

Atlas of PET/CT Imaging in Oncology. Czernin J, Dahlbom M, Ratib O, Schiepers C (2004) Berlin-Heidelberg: Springer-Verlag. ISBN-13: 9783540209522

Cardiac PET and PET/CT Imaging. Di Carli MF, Lipton MJ (2007) Berlin-Heidelberg: Springer-Verlag. ISBN-13: 9780387352756

Diagnostic Nuclear Medicine. Sandler MP, Coleman MP, Paton JA, Wackers FJ, Gottschalk A (2004) Philadelphia: Lippincott Williams & Wilkins. ISBN-13: 9780781732529

Nuclear Cardiology: Practical Applications. Heller GV, Hendel RC (2004) New York: McGraw-Hill. ISBN-13: 9780071386357

Nuclear Medicine: in Clinical Diagnosis and Treatment. Ell PJ, Gambhir SS (2004) Edinburgh: Churchill Livingstone. ISBN-13: 9780443073120

Nuclear Medicine: The Requisites. Ziessman HA, O'Malley JP, Thrall JH (2007) New York: Elsevier. ISBN-13: 9780323029469

Pediatric Nuclear Medicine/PET. Treves ST (2007) New York: Springer-Verlag. ISBN-13: 9780387323213

PET and PET/CT: A clinical guide. Lin EC, Alavi A (2005) New York: Thieme. ISBN-13: 9781588904003

Physics and Radiobiology of Nuclear Medicine. Saha GB (2006) Berlin-Heidelberg: Springer-Verlag. ISBN-13: 9780387307541

The Pathophysiologic Basis of Nuclear Medicine. Elgazzar AH (2006) Berlin-Heidelberg: Springer-Verlag. ISBN-13: 9783540239925

Weblinks

http://biomedcentral.com/bmcnuc/med
http://bnms.org.uk
http://brighamrad.harvard.edu/education/online/introduction.html
http://eamn.org
http://gamma.wustl.edu/home.htlm
http://nucmedinfo.com
http://semn.es
http://snmjournals.org
http://snm.org
http://springerlink.com

Articles

Brain

Claus JJ, van Harskamp F, Breteler MM, Krenning EP, de Koning I, van der Cammen TJ, Hofman A, Hasan D. The diagnostic value of SPECT with Tc 99m HMPAO in Alzheimer's disease: a population-based study. Neurology 1994; 44:454–461

Conrad GR, Sinha P. Scintigraphy as a confirmatory test of brain death. Semin Nucl Med 2003; 33(4):312–323

Costa DC, Motteux IM, McCready AC. Diagnosis of brain death with technetium 99m hexamethylpropylene amine oxime. Eur J Nucl Med 1991; 18(7):503–506

de la Riva A, Gonzalez FM, Llamas-Elvira JM, et al. Diagnosis of brain death: superiority of perfusion studies with 99Tcm-HMPAO over conventional radionuclide cerebral angiography. Br J Radiol 1992; 65(772):289–294

Donohoe KJ, Frey KA, Gerbaudo VH, Mariani G, Nagel JS, Shulkin B. Procedure guideline for brain death scintigraphy. J Nucl Med 2003; 44(5):846–851

Dougall NJ, Bruggink S, Ebmeier KP. Systematic review of the diagnostic accuracy of ^{99m}Tc-HMPAO-SPECT in dementia Am J Geriatr Psychiatry 2004; 12(6):554–570

Gordon I. Cerebral blood flow imaging in paediatrics: a review. Nucl Med Commun 1996; 17(12):1021–1029

Kurtek RW, Lai KK, Tauxe WN, Eidelman BH, Fung JJ. Tc-99m hexamethylpropylene amine oxime scintigraphy in the diagnosis of brain death and its implications for the harvesting of organs used for transplantation. Clin Nucl Med 2000; 25(1):7–10

Uchida Y, Minoshima S, Okada S, Kawata T, Ito H. Diagnosis of dementia using perfusion SPECT imaging at the patient's initial visit to a cognitive disorder clinic. Clin Nucl Med 2006; 31(12):764–773

Weckesser M, Schober O. Brain death revisited: utility confirmed for nuclear medicine. Eur J Nucl Med 1999; 26(11):1387–1391

Movement Disorders

Booij J, Speelman JD, Horstink MW, Wolters EC. The clinical benefit of imaging striatal dopamine transporters with [^{123}I]FP-CIT SPET in differentiating patients with presynaptic parkinsonism from those with other forms of parkinsonism. Eur J Nucl Med 2001; 28(3):266–272

Catafau AM, Tolosa E; DaTSCAN Clinically Uncertain Parkinsonian Syndromes Study Group. Impact of dopamine transporter SPECT using ^{123}I-Ioflupane on diagnosis and management of patients with clinically uncertain Parkinsonian syndromes. Mov Disord 2004; 19(10):1175–1182

Filippi L, Manni C, Pierantozzi M, Brusa L, Danieli R, Stanzione P, Schillaci O. 123I-FP-CIT in progressive supranuclear palsy and in Parkinson's disease: a SPECT semiquantitative study. Nucl Med Commun 2006; 27(4):381–386

Lorberboym M, Djaldetti R, Melamed E, Sadeh M, Lampl Y. 123I-FP-CIT SPECT imaging of dopamine transporters in patients with cerebrovascular disease and clinical diagnosis of vascular parkinsonism. J Nucl Med 2004; 45(10):1688–1693

Marshall V, Grosset D. Role of dopamine transporter imaging in routine clinical practice. Mov Disord 2003; 18(12):1415–1423

Marshall VL, Patterson J, Hadley DM, Grosset KA, Grosset DG. Two-year follow-up in 150 consecutive cases with normal dopamine transporter imaging. Nucl Med Commun 2006; 27(12):933–937

McKeith I, O'Brien J, Walker Z, Tatsch K, Booij J, Darcourt J, Padovani A, Giubbini R, Bonuccelli U, Volterrani D, Holmes C, Kemp P, Tabet N, Meyer I, Reininger C; DLB Study Group. Sensitivity and specificity of dopamine transporter imaging with 123I-FP-CIT SPECT in dementia with Lewy bodies: a phase III, multicentre study. Lancet Neurol 2007; 6(4):305–313

Schillaci O, Pierantozzi M, Filippi L, Manni C, Brusa L, Danieli R, Bernardi G, Simonetti G, Stanzione P. The effect of levodopa therapy on dopamine transporter SPECT imaging with (^{123})I-FP-CIT in patients with Parkinson's disease. Eur J Nucl Med Mol Imaging 2005; 32(12):1452–1456

Spiegel J, Mollers MO, Jost WH, Fuss G, Samnick S, Dillmann U, Becker G, Kirsch CM. FP-CIT and MIBG scintigraphy in early Parkinson's disease. Mov Disord 2005; 20(5):552–561

Coronary Disease

Cerqueira MD. Nuclear cardiology: finally a one-stop shop for diagnosis, risk stratification, and management of coronary artery disease. Clin Cardiol 2006; 29(9 Suppl 1):I26–33

Elhendy A, Bax JJ, Poldermans D. Dobutamine stress myocardial perfusion imaging in coronary artery disease. J Nucl Med 2002; 43(12):1634–1646

Hendel RC, Jamil T, Glover DK. Pharmacologic stress testing: new methods and new agents. J Nucl Cardiol 2003; 10(2):197–204

Heo J, Iskandrian AS. Technetium-labeled myocardial perfusion agents. Cardiol Clin 1994; 12(2):187–198

Iskandrian AS. Adenosine myocardial perfusion imaging. J Nucl Med 1994; 35(4):734–736

Kontos MC, Tatum JL. Imaging in the evaluation of the patient with suspected acute coronary syndrome. Semin Nucl Med 2003; 33(4):246–258

Metz LD, Beattie M, Hom R, Redberg RF, Grady D, Fleischmann KE. The prognostic value of normal exercise myocardial perfusion imaging and exercise echocardiography: a meta-analysis. J Am Coll Cardiol 2007; 49(2):227–237

Russell RR 3rd, Zaret BL. Nuclear cardiology: present and future. Curr Probl Cardiol 2006; 31(9):557–629

Tamaki N, Morita K. SPET in cardiology. Diagnosis, prognosis, and management of patients with coronary artery disease. Q J Nucl Med Mol Imaging 2005; 49(2):193–203

Udelson JE, Shafer CD, Carrio I. Radionuclide imaging in heart failure: assessing etiology and outcomes and implications for management. J Nucl Cardiol 2002; 9(5 Suppl):40S–52S

Gastrointestinal Bleeding

Feingold DL, Caliendo FJ, Chinn BT, et al. Does hemodynamic instability predict positive technetium-labeled red blood cell scintigraphy in patients wit acute lower gastrointestinal bleeding? A review of 50 patients. Dis Colon Rectum 2005; 48(5):1001–1004

Ford PV, Bartold SP, Fink-Bennett DM, Jolles PR, Lull RJ, Maurer AH, Seabold J. Procedure guideline for gastrointestinal bleeding and Meckel's diverticulum scintigraphy. Society of Nuclear Medicine. J Nucl Med 1999; 40(7):1226–1232

Howarth DM, Tang K, Lees W. The clinical utility of nuclear medicine imaging for the detection of occult gastrointestinal haemorrhage. Nucl Med Commun 2002; 23(6):591–594

Infante JR, Gonzalez FM, Vallejo JA, Torres M, Pacheco C, Latre JM. False-positive results of a gastrointestinal bleeding study caused by an ectopic kidney. Clin Nucl Med 2000; 25(8):645–646

Kan JH, Funaki B, O'Rourke BD, Ward MB, Appelbaum DE. Delayed ^{99m}Tc-labeled erythrocyte scintigraphy in patients with lower gastrointestinal tract hemorrhage: effect of positive findings on clinical management. Acad Radiol 2003; 10(5):497–501

Lefkovitz Z, Cappell MS, Kaplan M, Mitty H, Gerard P. Radiology in the diagnosis and therapy of gastrointestinal bleeding. Gastroenterol Clin North Am 2000; 29(2):489–512

Olds GD, Cooper GS, Chak A, Sivak M, Chiteale AA, Wong RCK. The yield of bleeding scans in acute lower gastrointestinal hemorrhage. J Clin Gastroenterol 2005; 39(4):273–277

Ponzo F, Zhuang H, Liu FM, Lacorte LB, Moussavian B, Wang S, Alavi A. Tc-99m sulfur colloid and Tc-99m tagged red blood cell methods are comparable for detecting lower gastrointestinal bleeding in clinical practice. Clin Nucl Med 2002; 27(6):405–409

Zettinig G, Staudenherz A, Leitha T. The importance of delayed images in gastrointestinal bleeding scintigraphy. Nucl Med Commun 2002; 23(8):803–808

Zuckier LS. Acute gastrointestinal bleeding. Semin Nucl Med 2003; 33(4):297–311

Inflammatory Bowel Disease

Alberini JL, Badran A, Freneaux E, Hadji S, Kalifa G, Devaux JY, Dupont T. Technetium-99m HMPAO-labeled leukocyte imaging compared with endoscopy, ultrasonography, and contrast radiology in children with inflammatory bowel disease. J Pediatr Gastroenterol Nutr 2001; 32(3):278–286

Bennink R, Peeters M, D'Haens G, Rutgeerts P, Mortelmans L. Tc-99m HMPAO white blood cell scintigraphy in the assessment of the extent and severity of an acute exacerbation of ulcerative colitis. Clin Nucl Med 2001; 26(2):99–104

Charron M. Pediatric inflammatory bowel disease imaged with Tc-99m white blood cells. Clin Nucl Med 2000; 25(9):708–715

Grahnquist L, Chapman SC, Hvidsten S, Murphy MS. Evaluation of ^{99m}Tc-HMPAO leukocyte scintigraphy in the investigation of pediatric inflammatory bowel disease. J Pediatr 2003; 143(1):48–53

Gyorke T, Duffek L, Bartfai K, Mako E, Karlinger K, Mester A, Tarjan Z. The role of nuclear medicine in inflammatory bowel disease. A review with experiences of aspecific bowel activity using immunoscintigraphy with ^{99m}Tc anti-granulocyte antibodies. Eur J Radiol 2000; 35(3):183–192

Lachter J, Isseroff HN, Yasin K, Keidar Z, Israel O. Radiolabeled leukocyte imaging in inflammatory bowel disease: a prospective blinded evaluation. Hepatogastroenterology 2003; 50(53):1439–1441

Martin-Comin J, Prats E. Clinical applications of radiolabeled blood elements in inflammatory bowel disease. Q J Nucl Med 1999; 43(1):74–82

Martin-Comin J. Radiolabelled white blood cells in inflammatory bowel diseases. Nucl Med Commun 2002; 23(11):1039–1040

Peters AM. Nuclear medicine imaging in infection and inflammation. J R Coll Physicians Lond 1998; 32(6):512–519

Stokkel MP, Reigman HE, Pauwels EK. Scintigraphic head-to-head comparison between ^{99m}Tc-WBCs and ^{99m}Tc-LeukoScan in the evaluation of inflammatory bowel disease: a pilot study. Eur J Nucl Med Mol Imaging 2002; 29(2):251–254

Pulmonary Thromboembolism

Giordano A, Angiolillo DJ. Current role of lung scintigraphy in pulmonary embolism. Q J Nucl Med 2001; 45(4):294–301

Hagen PJ, Hartmann IJ, Hoekstra OS, Stokkel MP, Teule GJ, Prins MH. How to use a gestalt interpretation for ventilation-perfusion lung scintigraphy. J Nucl Med 2002; 43(10):1317–1323

Hartmann IJ, Hagen PJ, Stokkel MP, Hoekstra OS, Prins MH. Technegas versus (81m)Kr ventilation-perfusion scintigraphy: a comparative study in patients with suspected acute pulmonary embolism. J Nucl Med 2001; 42(3):393–400

Hatabu H, Uematsu H, Nguyen B, Miller WT Jr, Hasegawa I, Gefter WB. CT and MR in pulmonary embolism: A changing role for nuclear medicine in diagnostic strategy. Semin Nucl Med 2002; 32(3):183–192

Itti E, Nguyen S, Robin F, Desarnaud S, Rosso J, Harf A, Meignan. Distribution of ventilation/perfusion ratios in pulmonary embolism: an adjunct to the interpretation of ventilation/perfusion lung scans. J Nucl Med 2002; 43(12):1596–1602

Meignan MA. Lung ventilation/perfusion SPECT: the right technique for hard times. J Nucl Med 2002; 43(5):648–651

Rizzo-Padoin N, Farina A, Le Pen C, Duet M, Mundler O, Leverge R. A comparison of radiopharmaceutical agents used for the diagnosis of pulmonary embolism. Nucl Med Commun 2001; 22(4):375–381

Schumichen C. V/Q-scanning/SPECT for the diagnosis of pulmonary embolism. Respiration 2003; 70(4):329–342

Wilson HT, Meagher TM, Williams S. Combined helical computed tomographic pulmonary angiography and lung perfusion scintigraphy for investigating acute pulmonary embolism. Clin Radiol 2002; 57(1):33–36

Worsley DF, Alavi A. Radionuclide imaging of acute pulmonary embolism. Semin Nucl Med 2003; 33(4):259–278

Parathyroid Imaging

Coakley AJ. Parathyroid imaging. Nucl Med Commun 1995; 16(7):522–533

de Jonge FA, Pauwels EK, Hamdy NA. Scintigraphy in the clinical evaluation of disorders of mineral and skeletal metabolism in renal failure. Eur J Nucl Med 1991; 18(10):839–855

Giordano A, Rubello D, Casara D. New trends in parathyroid scintigraphy. Eur J Nucl Med 2001; 28(9):1409–1420

Gotthardt M, Lohmann B, Behr TM, et al. Clinical value of parathyroid scintigraphy with technetium-99m methoxyisobutylisonitrile: discrepancies in clinical data and a systematic metaanalysis of the literature. World J Surg 2004; 28(1):100–107. Epub 2003 Nov 26

Hiromatsu Y, Ishibashi M, Nishida H, Okuda S, Miyake I. Technetium-99m tetrofosmin parathyroid imaging in patients with primary hyperparathyroidism. Intern Med 2000; 39(2):101–106

Kettle AG, O'Doherty MJ. Parathyroid imaging: how good is it and how should it be done? Semin Nucl Med 2006; 36(3):206–211

McBiles M, Lambert AT, Cote MG, Kim SY. Sestamibi parathyroid imaging. Semin Nucl Med 1995; 25(3):221–234

Mitchell BK, Kinder BK, Cornelius E, Stewart AF. Primary hyperparathyroidism: preoperative localization using technetium-sestamibi scanning. J Clin Endocrinol Metab 1995; 80(1):7–10

Palestro CJ, Tomas MB, Tronco GG. Radionuclide imaging of the parathyroid glands. Semin Nucl Med 2005; 35(4):266–276

Smith JR, Oates ME. Radionuclide imaging of the parathyroid glands: patterns, pearls, and pitfalls. Radiographics. 2004; 24(4):1101–1115

Diuretic Renography

Boubaker A, Prior J, Antonescu C, Meyrat B, Frey P, Delaloye AB. F+0 renography in neonates and infants younger than 6 months: an accurate method to diagnose severe obstructive uropathy. J Nucl Med 2001; 42(12):1780–1788

Dubovsky EV, Russell CD, Bischof-Delaloye A, Bubeck B, Chaiwatanarat T, Hilson AJ, Rutland M, Oei HY, Sfakianakis GN, Taylor A Jr. Report of the Radionuclides in Nephrourology Committee for evaluation of transplanted kidney (review of techniques). Semin Nucl Med 1999; 29(2):175–188

Eskild-Jensen A, Gordon I, Piepsz A, Frokiaer. Congenital unilateral hydronephrosis: a review of the impact of diuretic renography on clinical treatment. J Urol 2005; 173(5):1471–1476

Gordon I. Assessment of pediatric hydronephrosis using output efficiency. J Nucl Med 1997; 38(9):1487–1489

Koelliker SL, Cronan JJ. Acute urinary tract obstruction. Imaging update. Urol Clin North Am 1997; 24(3):571–582

Koff SA, Binkovitz L, Coley B, Jayanthi V. Renal pelvis volume during diuresis in children with hydronephrosis: implications for diagnosing obstruction with diuretic renography. J Urol 2005; 174(1):303–307

O'Reilly PH. Obstructive uropathy. Q J Nucl Med 2002; 46(4):295–303

Piepsz A, Ham HR. Pediatric applications of renal nuclear medicine. Semin Nucl Med 2006; 36:16–35

Taylor A Jr, Nally JV. Clinical applications of renal scintigraphy. AJR Am J Roentgenol 1995; 164(1):31–41

Wong DC, Rossleigh MA, Farnsworth RH. F+0 diuresis renography in infants and children. J Nucl Med 1999; 40(11):1805–1811

PET in Lymphoma

Baudard M, Comte F, Conge AM, Mariano-Goulart D, Klein B, Rossi JF. Importance of [^{18}F]fluorodeoxyglucose-positron emission tomography scanning for the monitoring of responses to immunotherapy in follicular lymphoma. Leuk Lymphoma 2007; 48(2):381–388

Brepoels L, Stroobants S, Verhoef G. PET and PET/CT for response evaluation in lymphoma: current practice and developments. Leuk Lymphoma 2007; 48(2):270–282

Burton C, Ell P, Linch D. The role of PET imaging in lymphoma. Br J Haematol 2004; 126(6):772–784

Collins CD. PET in lymphoma. Cancer Imaging 2006; 6: S63–70

Jerusalem G, Hustinx R, Beguin Y, Fillet G. Evaluation of therapy for lymphoma. Semin Nucl Med 2005; 35(3):186–196

Juweid ME, Stroobants S, Hoekstra OS, et al. Imaging Subcommittee of International Harmonization Project in Lymphoma. Use of positron emission tomography for response assessment of lymphoma: consensus of the Imaging Subcommittee of International Harmonization Project in Lymphoma. J Clin Oncol 2007; 25(5):571–578

Kazama T, Faria SC, Varavithya V, Phongkitkarun S, Ito H, Macapinlac HA. FDG PET in the evaluation of treatment for lymphoma: clinical usefulness and pitfalls. Radiographics 2005; 25(1):191–207

Kirby AM, George Mikhaeel N. The role of FDG PET in the management of lymphoma: practical guidelines. Nucl Med Commun 2007; 28(5):355–357

Kumar R, Maillard I, Schuster SJ, Alavi A. Utility of fluorodeoxyglucose-PET imaging in the management of patients with Hodgkin's and non-Hodgkin''s lymphomas. Radiol Clin North Am 2004; 42(6):1083–1100

Mikhaeel NG. Use of FDG-PET to monitor response to chemotherapy and radiotherapy in patients with lymphomas. Eur J Nucl Med Mol Imaging 2006; 33 Suppl 1:22–26

PET in Solitary Pulmonary Nodule

Aquino SL, Kuester LB, Muse VV, Halpern EF, Fischman AJ. Accuracy of transmission CT and FDG-PET in the detection of small pulmonary nodules with integrated PET/CT. Eur J Nucl Med Mol Imaging 2006; 33(6):692–696

Bruzzi JF, Munden RF. PET/CT imaging of lung cancer. J Thorac Imaging 2006; 21(2):123–136

Bunyaviroch T, Coleman R. PET evaluation of lung cancer. J Nucl Med 2006; 47(3):451–469

Coleman RE. PET in lung cancer. J Nucl Med 1999; 40(5):814–820

Goerres GW, von Schulthess GK, Steinert HC. Why most PET of lung and head-and-neck cancer will be PET/CT. J Nucl Med 2004; 45 Suppl 1:66S–71S

Jeong YJ, Yi CA, Lee KS. Solitary pulmonary nodules: detection, characterization, and guidance for further diagnostic workup and treatment. AJR Am J Roentgenol 2007; 188(1):57–68

Kim SK, Allen-Auerbach M, Goldin J, Fueger BJ, Dahlbom M, Brown M, et al. Accuracy of PET/CT in characterization of solitary pulmonary lesions. J Nucl Med 2007; 48(2):214–220

Kuehl H, Veit P, Rosenbaum SJ, Bockisch A, Antoch G. Can PET/CT replace separate diagnostic CT for cancer imaging? Optimizing CT protocols for imaging cancers of the chest and abdomen. J Nucl Med 2007; 48 Suppl 1:45S–57S

Mavi A, Lakhani P, Zhuang H, Gupta NC, Alavi A. Fluorodeoxyglucose-PET in characterizing solitary pulmonary nodules, assessing pleural diseases, and the initial staging, restaging, therapy planning, and monitoring response of lung cancer. Radiol Clin North Am 2005; 43(1):1–21, ix

Yi CA, Lee KS, Kim BT, Choi JY, Kwon OJ, Kim H, Shim YM, Chung MJ. Tissue characterization of solitary pulmonary nodule: comparative study between helical dynamic CT and integrated PET/CT. J Nucl Med 2006; 47(3):443–450

Pediatric Radiology

9

PEDRO DALTRO, L. CELSO HYGINO CRUZ JR, RENATA DO A. NOGUEIRA, and MIRRIAM T. C. PORTO

Introduction

The old medical saying "a kid is not a small grown-up" is perfect to illustrate the importance of pediatric radiology within the field of radiology. As Dr. Lefèbvre (the father of the European Society of Pediatric Radiology (ESPR)) said in 1958: "In pediatrics, losing time entails the risk of losing a life or permanent disability for an entire life… Radiologists who perform children's examinations must be well informed and competent."

All important medical centers should have a pediatric radiologist because there are important anatomic differences between children and adults; furthermore, different diseases, with their own specific characteristics affect children. Lastly, children are especially vulnerable to the effects of ionizing radiation, so the imaging techniques of choice used are often different, too. Like all radiologists, those working in pediatrics must keep abreast of the continual advances in imaging techniques and knowledge about diseases as well as new developments in treatment.

Pediatric radiology can be said to have become firmly established in 1945 with the appearance of the first edition of John Caffey's seminal book Pediatric X-ray Diagnosis (Year Book Publishers, Chicago). This book set guidelines for the imaging of pediatric patients and was and is referred to as "the Book" because it was the first reference work available.

In the second half of the 20th century, pediatric radiology underwent great developments in the U.S., mainly in Boston under the tutelage of Dr. Edward B.D. Neuhauser. Dr. Neuhauser's department was then known as a "leading light of pediatric radiology". At the same time, some European physicians also studied and worked to improve pediatric radiology: Dr. Lefèbvre, J Sauvegrain, Cl Fauré, H.Kaufman, U. Rudhe and others. Europe has now outstanding professors in the area of pediatric radiology all over the continent.

PEDRO DALTRO
Honorary Member of |ESPR
Ex- President of SLARP

Case 1
Hip Dysplasia

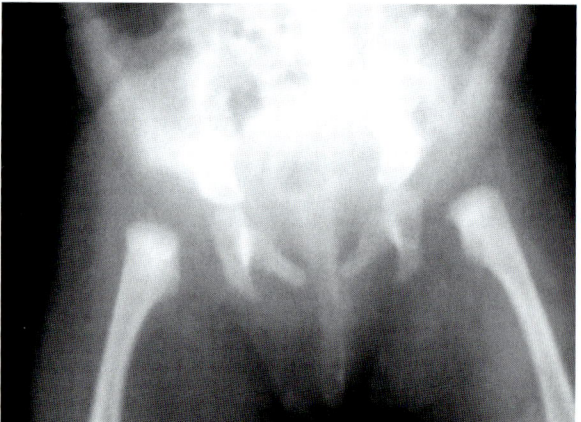

Fig. 9.1.1

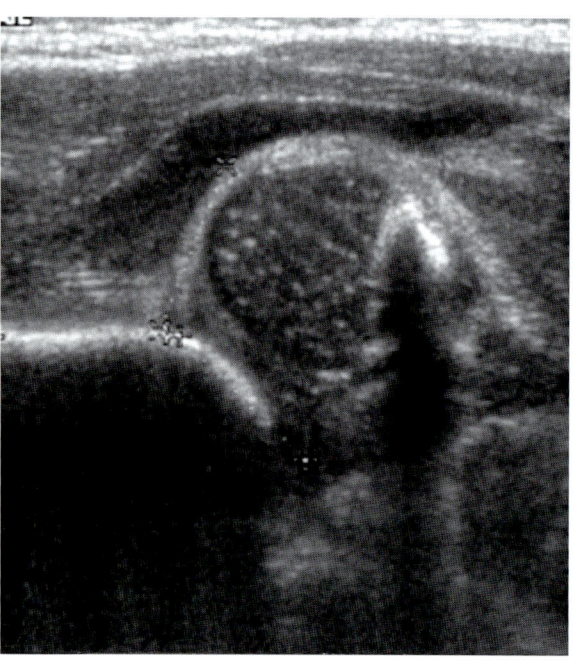

Fig. 9.1.2

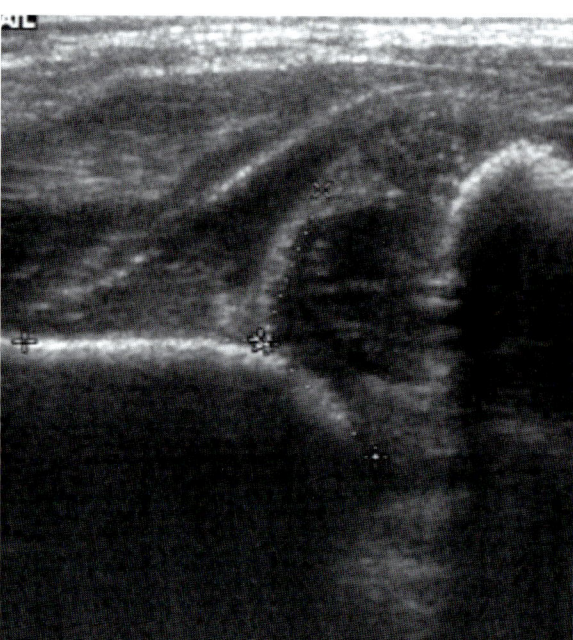

Fig. 9.1.4

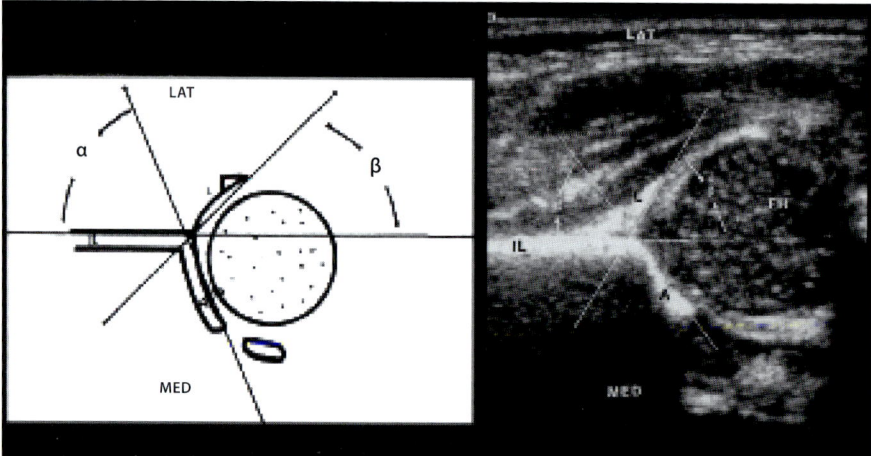

Fig. 9.1.3

A breech-delivered newborn girl presented a distinctive bilateral clicking sound while the head of the femur was moved in and out of the hip joint during the Ortolani test.

Comments

Developmental dysplasia of the hip is considered to form part of generalized pelvic instability (ligament and joint instability); it has an overall frequency of 0.1%. According to some studies, more than 60% of all newborns with suspected hip dysplasia become stable by the age of 1 week and 88% are stable by the age of 2 months. The remaining 12% of the children with positive Ortolani test shows residual hip instability.

Hip dysplasia may be associated with neuromuscular disorders such as cerebral palsy, myelomeningocele, arthrogryposis, or Larsen syndrome. Early diagnosis is essential to avoid evolution to acetabular dysplasia. Hip dysplasia may be difficult to diagnose in older babies and late diagnosis is associated with worse treatment outcome.

Plain-film findings: delayed ossification in the femoral heads; lateral and upward displacement of the femur; flat acetabular roof; development of a pseudoacetabulum in longstanding cases; vertical Perkins' line passes medial to the medial portion of the femoral metaphysis

Ultrasound findings (Graf's technique): Ultrasound is the first method of evaluation because it can detect minimal degrees of laxity in the joint. Dynamic study with posterior and abduction stresses to the hip is able to detect subluxation or dislocation. Four basic hip types have been described according to alpha and beta angle measurements and the development of the acetabulum. Measurement of the hip angles shows great overlap between normal and abnormal hips. Type 1 is considered normal (alpha angle greater than 60 degrees). Type 4 includes the greatest grade of hip dysplasia.

Imaging Findings

Right and left hip ultrasound in the coronal flexion view (Figs. 9.1.1 and 9.1.2) showed femoral head displacement out of the acetabulum. Plain-film radiography (Fig. 9.1.3) demonstrated lateral hip dislocation to vertical Perkins' lines.

Case 2
■
Hypertrophic Pyloric Stenosis

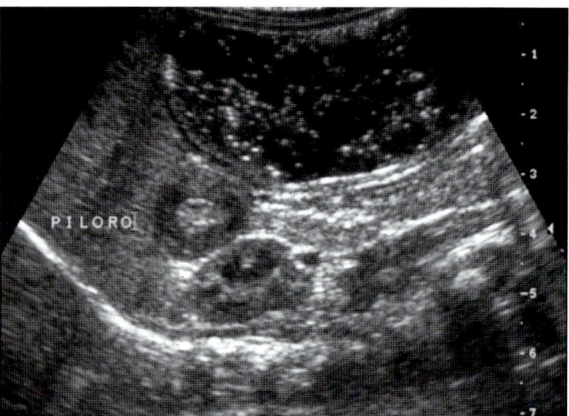

Fig. 9.2.1

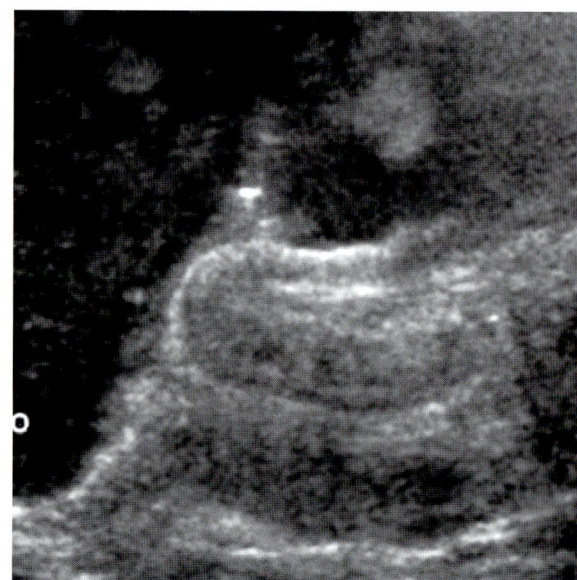

Fig. 9.2.2

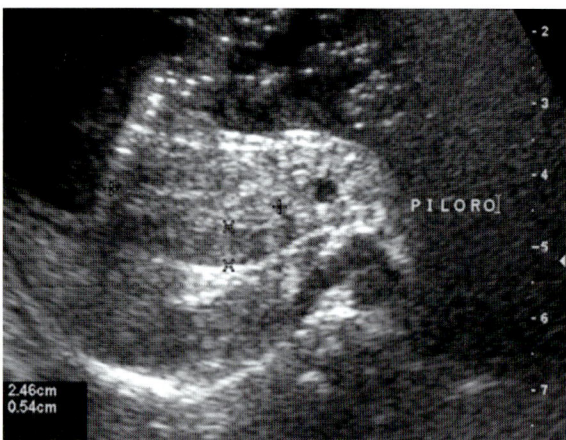

Fig. 9.2.3

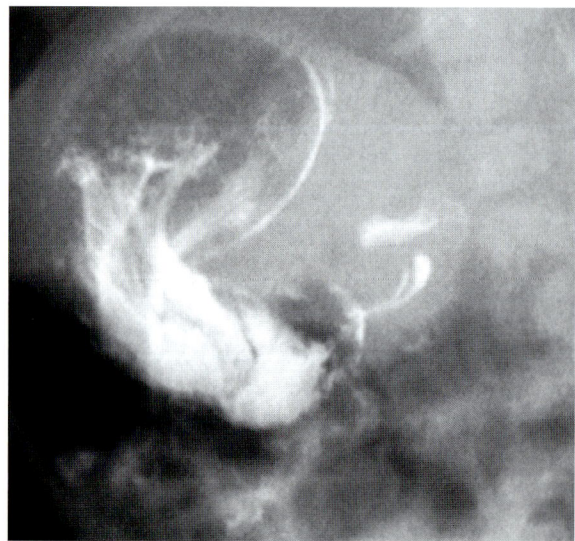

Fig. 9.2.4

A firstborn 4-week-old boy presented with non-bilious vomiting that was initially mild but worsened to projectile vomiting.

Hypertrophic pyloric stenosis (HPS) is the most common GI disease of infancy that requires surgery. Male-to-female ratio is 4–6:1. Symptoms of HPS may begin during the first weeks of life (three weeks is the peak age) but in rare cases may be delayed up to 5 months. Vomiting is the principal symptom, progressing from simple regurgitation to projectile vomiting. Constipation, weight loss, dehydration, and hypochloremic alkalosis may be found too. Physical examination may reveal a palpable pyloric mass (olive) and visible peristalsis. The etiology of HPS is unknown but a genetic component is suspected as it is far more common in families with another sibling affected. Hypertrophy and hyperplasia of the circular muscle layer of the pylorus is found in biopsies.

Ultrasound is the imaging method of choice allowing faster diagnosis and treatment. Plain-film findings include gastric distention and paucity of distal bowel gas. Upper gastrointestinal series are usually ordered after a negative ultrasound or if there is doubt about other causes of obstruction, such as malrotation or midgut volvulus.

For the ultrasound examination, the patient is placed in the supine and right lateral decubitus position and the stomach is filled with dextrose-water solution or breast milk.

The antropyloric region is evaluated in the longitudinal and transverse section.

On transverse scans of HPS patients, the pylorus looks like a doughnut, with the echolucent hypertrophied muscle surrounding the echogenic gastric mucosa. The pyloric muscle thickness should be measured on both transverse and longitudinal scans. The diagnosis of HPS can be made if the pyloric muscle thickness is greater than 3 mm and the channel length is larger than 18 mm. Pyloric muscle length greater than 14 mm and pyloric transverse diameter larger than 9 mm can help to confirm the diagnosis.

Abdominal ultrasound performed with convex and linear transducers showed a full stomach and the doughnut appearance of the pylorus characteristic of pyloric stenosis (Fig. 9.2.1). Longitudinal scan demonstrated a thickened pyloric muscle (5 cm) and elongated pyloric channel (25 mm) (Figs. 9.2.2–9.2.3).

In the upper gastrointestinal series, the pyloric canal was narrowed and elongated (Fig. 9.2.4).

Case 3
■ Intussusception

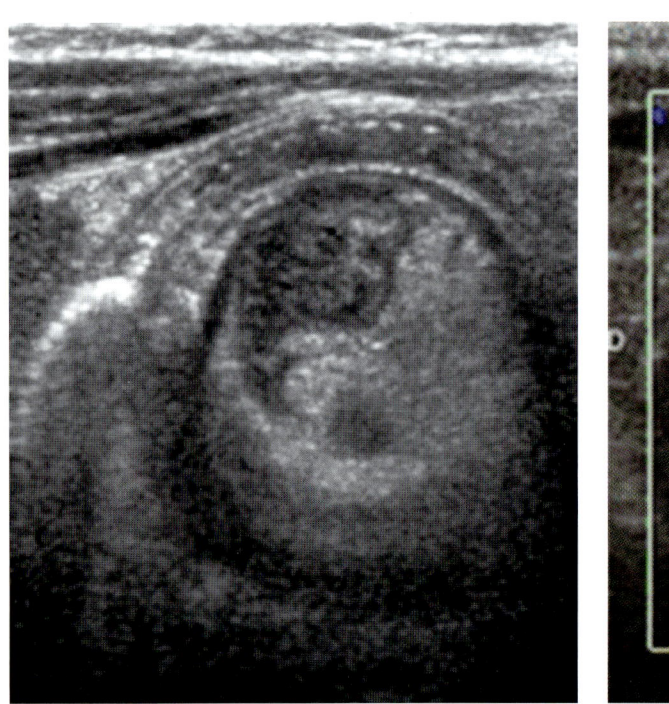

Fig. 9.3.1

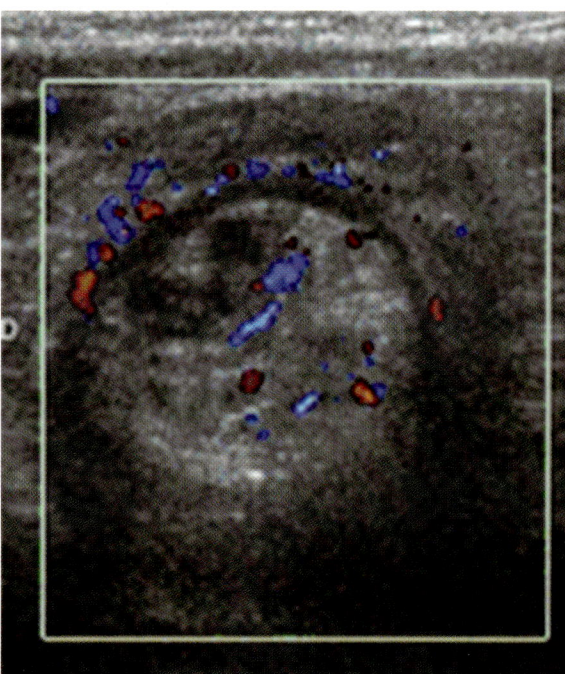

Fig. 9.3.2

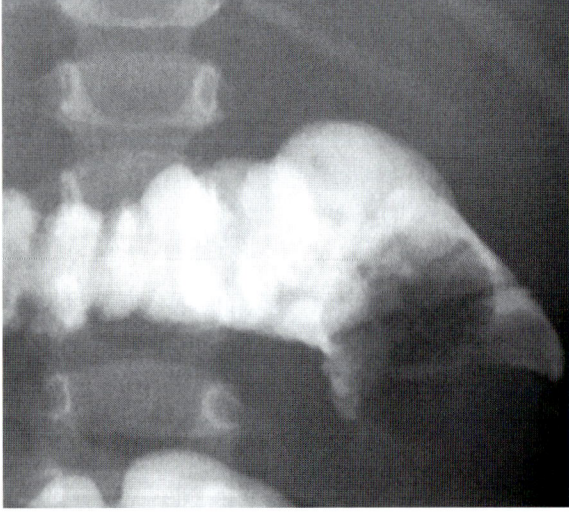

Fig. 9.3.3

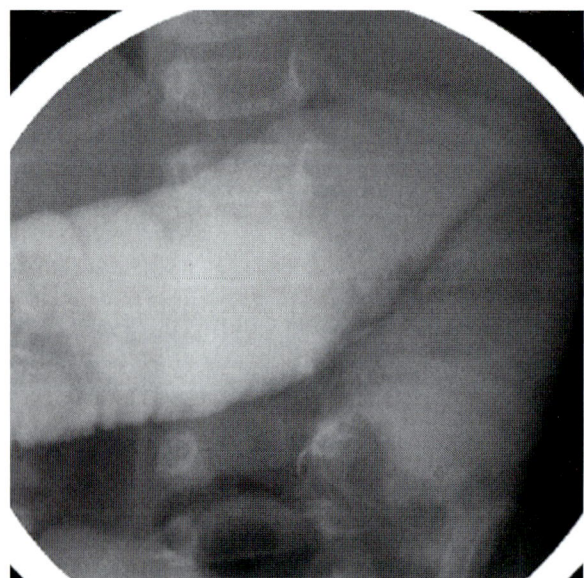

Fig. 9.3.4

A 9-month-old boy presented with irritability, vomiting, crampy abdominal pain, and rectal bleeding with red currant jelly stool.

Comments

Intussusception, the invagination or telescoping of one portion of the intestine into the contiguous distal segment, is a common abdominal emergency in children. The proximal segment is known as the intussusceptum while the distal portion is the intussuspiens.

Idiopathic intussusception is the most common cause of small intestinal obstruction in the infant-toddler age group. Considering diagnoses made in the group from 2 months to 3 years age, 50% of all intussusceptions are diagnosed during the first year of life and 24% during the second year. Males are affected more than twice as often as females.

Over 90% of intussusceptions are ileocolic, with enteroenteric and colocolic intussusceptions being uncommon. Ileocolic intussusception are usually seen in the right side of the abdomen, usually having a lead point. Ileoileal intussusception occurs more frequently in neonates and older children (>5 years old), and the bowel segment involved is shorter than in ileocolic intussusception. Imaging-guided pressure reduction is the treatment of choice and US-guided pneumatic reduction is a reliable and effective technique for the nonsurgical reduction of pediatric intussusception.

Ultrasound image shows a mass with alternating rings of hyper- and hypo-echogenicity; demonstrating the typical "pseudo-kidney" appearance on longitudinal images. Color Doppler ultrasound detects vascular changes in the "pseudo-kidney". The most common plain-film findings are: paucity of right lower quadrant gas; non-visualization of air-filled cecum; meniscus of soft-tissue mass outlined in air-filled colon, and small bowel obstruction.

Imaging Findings

Ultrasound performed with convex and linear transducers showed the crescent-in-doughnut sign characteristic of intussusception in axial (Fig. 9.3.1) and longitudinal (Fig. 9.3.2) scans. Radiographs after water-soluble contrast-medium enema showed the head of the ileocolic intussusception in the ascending colon (Figs. 9.3.3 and 9.3.4).

Case 4
■
Round Pneumonia

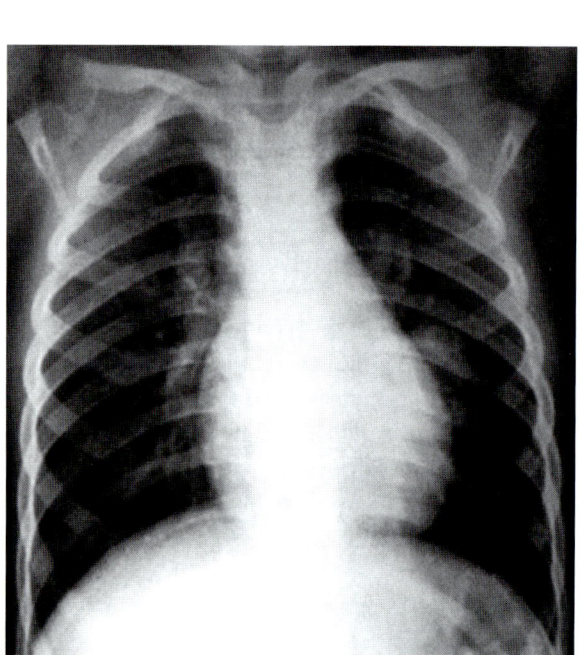

Fig. 9.4.1

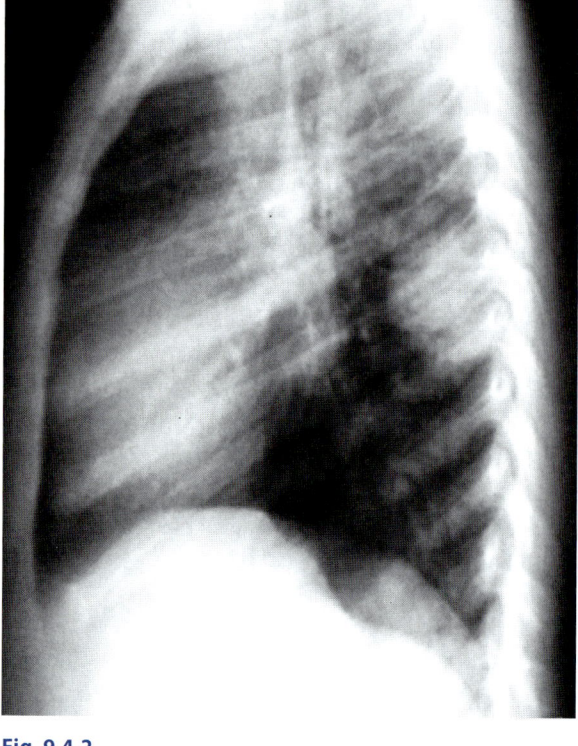

Fig. 9.4.2

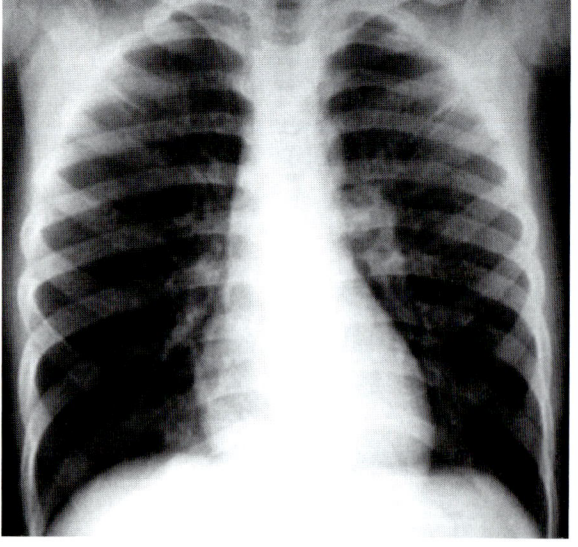

Fig. 9.4.3

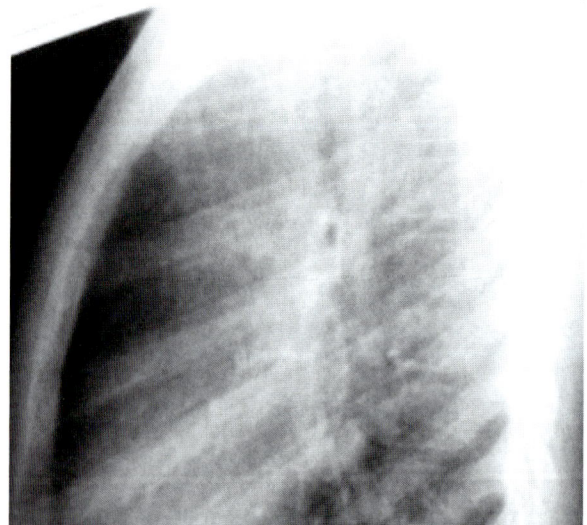

Fig. 9.4.4

A 5-year-old-age boy presented at the ER with cough, fever, and chest pain.

Less than 1% of pneumonia presents as round pulmonary lesions. Round pneumonia corresponds to the initial phase of pneumonia. It can be often misinterpreted as either neoplastic lung disease or a focal inflammatory process. The focal infection begins in a segmental bronchus and spreads centripetally through the lymphatic channels and the pores of Kohn until it reaches the pleural surface, producing a spherical appearance.

Large-sized round pneumonias are associated with fever and elevated white blood cell count, although most small round pneumonias are associated with normal blood results and no fever.

Round pneumonia affections children much more frequently than adults. The most common causative organisms are Streptococcus pneumoniae, Klebsiella pneumoniae , Mycobacterium tuberculosis or Haemophilus influenzae. The differential diagnosis of round pneumonias in children older than 8 years should raise the suspicion of associated immunodeficiency syndrome (with atypical infectious agents, such as fungi) or malignant diseases such as neuroblastoma.

The most common presentation of round pneumonia in plain chest films is a spherical lung opacity with irregular borders and air bronchogram within the mass. Round pneumonia has a very short doubling time of growth. It is usually localized in the posterior lower lobes. The lesion most commonly disappears rapidly after antibiotic treatment. Comparison to recent norma chest radiographs, if available, is key to establishing the diagnosis. Prompt recognition of this disease is important to avoid unnecessary repetition of chest radiographs or CT, entailing extra radiation exposure. If a child has symptoms of pulmonary infection and a "round density" is visualized on chest radiographs, additional imaging such as CT is not necessary.

Plain chest film showed a round lung opacity with irregular borders (Figs. 9.4.1 and 9.4.2) that was not evident in a plain chest film performed 2 months before. Follow-up chest radiographs obtained 10 days later, after finishing antibiotic treatment, demonstrated nearly complete resolution of the round mass (Figs. 9.4.3 and 9.4.4).

Case 5
■
Congenital Cystic Adenomatoid Malformation

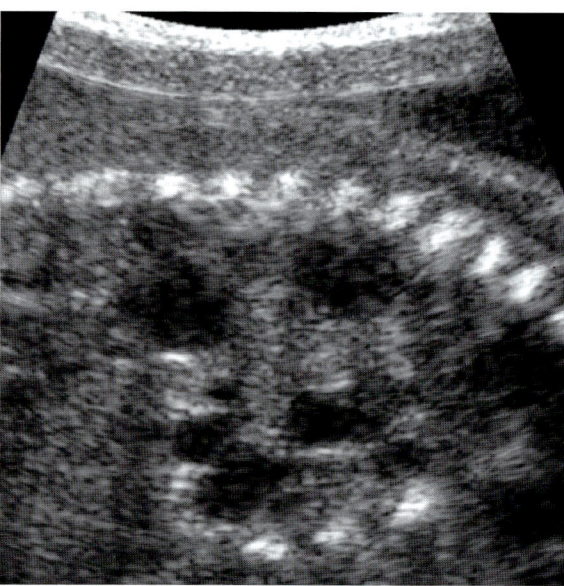

Fig. 9.5.1

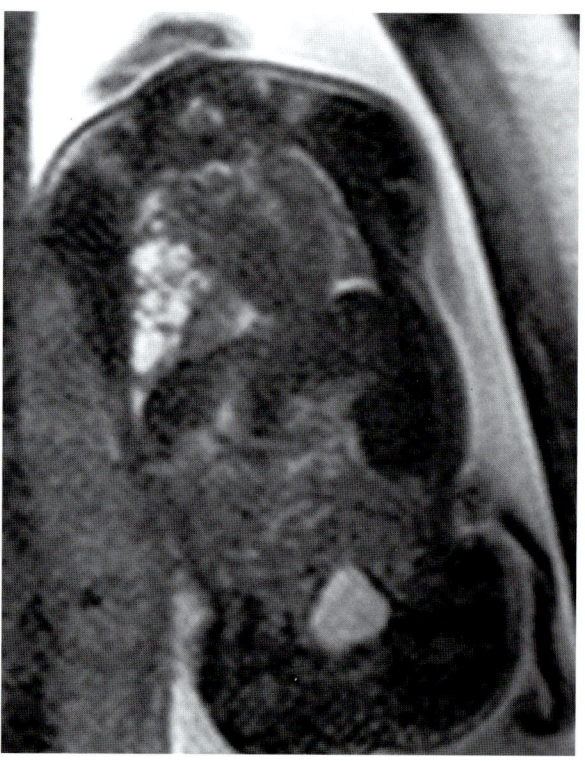

Fig. 9.5.2

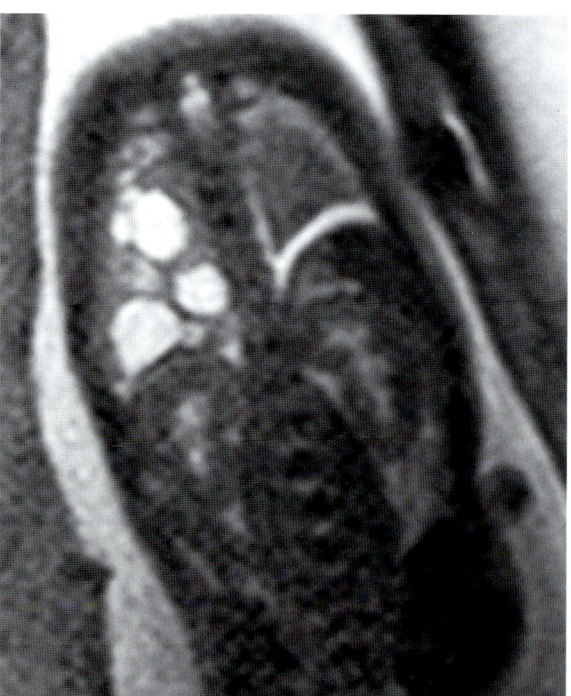

Fig. 9.5.3

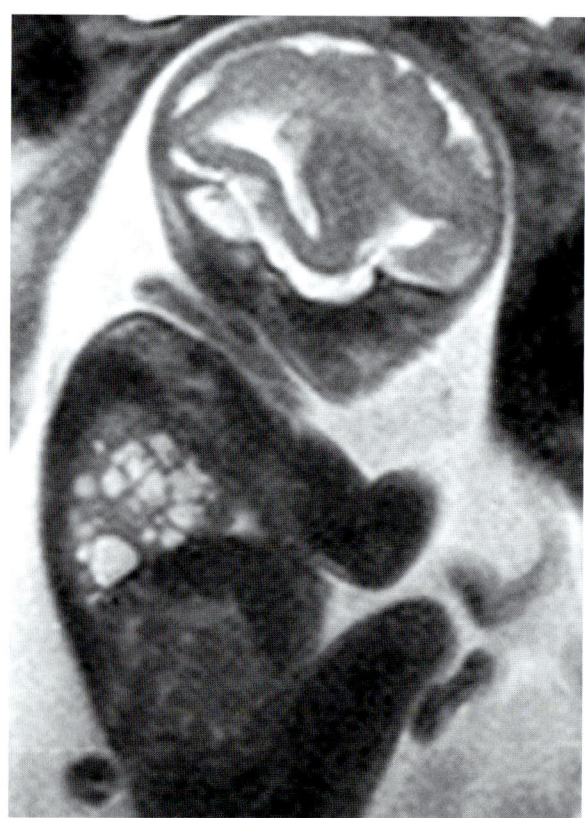

Fig. 9.5.4

Prenatal ultrasound detected a heterogeneous echogenic in the right lung of the fetus.

Comments

Congenital cystic adenomatoid malformation (CCAM) accounts for 25% of all congenital lung malformations. It most commonly presents with respiratory distress in newborns. It is a congenital lung mass of adenomatoid proliferation. These lesions are often diagnosed on prenatal sonography or MRI, allowing prenatal treatment.

Newborns may be asymptomatic at birth, and sometimes CCAM presents later in life, with recurrent pulmonary infections or hemoptysis. The Stoker classification of CCAM distinguishes between: Type I, consisting of large cysts; type II consisting of small cysts; and type III showing lesions resembling a homogeneous mass, with cysts only seen at microscopy. Resection remains the treatment of choice to avoid the risks of recurrent infection and a small risk for malignant degeneration. The differential diagnosis of CCAM must be made with pulmonary sequestration, congenital diaphragmatic hernia, and complicated pneumonia with cavitary necrosis.

Prenatal sonography may detect CCAM as an echogenic fetal lung mass with or without cystic components. Its imaging appearance is variable depending on the type of CCAM and is determined by the size and number of cysts. The most common presentation is a mass with a variable number of solid and cystic components, but it may be completely cystic or completely solid (CCAM type III). Cysts may be uniform or variable in size. As congenital cystic adenomatoid malformation communicates with the bronchial tree, it typically contains air soon after birth (hours to days). Lesions are typically solitary with no lobar predilection (differential diagnosis with congenital lobar emphysema). Even in asymptomatic patients with prenatal diagnosis, chest radiography and lung CT are mandatory to complete the evaluation of CCAM.

Imaging Findings

Prenatal ultrasound detected a heterogeneous echogenic lesion with cystic areas in the right lung of the fetus (Fig. 9.5.1). On prenatal MRI, the mass showed multiple confluent hyperintense locules, giving the appearance of a multiseptated cystic mass, as is shown here in the coronal (Figs. 9.5.2 and 9.5.3) and sagittal HASTE (Fig. 9.5.4) images. At delivery, respiratory distress was observed.

Case 6
■ Neuroblastoma

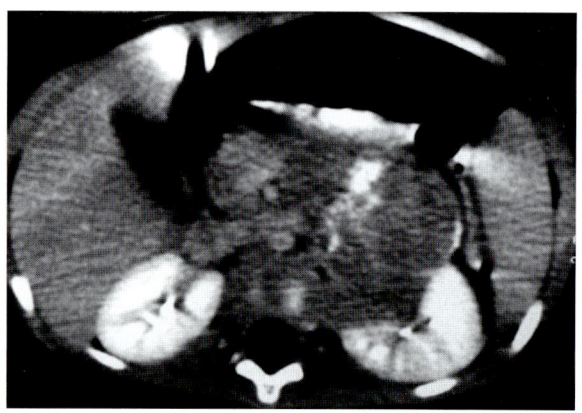

Fig. 9.6.1

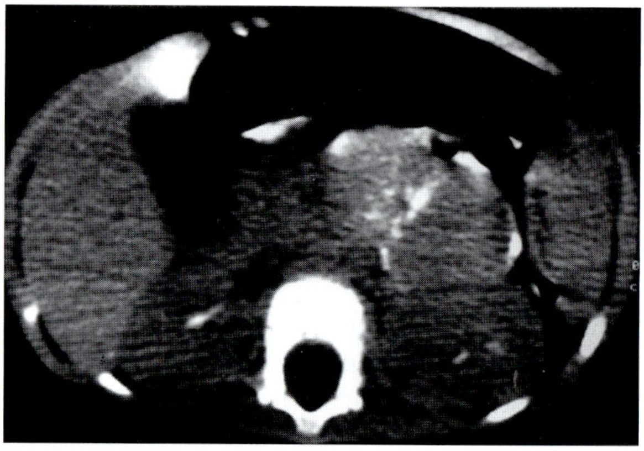

Fig. 9.6.2

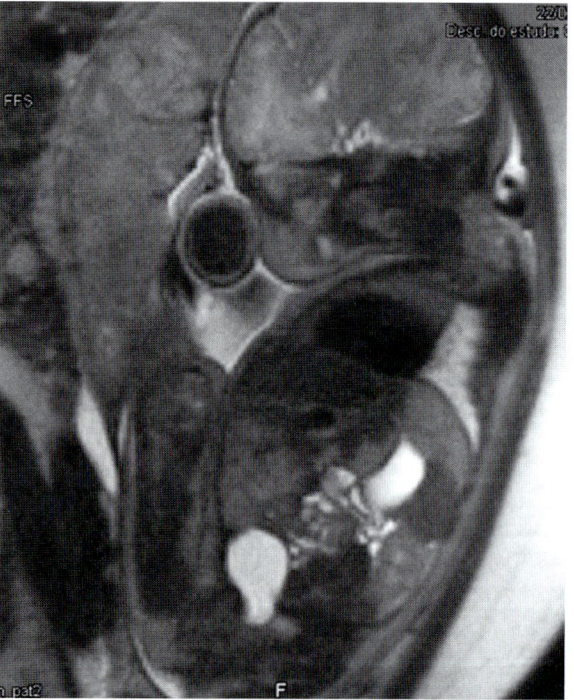

Fig. 9.6.3

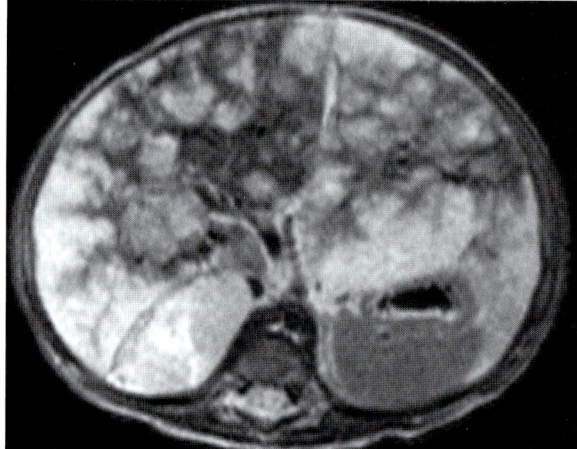

Fig. 9.6.4

Case I: A 4-year-old boy presented with a painful fixed abdominal mass that crossed the midline.

Case II: An abdominal mass was detected at prenatal ultrasound – not shown – in a male fetus.

Neuroblastoma is the most common solid intra-abdominal tumor within the first year of life, and the third most common pediatric malignancy. Its clinical incidence is about 1 in 8000–10000 children and the male-to-female ratio is 1.3–2:1. It usually appears in younger patients than Wilms tumor does. Around 97% of all cases of neuroblastoma are diagnosed in children younger than 8 years of age. Neuroblastoma can be detected prenatally by obstetric ultrasound.

Comments

Neuroblastoma results from the malignant growth of precursors of the sympathetic nervous system derived from neural crest cells. It has a variable presentation depending on the primary site of origin and metastatic spread. The rate of spontaneous resolution varies widely among different published series. Physical findings in advanced disease include an enlarged liver, subcutaneous tumor deposits, and orbital swelling from retrobulbar metastases. Extension from the retroperitoneum into the spinal canal may result in paraplegia. Bone marrow invasion may cause anemia and thrombocytopenia. Cortical bone metastases may cause severe pain.

The INSS (International Neuroblastoma Staging System) is the established clinical, radiographic, and surgical staging system for neuroblastomas.

The differential diagnosis includes Wilms tumor, lymphoma, and nonneoplastic lesions. The diagnosis of neuroblastoma may be difficult in 10% of the cases, especially in tumors that do not produce catecholamine metabolic products.

Abdominal plain film may detect microcalcifications within the mass and chest radiographs may show pulmonary metastases on rare occasions. Ultrasound is noninvasive and provides information about the laterality, consistency, and size of the mass. Abdominal computed tomography will distinguish between renal, adrenal, and paraspinal primary origin, as well as provide information about regional lymph-node or vessel invasion and distant metastatic disease. Magnetic resonance imaging allows intraspinal extension to be detected and is also a very sensitive detector of bone involvement, obviating the use of bone scans.

Case I: Unenhanced computed tomography demonstrated a retroperitoneal mass with internal foci of calcification (Fig. 9.6.1). Contrast-enhanced CT showed heterogeneous enhancement of the mass (Fig. 9.6.2).

Imaging Findings

Case II: Fetal MRI shows a mass in the adrenal gland (Fig. 9.6.3) and metastatic lesions in the liver (Fig. 9.6.4). After birth, the boy was asymptomatic.

Case 7
■
Wilms Tumor

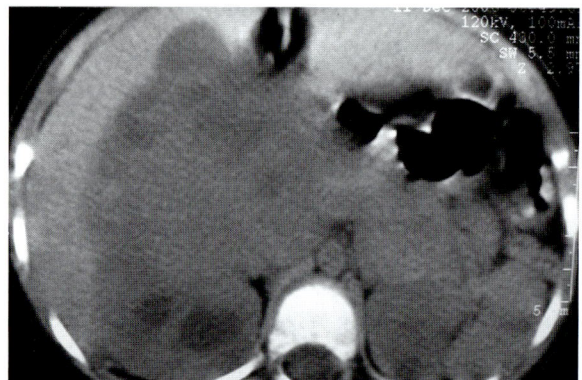

Fig. 9.7.1

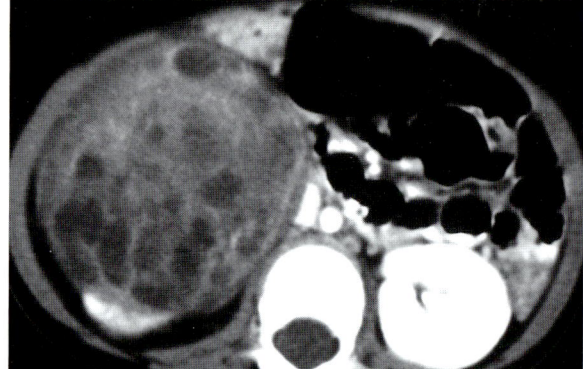

Fig. 9.7.2

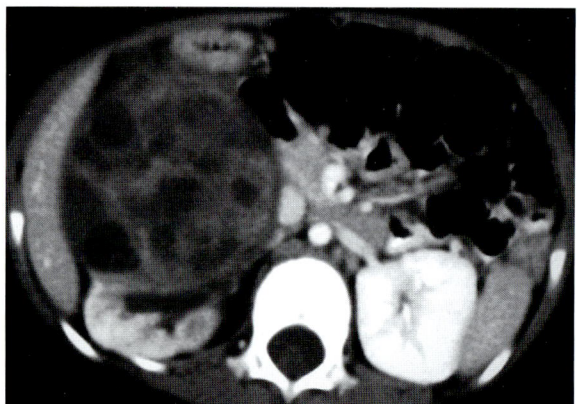

Fig. 9.7.3

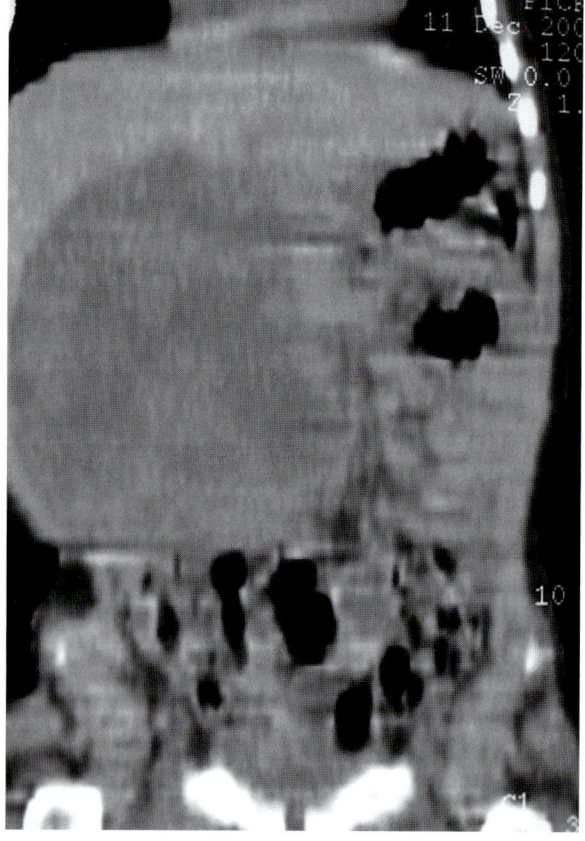

Fig. 9.7.4

A 3-year-old boy presented with a palpable abdominal mass, hematuria, abdominal pain, and hypertension.

Wilms tumor (malignant nephroblastoma) is the most frequent abdominal malignancy found in children and the third most common malignant childhood disease. It is typically found in the first years of life, with more than 80% of cases in the 0–14 age range presenting under 5 years of age. Up to 5–10% of cases are bilateral. Most cases are sporadic, but probably 1–2% of the cases have a familial incidence.

The presence of genitourinary anomalies, such as cryptorchidism or hypospadias, and associated syndromes, including sporadic aniridia, Beckwith-Wiedemann or Denys-Drash syndromes, suggests Wilms tumor.

The diagnostic evaluation of a child with suspected nephroblastoma has three purposes:

1-to confirm the tumor's location and origin in the kidney and to distinguish it from other abdominal masses such as a neuroblastoma or hepatic tumors;

2-to evaluate the extension of the tumor, specifically, to identify local tumor spread and renal vein involvement;

3-to rule out metastatic or bilateral disease.

Wilms tumor is often a large heterogeneous tumor mass that bulges the renal capsule, displaces adjacent organs, and may appear quite exophytic. It commonly invades the renal and inferior vena cava veins. It usually grows predominantly by local extension, compressing the surrounding renal parenchyma and giving the appearance of a sharply margined mass, often with a prominent pseudocapsule. Less commonly, small internal areas of fat density or calcification may be noted. Wilms tumors are usually hypovascular, showing poor enhancement in post-contrast series. Lung metastasis occurs in approximately 20% of cases.

Ultrasound is often the first initial imaging examination, but it is often difficult to image the entire mass in a single US slice. Doppler-ultrasound may help to detect tumor thrombus extension or vein compression. CT is the most common imaging technique used to establish the diagnosis and for staging. However, the diagnostic accuracy of MRI is similar to that of CT, and MRI has the important advantage of sparing the child ionizing radiation. The multiplanar capabilities of MRI enable the organ of origin to be determined in large abdominal masses. The most common MR presentation of Wilms tumor is a large heterogeneous mass with low signal intensity on T1-weighted images and high signal on T2-weighted images.

Unenhanced computed tomography (CT) demonstrated a large heterogeneous tumor displacing the right kidney anteriorly (Fig. 9.7.1) and contrast-enhanced CT showed enhancement of the tumor and kidney parenchyma (Figs. 9.7.2 and 9.7.3). Figure 9.7.4 shows a coronal reconstruction of the large mass.

Case 8
■
Medulloblastoma

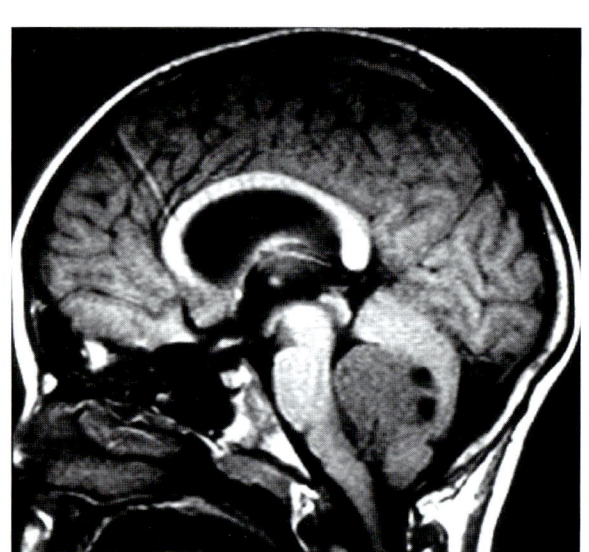

Fig. 9.8.1

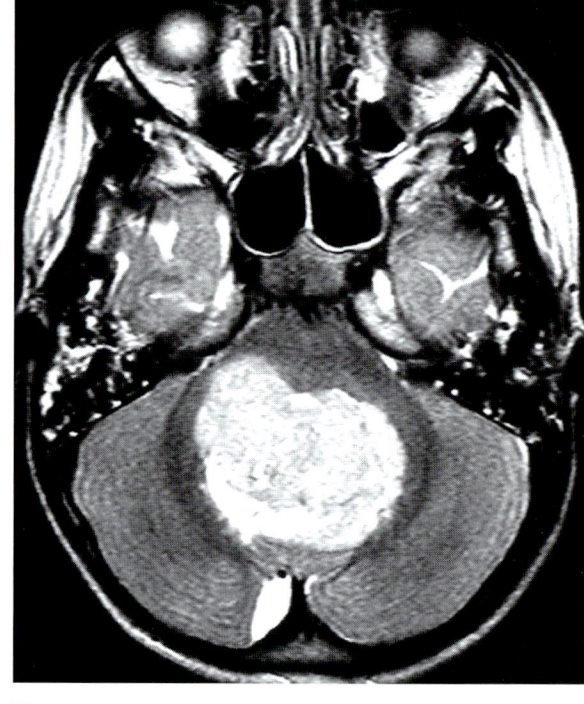

Fig. 9.8.2

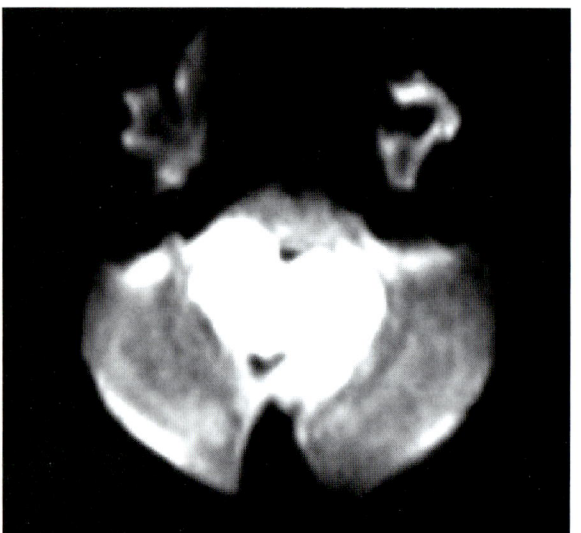

Fig. 9.8.3

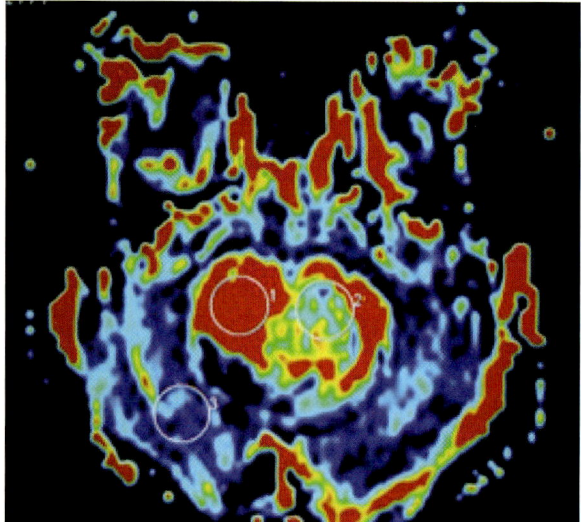

Fig. 9.8.4

A 7-year-old boy presented with headache, ataxia, nausea, and vomiting.

Comments

Medulloblastoma is the most common primary central nervous system tumor. It arises most commonly in childhood, accounting for about 15 to 20% of all childhood brain tumors and accounts for 6%–8% of all central nervous system tumors. It is rare in the adult population, although it may occur in the 3rd and 4th decades of life. It is most commonly located within the fourth ventricle, arising from the superior medullary velum and in the majority of the cases it arises in the midline cerebellar vermis. Most patients have symptoms for less than 3 months. Common symptoms are unsteadiness, headaches, and vomiting. Patients may also suffer clumsiness and have problems with tasks like handwriting. The diagnosis is usually made within one to three months of the onset of symptoms, as this is a fast-growing tumor. This tumor has a tendency to spread to other areas of the brain and spinal cord. Evidence of leptomeningeal metastatic spread is present in 33% of all cases at the time of diagnosis.

Computed tomographic reveals a hyperattenuated, well-defined, enhancing lesion, surrounded by vasogenic edema and usually associated to obstructive hydrocephalus. Cystic and/or necrotic degeneration within the tumor may be present. Calcification is seen in up to 20% of cases. Hemorrhage is rare. On MR imaging, the lesion is hypointense on T1-weighted images and hyperintense on T2-weighted images, often enhancing heterogeneously after intravenous contrast infusion. Diffusion-weighted imaging reveals restricted diffusion due to the high tumor cellularity. Perfusion MR imaging may demonstrate a hyperperfusion neoplasm. MR spectroscopy also helps to establish the diagnosis, as this tumor typically shows elevated choline peaks, reduced N-acetyl aspartate and creatine peaks, and occasionally elevated lipid and lactic acid peaks.

Imaging Findings

Sagittal T1-weighted MR image (Fig. 9.8.1) shows an expanding fourth ventricle mass distorting the cerebellum and displacing the brainstem forward. Axial T2-weighted image (Fig. 9.8.2) demonstrates a hyperintense round expansive lesion filling the fourth ventricle and causing obstructive hydrocephalus – better seen in Figure 9.8.1. Medulloblastoma is a highly cellular neoplasm with a high nucleocytoplasm ratio, presenting with hyperintense signal intensity on diffusion-weighted axial images (Fig. 9.8.3) due to restricted water mobility. Relative cerebral blood volume map (Fig. 9.8.4) demonstrates a hyperperfusion lesion, indicating the presence of tumor neoangiogenesis.

Case 9
Corpus Callosum Agenesis

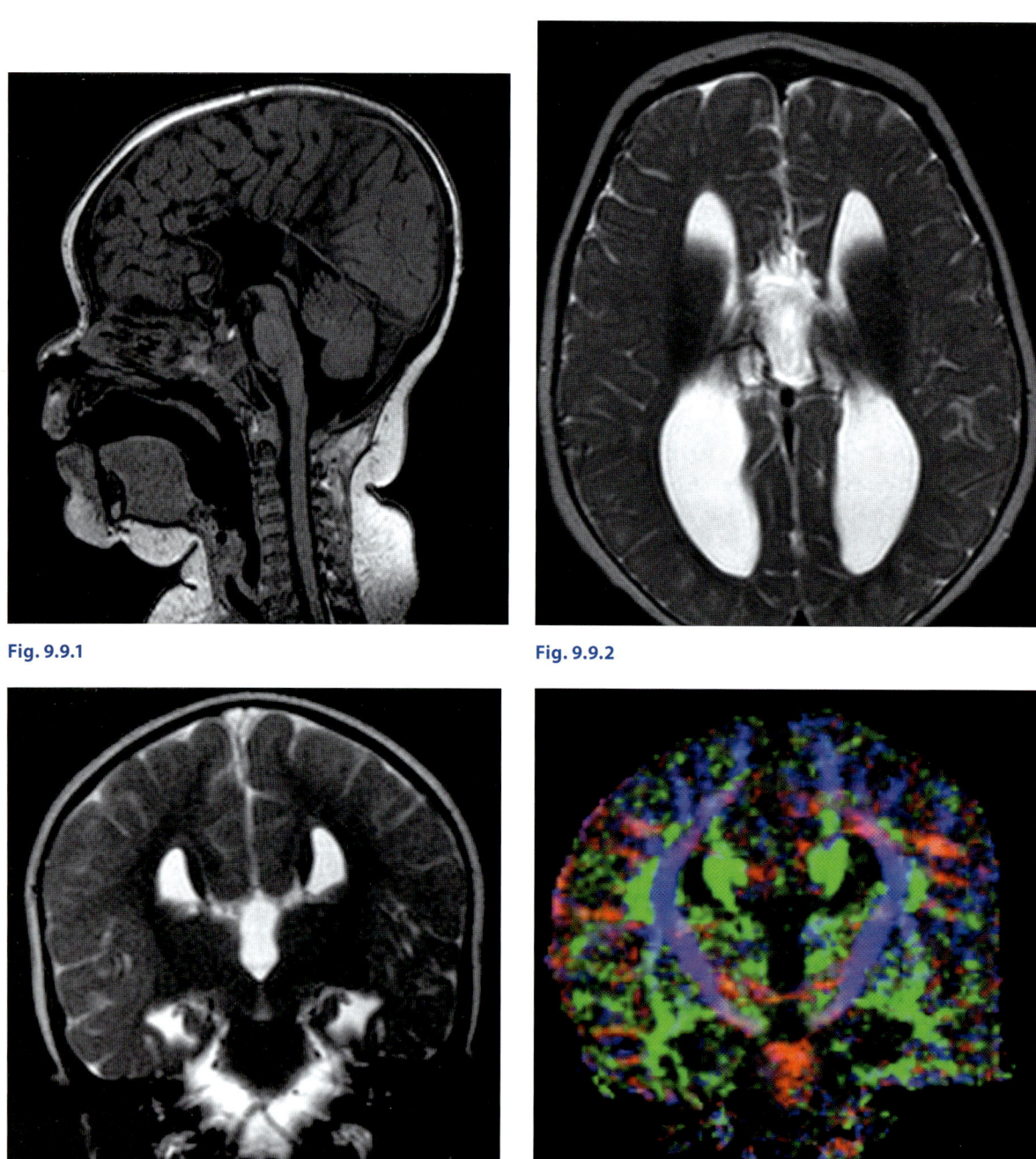

Fig. 9.9.1

Fig. 9.9.2

Fig. 9.9.3

Fig. 9.9.4

15-month-old boy presented with developmental delay and seizures. No complications were observed during gestation or delivery.

Agenesis of the corpus callosum (ACC) is a rare birth defect occurring in 1 of 4000 individuals. The corpus callosum can be partially or completely absent. Thus, the term dysgenesis has also been used to describe the spectrum of callosal anomalies. Once thought to be extremely rare, ACC has been detected with increasing frequency with the widespread clinical use of brain MRI. ACC can occur in association with other cerebral abnormalities, including Chiari malformation, Dandy-Walker syndrome, schizencephaly, and holoprosenephaly. It can also be seen together with anomalies of other organ systems, particularly the musculoskeletal and genitourinary systems, as well as with midline facial defects. A disturbance in embryogenesis results in the failure of the callosal axons to cross the midline. These arrested axons form the longitudinally oriented white matter tracts of Probst's bundles that are located medial to the lateral ventricles.

Although ACC has been found in asymptomatic individuals, it is generally considered a potential marker for neurologic impairment. The effects of the disorder range from subtle or mild to severe, depending on associated brain abnormalities. Intelligence may be normal with only mild compromise of skills requiring matching of visual patterns; however, children with the most severe brain malformations may have intellectual retardation, seizures, hydrocephalus, and spasticity.

MRI is the imaging modality of choice because of its greater sensitivity for depicting the dysgenesis of the corpus callosum and associated cerebral anomalies. Sagittal T1-weighted images clearly demonstrate the extent of callosal dysgenesis and the radial disposition of the gyri. Axial images show widely separated parallel lateral ventricles associated to colpocephaly (dilatation of the occipital horns). The nondecussated longitudinal callosal fascicle (Probst's bundles) is observed in the superomedial aspect of lateral ventricle and is best seen on the axial and coronal images. Coronal images can also demonstrate a "trident-shaped" appearance of the frontal horns, "keyhole" temporal horns, and vertical hippocampi. Cortical dysplasias and heterotopias are easily demonstrated with inversion-recovery 3D sequences. Diffusion-tensor MR imaging is useful in the evaluation of the white matter configuration in callosal dysgenesis and has contributed to the understanding of the main fiber tracts in this entity.

Brain MRI demonstrated agenesis of the corpus callosum. Sagittal T1-weighted image (Fig. 9.9.1) shows the absence of the corpus callosum along the midline, associated to radially arrayed gyri pointing toward a high-riding third ventricle. Axial T2-weighted image (Fig. 9.9.2) demonstrates parallel lateral ventricles with pointed frontal horns and dilatation of the posterior aspects of the ventricles, characteristic of colpocephaly. Coronal T2-weighted image (Fig. 9.9.3) reveals pointed frontal horns and "keyhole" temporal horns associated to vertical hippocampi. Probst´s bundles are present: these compact white matter tracts course longitudinally and cause invagination in the superomedial aspects of the widely spaced lateral ventricles. Coronal diffusion-tensor MR imaging (Fig. 9.9.4) demonstrates the principal fiber tracts and their orientation based on a color-coded map, where red refers to a horizontal direction, green a longitudinal direction, and blue a superior-inferior orientation. Aberrant fiber connections (Probst's bundles) are easily identified as green fiber tracts in both cerebral hemispheres.

Case 10
Tethered Cord

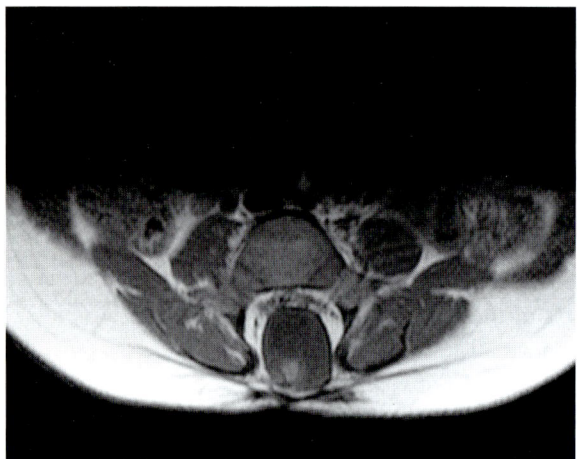

Fig. 9.10.1

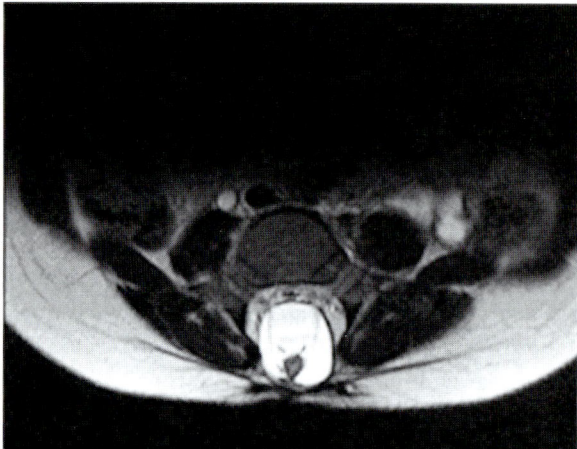

Fig. 9.10.2

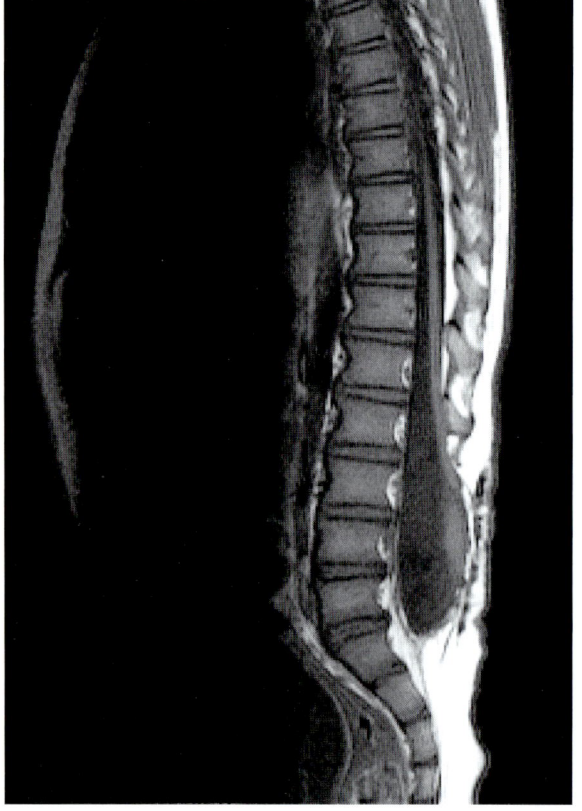

Fig. 9.10.3

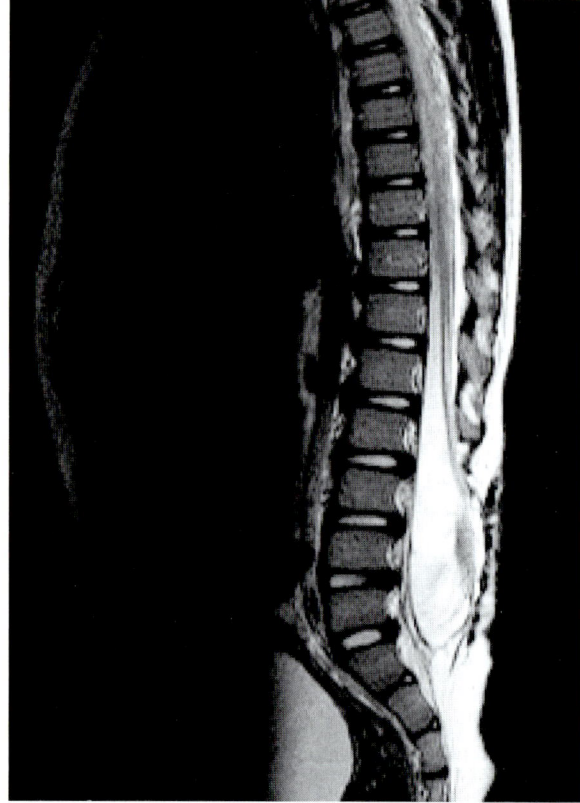

Fig. 9.10.4

A 5-year-old boy presented with low back pain and weakness of the lower limbs associated to slight muscular atrophy and urinary incontinence. Physical examination found abnormal lower-limb reflex, a simple dimple in the soft tissue of the lumbar region, and mild scoliosis.

Comments

A failure in the involution of the filum terminale can lead to a tethered cord. This spinal abnormality can be associated to other neurological and orthopedic deformities, as well as bowel and bladder disturbances, motor and sensory abnormalities in the lower limbs, gait disturbances, and scoliosis. VACTERL syndrome (Vertebrae, anus, cardiovascular tree, esophagus, renal system, and limb buds) may also be associated. Symptoms usually appear at school age, around 4 to 6 years old, and during the adolescent growth spurt. There is no gender predilection. Symptoms are generally progressive and early surgery may alter the clinical outcome, with improvement or stabilization of neurological symptoms such as motor weakness, sensory dysfunction, pain, and bladder dysfunction.

Findings at plain-film radiography can be normal or can reveal spinal dysraphism or incomplete posterior fusion. CT findings can also demonstrate associated bone abnormalities, enlargement of the dural sac, and posterior and inferior positioning of the filum terminale. Ultrasound can dynamically demonstrate the reduction or absence of spinal cord motion, as well as the low-lying conus and a thickened filum terminale. MR is the imaging modality of choice in patients with clinical suspicion of tethered cord. Its multiplanar capabilities permit a complete analysis of the spinal abnormalities and associated alterations, such as lipomas and meningoceles.

Imaging Findings

Magnetic resonance revealed dysraphism of the lumbar spine and spina bifida. Sagittal T1-weighted (Fig. 9.10.1) and T2-weighted (Fig. 9.10.2) images demonstrated an elongated, thinning spinal cord; a thickened filum terminale; and a low-lying (ending below L2 inferior endplate), dorsally positioned conus in contact with the dural sac. Note the enlargement of the inferior portion of the dural sac and the spinal dysraphism. Axial T1-weighted (Fig. 9.10.3) and T2-weighted (Fig. 9.10.4) images also showed the widening dural sac and the inferior-posterior location of the dorsally displaced filum terminale.

Further Readings

Books

Caffey´s Pediatric Diagnostic Imaging. Kuhn JP, Slovis TL, Haller JO (2003) Philadelphia: Mosby, 2003. ISBN-13: 9780323011099

Diagnostic Imaging: Pediatric. Donnelly LF (2005) Salt Lake City: AMIRSYS. (Philadelphia: Elsevier). ISBN-13: 9781416023333

Fundamentals of Pediatric Radiology. Donnelly LF (2001) Philadelphia: W.B. Saunders. ISBN-13: 9780721690612

Imaging of the newborn infant, and young child. 5th ed. Swischuk LE (2003) Philadelphia: Lippincott Williams & Wilkins. ISBN-13: 9780781734585

Pediatric Body CT. Siegel MJ (1999) Philadelphia: Lippincott Williams & Wilkins. ISBN-13: 9780781712491

Pediatric Chest Imaging. Lucaya J, Strife JL (2002) Springer-Verlag, Berlin-Heidelberg. ISBN-13: 9783540675273

Pediatric Neuroimaging. Barkovich AJ (2005) Philadelphia: Lippincott Williams & Wilkins. ISBN-13: 9780781717403

Pediatric Sonography. 3rd ed. Siegel MJ (2002) Philadelphia: Lippincott Williams & Wilkins. ISBN-13: 9780781727532

Pediatric Uroradiology. Fotter R (2001) Springer-Verlag, Berlin-Heidelberg. ISBN-13: 9783540436850

Pratical Pediatric Imaging: Diagnostic Radiology of Infants and Children. 3rd ed. Kirks DR, Griscom NT (1997) Philadelphia: Lippincott-Raven. ISBN-13: 9780316494731

Web-Links

http://auntminnie.com/index.asp?sec=def

http://hawaii.edu/medicine/pediatrics/pemxray/pemxray.html

http://pediatricradiology.com/

http://pediatric-radiology.com/

http://pediatricradiologyinfo.com/

http://pedrad.info/

http://pedsradiology.com/

http://radiologyeducation.com/

http://rsna.org/Education/archive/bestcases.cfm

http://.uhrad.com/pedsarc.htm

Articles

Accardo J, Kammann H, Hoon AH Jr. Neuroimaging in cerebral palsy. J Pediatr 2004; 145(2 Suppl):S19–27

Adamsbaum C, Moutard ML, Andre C, Merzoug V, Ferey S, Quere MP, Lewin F, Fallet-Bianco C. MRI of the fetal posterior fossa. Pediatr Radiol 2005; 35(2):124–140. Epub 2004 Nov 23

Amini A, Liu JK, Kestle JR. Disseminated medulloblastoma. J Neurooncol 2006; 80(2):157–158. Epub 2006 Sep 26

Applegate KE, Anderson JM, Klatte EC. Intestinal malrotation in children: a problem-solving approach to the upper gastrointestinal series. Radiographics 2006; 26(5):1485–1500

Argyropoulou MI, Kiortsis DN. MRI of the hypothalamic-pituitary axis in children. Pediatr Radiol 2005; 35(11):1045–1055. Epub 2005 Jun 1

Arthur R. Magnetic resonance imaging in preterm infants. Pediatr Radiol 2006; 36(7):593–607. Epub 2006 May 19

Atkinson DS Jr. Computed tomography of pediatric stroke. Semin Ultrasound CT MR 2006; 27(3):207–218

Avni FE, Garel L, Cassart M, Massez A, Eurin D, Didier F, Hall M, Teele RL. Perinatal assessment of hereditary cystic renal diseases: the contribution of sonography. Pediatr Radiol 2006; 36(5):405–414. Epub 2006 Feb 4. Erratum in: Pediatr Radiol 2006; 36(7):731

Bacon S, Clinkard J, Taylor RE. Paediatric medulloblastoma associated with poor prognosis and short volume doubling time. Br J Radiol 2005; 78(935):1059–1060

Barkovich AJ, Simon EM, Walsh CA. Callosal agenesis with cyst: a better understanding and new classification. Neurology 2001; 56:220–227

Bedeschi MF, Bonaglia MC, Grasso R, Pellegri A, Garghentino RR, Battaglia MA, Panarisi AM, Di Rocco M, Balottin U, Bresolin N, Bassi MT, Borgatti R. Agenesis of the corpus callosum: clinical and genetic study in 63 young patients. Pediatr Neurol 2006; 34(3):186–193

Boesch RP, Daines C, Willging JP, Kaul A, Cohen AP, Wood RE, Amin RS. Advances in the diagnosis and management of chronic pulmonary aspiration in children. Eur Respir J 2006; 28(4):847–861

Bousvaros A, Kirks DR, Grossman H. Imaging of neuroblastoma: an overview. Pediatr Radiol 1986; 16(2):89–106

Brisse H, Ollivier L, Edeline V, Pacquement H, Michon J, Glorion C, Neuenschwander S. Imaging of malignant tumours of the long bones in children: monitoring response to neoadjuvant chemotherapy and preoperative assessment. Pediatr Radiol 2004; 34(8):595–605. Epub 2004 Apr 22

Burrows PE, Dubois J, Kassarjian A. Pediatric hepatic vascular anomalies. Pediatr Radiol 2001; 31(8):533–545

Bush A, Davies J. Early detection of lung disease in preschool children with cystic fibrosis. Curr Opin Pulm Med 2005; 11(6):534–538

Byrne AT, Geoghegan T, Govender P, Lyburn ID, Colhoun E, Torreggiani WC. The imaging of intussusception. Clin Radiol 2005; 60(1):39–46. Erratum in: Clin Radiol 2005; 60(3):412

Cass DL, Crombleholme TM, Howell LJ, Stafford PW, Ruchelli ED, Adzick NS. Cystic lung lesions with systemic arterial blood supply: a hybrid of congenital cystic adenomatoid malformation and bronchopulmonary sequestration. J Pediatr Surg 1997; 32(7):986–990

Cleveland RH. A radiologic update on medical diseases of the newborn chest. Pediatr Radiol 1995; 25(8):631–637

Corness JA, McHugh K, Roebuck DJ, Taylor AM. The portal vein in children: radiological review of congenital anomalies and acquired abnormalities. Pediatr Radiol 2006; 36(2):87–96, quiz 170-1. Epub 2005 Nov 12

Cross JH. Neurocutaneous syndromes and epilepsy-issues in diagnosis and management. Epilepsia 2005; 46 Suppl 10:17–23

Crowley JJ, Sarnaik S. Imaging of sickle cell disease. Pediatr Radiol 1999; 29(9):646–661

Daltro P, Fricke BL, Kline-Fath BM, Werner H, Rodrigues L, Fazecas T, Domingues R, Donnelly LF. Prenatal MRI of congenital abdominal and chest wall defects. AJR Am J Roentgenol 2005; 184(3):1010–1016

Daltro P, Fricke BL, Kuroki I, Domingues R, Donnelly LF. CT of congenital lung lesions in pediatric patients. AJR Am J Roentgenol 2004; 183(5):1497–1506

Daneman A, Navarro O. Intussusception. Part 1: a review of diagnostic approaches. Pediatr Radiol 2003; 33(2):79–85. Epub 2002 Nov 19

Daneman A, Epelman M, Blaser S, Jarrin JR. Imaging of the brain in full-term neonates: does sonography still play a role? Pediatr Radiol 2006; 36(7):636–646. Epub 2006 May 16

Darge K, Trusen A, Gordjani N, Riedmiller H. Intrarenal reflux: diagnosis with contrast-enhanced harmonic US. Pediatr Radiol 2003; 33(10):729–731. Epub 2003 Aug 20

de Mello RR, Dutra MV, Ramos JR, Daltro P, Boechat M, de Andrade Lopes JM. Lung mechanics and high-resolution computed tomography of the chest in very low birth weight premature infants. Sao Paulo Med J 2003; 121(4):167–172. Epub 2003 Oct 29

de Mello RR, Dutra MV, Ramos JR, Daltro P, Boechat M, Lopes JM. Neonatal risk factors for respiratory morbidity during the first year of life among premature infants. Sao Paulo Med J 2006; 124(2):77–84

Diefenbach KA, Breuer CK. Pediatric inflammatory bowel disease. World J Gastroenterol 2006; 12(20):3204–3212

Dubois J, Garel L. Imaging and therapeutic approach of hemangiomas and vascular malformations in the pediatric age group. Pediatr Radiol 1999; 29(12):879–893

Ebel KD. Uroradiology in the fetus and newborn: diagnosis and follow-up of congenital obstruction of the urinary tract. Pediatr Radiol 1998; 28(8):630–635

Epelman M, Daneman A, Blaser SI, Ortiz-Neira C, Konen O, Jarrin J, Navarro OM. Differential diagnosis of intracranial cystic lesions at head US: correlation with CT and MR imaging. Radiographics 2006; 26(1):173–196

Erichsen D, Sellstrom H, Andersson H. Small bowel intussusception after blunt abdominal trauma in a 6-year-old boy: case report and review of 6 cases reported in the literature. J Pediatr Surg 2006; 41(11):1930–1932

Franken EA Jr, Smith JA, Smith WL. Tumors of the chest wall in infants and children. Pediatr Radiol 1977; 6(1):13–18

Frush DP. Pediatric CT: practical approach to diminish the radiation dose. Pediatr Radiol 2002; 32(10):714–717; discussion 751–754. Epub 2002 Aug 29

Garel C. New advances in fetal MR neuroimaging. Pediatr Radiol 2006; 36(7):621–625. Epub 2006 May 3

Garel C. The role of MRI in the evaluation of the fetal brain with an emphasis on biometry, gyration and parenchyma. Pediatr Radiol 2004; 34(9):694–699. Epub 2004 Jul 28

Garel C, Brisse H, Sebag G, Elmaleh M, Oury JF, Hassan M. Magnetic resonance imaging of the fetus. Pediatr Radiol 1998; 28(4):201–211

Garcia-Pena P, Lucaya J, Hendry GM, McAndrew PT, Duran C. Spontaneous involution of pulmonary sequestration in children: a report of two cases and review of the literature. Pediatr Radiol 1998; 28(4):266–270

Grattan-Smith JD, Jones RA. MR urography in children. Pediatr Radiol 2006; 36(11):1119–1132; quiz 1228-1229. Epub 2006 Jun 22

Gressens P, Luton D. Fetal MRI: obstetrical and neurological perspectives. Pediatr Radiol 2004; 34(9):682–684. Epub 2004 Jul 23

Haller JO, Cohen HL. Pediatric HIV infection: an imaging update. Pediatr Radiol 1994; 24(3):224–230

Haller JO, Ginsberg KJ. Tuberculosis in children with acquired immunodeficiency syndrome. Pediatr Radiol 1997; 27(2):186–188

Harris TM, Cohen MD. Abdominal magnetic resonance imaging. Pediatr Radiol 1989; 20(1–2):10–19

Hawass ND, Badawi MG, al-Muzrakchi AM, al-Sammarai AI, Jawad AJ, Abdullah MA, Bahakim H. Horseshoe lung: differential diagnosis. Pediatr Radiol 1990; 20(8):580–584

Helton KJ, Fouladi M, Boop FA, Perry A, Dalton J, Kun L, Fuller C. Medullomyoblastoma: a radiographic and clinicopathologic analysis of six cases and review of the literature. Cancer 2004; 101(6):1445–1454

Hedlund G. Congenital frontonasal masses: developmental anatomy, malformations, and MR imaging. Pediatr Radiol 2006; 36(7):647–662; quiz 726-727. Epub 2006 Mar 11

Hetts SW, Sherr EH, Chao S, Gobuty S, Barkovich AJ. Anomalies of the corpus callosum: an MR analysis of the phenotypic spectrum of associated malformations. AJR Am J Roentgenol 2006; 187(5):1343–1348

Hsu YR, Lee SY. Prenatal diagnosis of congenital cystic adenomatoid malformation. Chang Gung Med J 2004; 27(1):61–65

Jamieson DH. Imaging intracranial tuberculosis in childhood. Pediatr Radiol 1995; 25(3):165–170

Keller MS. Musculoskeletal sonography in the neonate and infant. Pediatr Radiol 2005; 35(12):1167–1173; quiz 1293. Epub 2005 Aug 3

Kim MJ, Lee KY. Bronchiolitis obliterans in children with Stevens-Johnson syndrome: follow-up with high resolution CT. Pediatr Radiol 1996; 26(1):22–25

Kirks DR. Air intussusception reduction: "the winds of change". Pediatr Radiol 1995; 25(2):89–91

Koch BL. Cystic malformations of the neck in children. Pediatr Radiol 2005; 35(5):463–477. Epub 2005 Mar 23

Kornreich L, Schwarz M, Karmazyn B, Cohen IJ, Shuper A, Michovitz S, Yaniv I, Fenig E, Horev G. Role of MRI in the management of children with diffuse pontine tumors: a study of 15 patients and review of the literature. Pediatr Radiol 2005; 35(9):872–879. Epub 2005 May 26

Lamego CM, Torloni H. Colorectal adenocarcinoma in childhood and adolescent. Report of 11 cases and review of the literature. Pediatr Radiol 1989; 19(8):504–508

Laor T. MR imaging of soft tissue tumors and tumor-like lesions. Pediatr Radiol 2004; 34(1):24–37. Epub 2003 Dec 12

Lee SK, Kim DI, Kim J, Kim DJ, Kim HD, Kim DS, Mori S. Diffusion-tensor MR imaging and fiber tractography: a new method of describing aberrant fiber connections in developmental CNS anomalies. Radiographics 2005; 25(1):53–65; discussion 66–68

Manson DE, Sikka S, Reid B, Roifman C. Primary immunodeficiencies: a pictorial immunology primer for radiologists. Pediatr Radiol 2000; 30(8):501–510

May JA, Krieger MD, Bowen I, Geffner ME. Craniopharyngioma in childhood. Adv Pediatr 2006; 53:183–209

McCahon E. Lung tumours in children. Paediatr Respir Rev 2006; 7(3):191–196. Epub 2006 Aug 4

McCarville MB, Hoffer FA, Gingrich JR, Jenkins JJ 3rd. Imaging findings of hemorrhagic cystitis in pediatric oncology patients. Pediatr Radiol 2000; 30(3):131–138

McCollough M, Sharieff GQ. Abdominal pain in children. Pediatr Clin North Am 2006; 53(1):107–137, vi

McHugh K. Renal and adrenal tumours in children. Cancer Imaging 2007; 7:41–751

Mendelson KG, Fallat ME. Pediatric injuries: prevention to resolution. Surg Clin North Am 2007; 87(1):207–228, viii

Mercado-Deane MG, Burton EM, Howell CG. Transverse colon volvulus in pediatric patients. Pediatr Radiol 1995; 25(2):111–112

Meyer JS, Mackenzie W. Malignant bone tumors and limb-salvage surgery in children. Pediatr Radiol 2004; 34(8):606–13. Epub 2004 Jun 19. Erratum in: Pediatr Radiol 2004; 34(12):1030

Moore GJ. Proton magnetic resonance spectroscopy in pediatric neuroradiology. Pediatr Radiol 1998; 28(11):805–814

Moskowitz SM, Gibson RL, Effmann EL. Cystic fibrosis lung disease: genetic influences, microbial interactions, and radiological assessment. Pediatr Radiol 2005; 35(8):739–757. Epub 2005 May 3

Navarro O, Daneman A. Intussusception. Part 3: Diagnosis and management of those with an identifiable or predisposing cause and those that reduce spontaneously. Pediatr Radiol 2004; 34(4):305–312; quiz 369. Epub 2003 Oct 8

Navarro O, Nunez-Santos E, Daneman A, Faria P, Daltro P. Malignant peripheral nerve-sheath tumor arising in a previously irradiated neuroblastoma: report of 2 cases and a review of the literature. Pediatr Radiol 2000; 30(3):176–180

Nazir Z, Qazi SH, Ahmed N, Atiq M, Billoo AG. Pulmonary agenesis--vascular airway compression and gastroesophageal reflux influence outcome. J Pediatr Surg 2006; 41(6):1165–1169

Neil JJ, Inder TE. Imaging perinatal brain injury in premature infants. Semin Perinatol 2004; 28(6):433–443

Nelson MD Jr, Maher K, Gilles FH. A different approach to cysts of the posterior fossa. Pediatr Radiol 2004; 34(9):720–732. Epub 2004 Jul 30

Neumann G, Benz-Bohm G, Rister M. Wegener's granulomatosis in childhood. Review of the literature and case report. Pediatr Radiol 1984; 14(5):267–271

Newman B. Congenital bronchopulmonary foregut malformations: concepts and controversies. Pediatr Radiol 2006; 36(8):773–791. Epub 2006 Mar 22

Nijs E, Callahan MJ, Taylor GA. Disorders of the pediatric pancreas: imaging features. Pediatr Radiol 2005; 35(4):358–373; quiz 457. Epub 2004 Nov 5

Nofech-Mozes Y, Rachmel A, Schonfeld T, Schwarz M, Steinberg R, Ashkenazi S. Difficulties in making the diagnosis of Hirschsprung disease in early infancy. J Paediatr Child Health 2004; 40(12):716–719

Oddone M, Granata C, Vercellino N, Bava E, Toma P. Multimodality evaluation of the abnormalities of the aortic arches in children: techniques and imaging spectrum with emphasis on MRI. Pediatr Radiol 2005; 35(10):947–960. Epub 2005 Jun 23

Osorio A, Kessler RM, Guruprasad H, Isaacson G. Isolated intrathoracic presentation of Mycobacterium avium complex in an immunocompetent child. Pediatr Radiol 2001; 31(12):848–851

Owens C. Pearls and pitfalls in HRCT in children. Paediatr Respir Rev 2006; 7 Suppl 1:S44–49. Epub 2006 Jun 5

Pedicelli G, Ciarpaglini LL, De Santis M, Leonetti C. Congenital bronchial atresia (CBA). A critical review of CBA as a disease entity and presentation of a case series. Radiol Med (Torino) 2005; 110(5–6):544–553

Pfluger T, Czekalla R, Koletzko S, Munsterer O, Willemsen UF, Hahn K. MRI and radiographic findings in Currarino's triad. Pediatr Radiol 1996; 26(8):524–527

Prayer D, Brugger PC, Prayer L. Fetal MRI: techniques and protocols. Pediatr Radiol 2004; 34(9):685–693. Epub 2004 Jul 28

Puderbach M, Kauczor HU. Assessment of lung function in children by cross-sectional imaging: techniques and clinical applications. Pediatr Radiol 2006; 36(3):192–204, quiz 280-281. Epub 2005 Nov 15

Reid JR. Complications of pediatric paranasal sinusitis. Pediatr Radiol 2004; 34(12):933–942. Epub 2004 Jul 27

Roebuck DJ, Olsen O, Pariente D. Radiological staging in children with hepatoblastoma. Pediatr Radiol 2006; 36(3):176–182. Epub 2005 Dec 10

Roebuck DJ, Perilongo G. Hepatoblastoma: an oncological review. Pediatr Radiol 2006; 36(3):183–186. Epub 2006 Jan 11

Rossi A, Cama A, Consales A, Gandolfo C, Garre ML, Milanaccio C, Pavanello M, Piatelli G, Ravegnani M, Tortori-Donati P. Neuroimaging of pediatric craniopharyngiomas: a pictorial essay. J Pediatr Endocrinol Metab 2006; 19 Suppl 1:299–319

Rutherford M, Srinivasan L, Dyet L, Ward P, Allsop J, Counsell S, Cowan F. Magnetic resonance imaging in perinatal brain injury: clinical presentation, lesions and outcome. Pediatr Radiol 2006; 36(7):582–592. Epub 2006 May 16

Rutherford M, Ward P, Allsop J, Malamatentiou C, Counsell S. Magnetic resonance imaging in neonatal encephalopathy. Early Hum Dev 2005; 81(1):13–25. Epub 2004 Nov 19

Safriel YI, Haller JO, Lefton DR, Obedian R. Imaging of the brain in the HIV-positive child. Pediatr Radiol 2000; 30(11):725–732

Samuel M, Burge DM. Management of antenatally diagnosed pulmonary sequestration associated with congenital cystic adenomatoid malformation. Thorax 1999; 54(8):701–706

Sargent MA. What is the normal prevalence of vesicoureteral reflux? Pediatr Radiol 2000; 30(9):587–593

Schmahmann S, Haller JO. Neonatal ovarian cysts: pathogenesis, diagnosis and management. Pediatr Radiol 1997; 27(2):101–105

Shemie SD, Pollack MM, Morioka M, Bonner S. Diagnosis of brain death in children. Lancet Neurol 2007; 6(1):87–92

Simon EM. MRI of the fetal spine. Pediatr Radiol 2004; 34(9):712–719. Epub 2004 Jul 28

Sittig SE, Asay GF. Congenital cystic adenomatoid malformation in the newborn: two case studies and review of the literature. Respir Care 2000; 45(10):1188–1195

Sivit CJ. Imaging the child with right lower quadrant pain and suspected appendicitis: current concepts. Pediatr Radiol 2004; 34(6):447–453. Epub 2004 Apr 23

Soper JR, De Silva M. Infantile myofibromatosis: a radiological review. Pediatr Radiol 1993; 23(3):189–194

Stanton M, Davenport M. Management of congenital lung lesions. Early Hum Dev 2006; 82(5):289–295. Epub 2006 Apr 3

Strouse PJ. Disorders of intestinal rotation and fixation ("malrotation"). Pediatr Radiol 2004; 34(11):837–851. Epub 2004 Sep 4

Tiddens HA. Chest computed tomography scans should be considered as a routine investigation in cystic fibrosis. Paediatr Respir Rev 2006; 7(3):202–208. Epub 2006 Aug 2

Tokumaru AM, Horiuchi K, Kaji T, Kohyama S, Sakata I, Kusano S. MRI findings of recurrent herpes simplex encephalitis in an infant. Pediatr Radiol 2003;33(10):725–728. Epub 2003 Jul 19

Triulzi F, Parazzini C, Righini A. Patterns of damage in the mature neonatal brain. Pediatr Radiol 2006; 36(7):608–620. Epub 2006 May 18

Tsitouridis I, Tsinoglou K, Morichovitou A, Stratilati S, Siouggaris N, Kontaki T. Scimitar syndrome versus meandering pulmonary vein: evaluation with three-dimensional computed tomography. Acta Radiol 2006; 47(9):927–932

Veyrac C, Couture A, Saguintaah M, Baud C. Brain ultrasonography in the premature infant. Pediatr Radiol 2006; 36(7):626–635. Epub 2006 May 3

Vezina LG. Neuroradiology of childhood brain tumors: new challenges. J Neurooncol 2005; 75(3):243–252

Volle E, Kaufmann HJ. Pulmonary alveolar microlithiasis in pediatric patients –review of the world literature and two new observations. Pediatr Radiol 1987; 17(6):439–442

Wilms G, Demaerel P, Sunaert S. Intra-axial brain tumours. Eur Radiol 2005; 15(3):468–484. Epub 2004 Dec 31

Wihlborg C, Babyn P, Ranson M, Laxer R. Radiologic mimics of juvenile rheumatoid arthritis. Pediatr Radiol 2001; 31(5):315–326

White KS, Grossman H. Wilms' and associated renal tumors of childhood. Pediatr Radiol 1991; 21(2):81–88

Wootton-Gorges SL, Thomas KB, Harned RK, Wu SR, Stein-Wexler R, Strain JD. Giant cystic abdominal masses in children. Pediatr Radiol 2005; 35(12):1277–1288. Epub 2005 Sep 9

Zar H, McIvor B, Furlan G, Jedeikin L, Pitcher R. Congenital lung mass in an asymptomatic patient. S Afr Med J 2006; 96(6):512–513

Zacharia TT, Jaramillo D, Poussaint TY, Korf B. MR imaging of abdominopelvic involvement in neurofibromatosis type 1: a review of 43 patients. Pediatr Radiol 2005; 35(3):317–322. Epub 2004 Oct 27

Zarewych ZM, Donnelly LF, Frush DP, Bisset GS 3rd. Imaging of pediatric mesenteric abnormalities. Pediatr Radiol 1999; 29(9):711–719

Zimmerman RA, Bilaniuk LT. Neuroimaging evaluation of cerebral palsy. Clin Perinatol 2006; 33(2):517–544

Ultrasound Imaging 10

PEDRO SEGUI and SIMONA ESPEJO

Ultrasonography (US) is the most widely used and fastest growing sectional imaging method. The current success of US is based on certain specific advantages over other imaging modalities:

- There are no known risks or contraindications to its use.
- The spatial resolution of a high-frequency US image is higher than that of other cross-sectional modalities such as computed tomography (CT) or magnetic resonance (MR). This resolution is particularly high when superficial structures are examined.
- The dynamic qualities of US are unique, enabling real-time observations of movements of muscles or tendons, pulsations, and peristalsis. The effects of compression, Valsalva's maneuver, and gravity can be appreciated.
- The Doppler effect can be used to make quantitative measurements of blood velocity and to map blood flow.
- Modern US scanners are small and provide high-quality images. Portable and hand-held units can be used in high-care units, operating rooms, and emergency units.
- US is extensively used to guide punctures and interventions.
- US examination allows direct communication with the patient and the information the patient provides, e.g., the area of maximum tenderness, is extremely helpful for a specific sonographic search.
- US is relatively inexpensive, especially when compared with modalities such as CT and MR.

US instruments have been used to image the human body for more than 50 years, but primitive real-time sonographic units did not appear until 1975. After improvements in gray-scale US were made, the addition of Doppler techniques greatly increased the capabilities of US. US technology is currently evolving at a more rapid pace than ever. Recent developments include tissue harmonic imaging, spatial compound imaging, extended field-of-view imaging, coded pulse excitation, electronic focusing of the image section or plane, three-dimensional and four-dimensional imaging, and many innovations in Doppler US techniques. Another innovation is intravascular microbubbled contrast agents, which were initially used for improvement of Doppler studies and have been recently introduced for characterization of focal masses.

Despite these technical innovations, it is important to note that the value of US is ultimately determined by the training and experience of the individual performing and interpreting the examination. The popularity of US and the availability of low-cost scanners have stimulated the rapid proliferation of US into unskilled hands, with the consequent results of poorly performed studies and increasing misdiagnosis that have begun to discredit this imaging modality.

A 66-year-old man with a three-day history of right upper quadrant pain was admitted to the hospital. He had severe leukocytosis but no fever. US examination showed signs of acute calculous cholecystitis. The patient underwent emergency open cholecystectomy. Acute inflammation and wall necrosis (gangrenous cholecystitis) without gallbladder perforation were observed at surgery and histological examination.

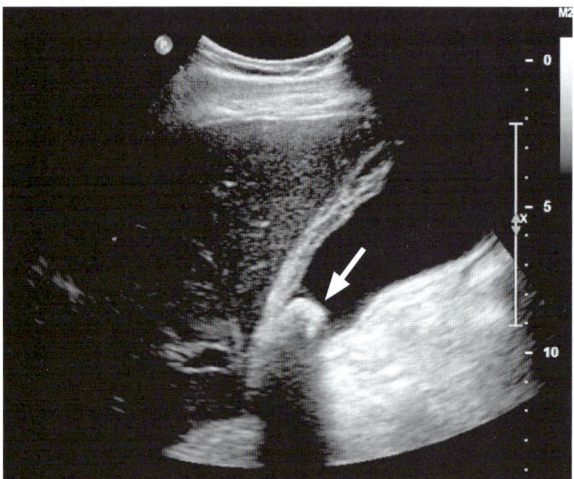

Fig. 10.1.1

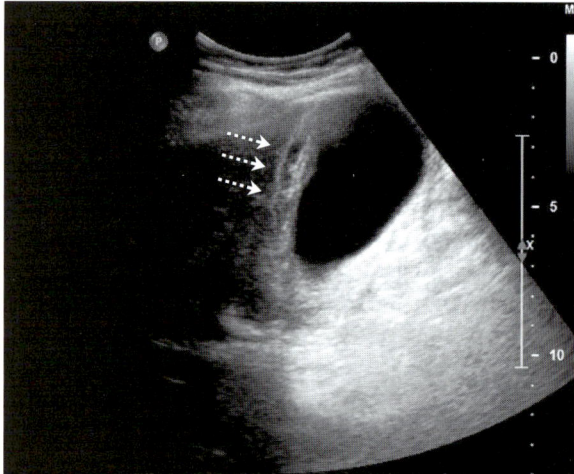

Fig. 10.1.2

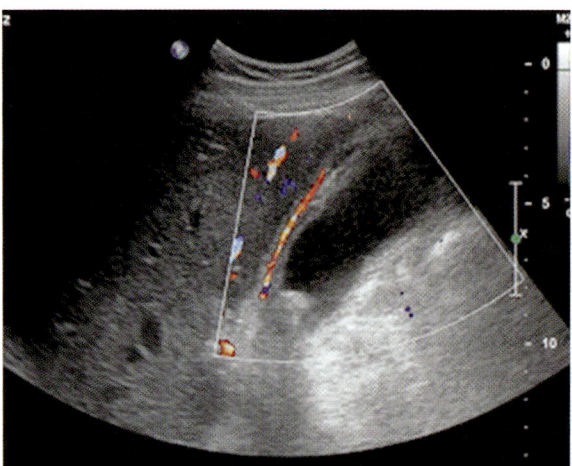

Fig. 10.1.3

Acute cholecystitis results from obstruction of the gallbladder neck or cystic duct with inflammation of the gallbladder wall. Approximately 95% of the cases result from obstruction due to gallstones. Acute cholecystitis manifests as persistent upper right quadrant pain that may radiate to the right scapula. Nausea, vomiting, fever, and leukocytosis are common.

Ultrasonography is usually the initial imaging procedure of choice in a patient with suspected acute cholecystitis. In uncomplicated cases, the ultrasound findings include gallstones (often impacted in the gallbladder neck or cystic duct), positive sonographic Murphy's sign, gallbladder larger than 4×10 cm in diameter, gallbladder wall thickening greater than 3 mm, and pericholecystic fluid. Of these findings, the first two are considered the most specific.

The sonographic Murphy's sign refers to localized tenderness directly over the gallbladder, and it is positive when pressure applied with the transducer elicits maximal tenderness over the gallbladder visualized at sonography. The combination of gallstones and Murphy's sign has a positive predictive value of over 90%. This sign may be absent in non-responsive patients, when pain medication has been administered, or in cases of gangrenous cholecystitis.

Thickening of the gallbladder wall occurs to some degree in most cases of acute cholecystitis. However, many causes of gallbladder wall thickening exist beyond cholecystitis, so this finding is less specific.

Pericholecystic fluid is found in approximately 20% of patients, and its presence implies a more advanced type of cholecystitis. It is usually seen as a focal collection adjacent to the gallbladder wall.

Gangrenous cholecystitis is a severe advanced form of acute cholecystitis, with increased morbidity and mortality rates. The sonographic hallmark is the presence of heterogeneous or striated thickening of the gallbladder wall, which is often irregular with localized disruptions or projections into the lumen. Murphy's sign may be absent. However, a striated appearance of the gallbladder wall is common and may be seen in uncomplicated cholecystitis and other conditions causing gallbladder edema.

A striated appearance of the gallbladder wall is common, but this may be seen in uncomplicated cholecystitis and other conditions causing gallbladder edema. Intraluminal membranes and wall disruptions are more specific but less frequent findings.

Emphysematous cholecystitis is a rare complication of acute cholecystitis and is associated with gas-forming bacteria. Up to 50% patients have diabetes. Gas may be intraluminal or intramural. Intraluminal gas can be recognized by the antidependent gas echoes within the lumen. Intramural gas may be more difficult to identify because it may mimic the calcified wall of a porcelain gallbladder.

Acalculous cholecystitis may occur in extremely ill patients. In these cases, US is often equivocal because these severely-ill patients have distended, thick-walled gallbladders even in the absence of inflammation, and Murphy's sign is unreliable in these patients. CT may be more specific, but the diagnosis is often difficult to make or exclude by any means.

Comments

Ultrasound image of the gallbladder in the sagittal (Fig. 10.1.1) and transverse planes (Fig. 10.1.2) demonstrated distension of the gallbladder, a gallstone impacted in the gallbladder neck (*arrow*), and thickened gallbladder wall with a striated appearance (dotted *arrows*). There was a positive sonographic Murphy sign. These findings can be found in acute uncomplicated cholecystitis or in gangrenous cholecystitis. Color Doppler ultrasound (Fig. 10.1.3) shows a hypervascular gallbladder wall, which is a nonspecific feature.

Imaging Findings

Case 2
■
Appendicitis

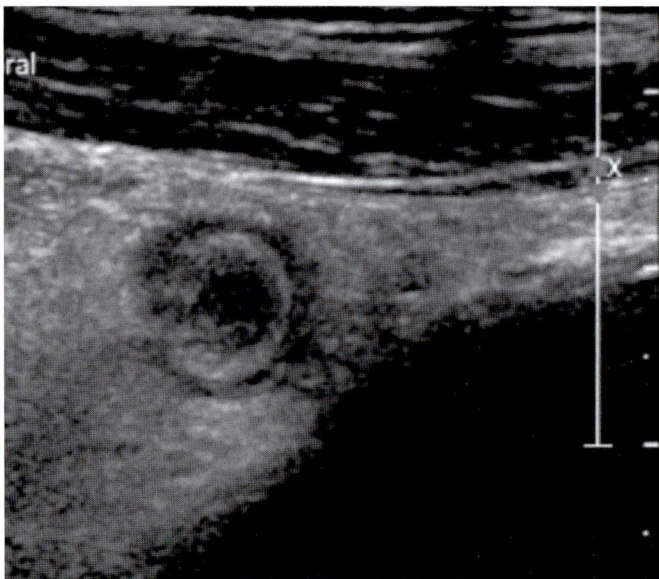

Fig. 10.2.1

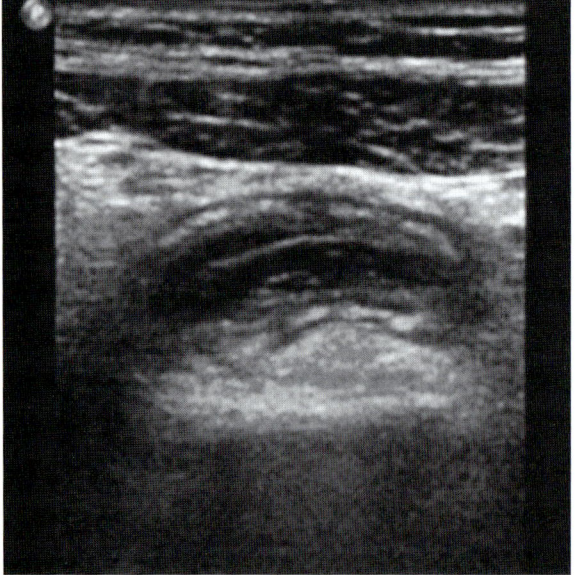

Fig. 10.2.2

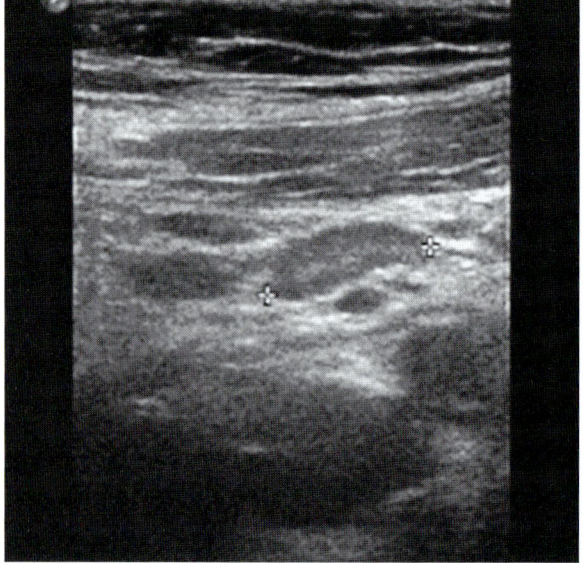

Fig. 10.2.3

A 12-year-old girl was admitted to the hospital with a one-day history of epigastric and right lower quadrant pain, fever, and vomiting. Physical examination revealed tenderness in the right lower quadrant. Laboratory studies yielded leukocytosis with neutrophilia. US examination showed acute appendicitis without signs of perforation. An inflamed nonperforated appendix was found at surgery. Histologic examination demonstrated acute phlegmonous appendicitis.

Comments

Acute appendicitis is the most common abdominal surgical emergency in the western world. The overall accuracy of clinical diagnosing of appendicitis is approximately 80%, with a mean false-negative appendectomy rate of 20% and a mean overall incidence of perforation of 20%. New imaging technology (helical CT, graded-compression US) has the potential to improve these clinical outcomes. US examination of the patient with suspected appendicitis usually starts with a curvilinear 3.5–5 MHz transducer. The linear transducer is used last for more detailed images.

The typical appearance of an inflamed appendix is a thick-walled, noncompressible sausage-like and blind-ended structure in a fixed position at the point of maximal tenderness. The appendix is considered enlarged when its outer anteroposterior diameter under compression measured in the transverse plane is 6 mm or larger. The average maximum diameter is 9 mm. Appendicoliths are found in 30% of inflamed appendices and appear as bright, echogenic foci with clean distal acoustic shadowing. The adjacent fat of the mesoappendix may become larger, hyperechoic, and less compressible, and, if inflammation progresses, this fatty tissue tends to increase in volume around the appendix. With perforation of the appendix, the distended appendix may no longer be visualized at US examination and the inflammatory changes in the perienteric fat are more obvious. Patients evaluated with a considerable delay from the onset of appendicitis may show a large mass of noncompressible fat around the appendix, interspersed with poorly marginated hypoechoic zones (appendiceal phlegmon) or a fluid collection (appendiceal abscess). A small amount of free intraperitoneal fluid is nonspecific and may be present in both nonperforated and perforated appendicitis, as well as in many other conditions. A large amount of peritoneal fluid in the presence of a inflamed appendix usually represents pus from a perforated appendix.

Color Doppler US is also useful. Circumferential color in the wall of the inflamed appendix is strongly supportive evidence of active inflammation. With gangrene, color Doppler may show decreased perfusion or none at all.

US and CT have similar positive and negative predictive values (both over 90%) for appendicitis. The choice between US and CT is largely dependent on institutional preference and on available expertise. Operator skill has particular importance in the US evaluation of the patient with right lower quadrant pain, and the learning curve required is considerable. Patient sex, age, and body habitus are important factors. US is usually the recommended initial imaging study in children, in young women, and during pregnancy. In patients with equivocal US findings, most of which are obese, CT is indicated.

Imaging Findings

Cross-sectional (Fig. 10.2.1) and long-axis (Fig. 10.2.2) US images of the right lower quadrant obtained with a linear transducer show a blind-ended, tubular structure measuring 10 mm in diameter with a laminated wall. The appendix was not compressible. Cross-sectional US image (Fig. 10.2.3) shows some oval, reactive lymph nodes (*arrows*) near the terminal illeum, a common finding in the context of acute appendicitis.

A 43-year-old man was admitted with left lower quadrant pain and fever of one day's duration. Physical examination revealed tenderness and guarding in the left lower abdomen. Laboratory tests showed leukocytosis with neutrophilia. US findings were suggestive of uncomplicated sigmoid diverticulitis. The patient underwent conservative management with antibiotics and was symptom free after a few days. Scheduled surgical resection (sigmoidectomy) was performed three months later. Histologic examination disclosed diverticulosis and chronic diverticulitis, without malignancy.

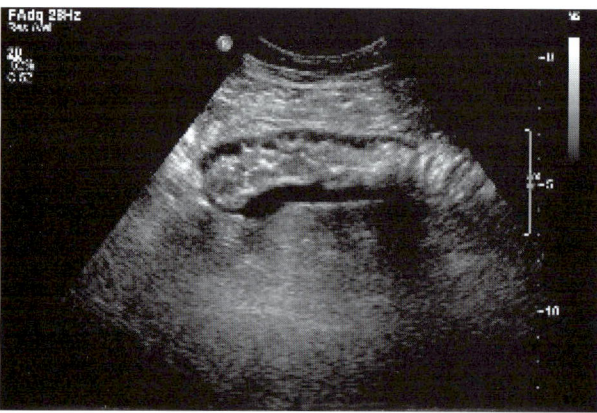

Fig. 10.3.1

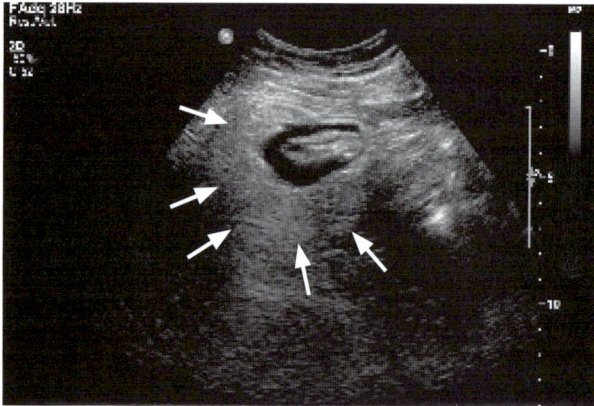

Fig. 10.3.2

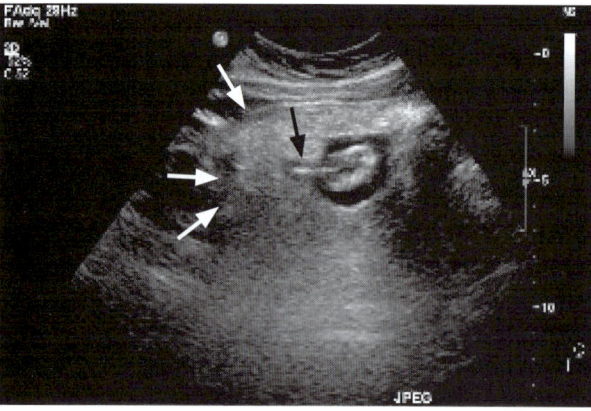

Fig. 10.3.3

Diverticulitis is a common cause of left-sided abdominal pain in the adult population. It is related to inflammatory changes involving acquired diverticula, most often in the descending and the sigmoid colon. Diverticulitis occurs in up to 25% of patients with known diverticulosis. The diagnosis is often made on clinical grounds: the classic presentation is localized pain and guarding in the left lower abdomen, fever, and leukocytosis. However, the diagnosis is not always clear, and there are a large number of erroneous clinical diagnoses. Differential diagnoses include urinary tract infection, renal colic, perforated pelvic ulcer, adnexitis, sigmoid carcinoma, and epiploic appendagitis. Diverticulitis is considered uncomplicated (simple) in the presence of peridiverticulitis or phlegmon and complicated when associated with obstruction, perforation, fistula, or abscess formation. This information can help in deciding whether medical or surgical management is indicated. Many authors recommend radiological evaluation of all patients with clinically suspected diverticulitis, both to confirm the diagnosis and to assess the location and extent of the inflammatory processes.

The normal descending colon and upper part of the sigmoid can be reliably identified on ultrasound in virtually all patients because of their consistent location in the left paracolic gutter. In diverticulosis the muscularis layer is often thickened, and fecalith-containing diverticula can be easily recognized as large, strongly hyperechoic, round-ovoid structures with acoustic shadow located on the outside contour of the colon.

In acute diverticulitis there is usually local thickening (> 3 mm) of the intestinal wall. The inflammatory pericolic fat that surrounds the fecalith is seen as a hyperechoic, noncompressible halo and shows local tenderness induced by graded compression. This inflamed fat must be present for the diagnosis of diverticulitis (intestinal wall thickening can be seen in diverticulosis). Later, a small (often < 1 cm) paracolic abscess develops, the fecalith disintegrates, usually with evacuation of pus through the weakened wall into the colonic lumen, and symptoms disappear in a few days. In about 20–30% of patients, diverticulitis takes a complicated course with a larger (> 2.5 cm) diverticular abscess (demonstrated as a well-defined hypoechoic mass localized in the pericolic environment, with or without an aeric component), fistula, or free perforation; these patients are less likely to respond to conservative treatment.

Right-sided diverticulitis is much less common. It involves congenital or true diverticula and occurs more commonly in young women. The bowel wall will show thickening, and the inflamed diverticula are identical in appearance to the acquired variety in the left hemicolon.

The differentiation between diverticulitis and perforated colonic neoplasm can be very difficult with any imaging technique. Once the inflammatory changes have subsided, contrast enema examination or colonoscopy to exclude carcinoma is warranted in every patient with diverticulitis undergoing conservative management.

US has yielded results similar to those of CT in diagnosing acute diverticulitis, with a sensitivity between 84 and 100%. US can be the initial imaging technique in patients referred for lower quadrant or pelvis pain, with CT reserved for initial imaging of patients with clinical suspicion of free intraperitoneal perforation or for reassessment of patients with a doubtful US. However, most institutions consider CT the technique of choice for diagnosing patients with clinical suspicion of acute diverticulitis.

Longitudinal (Fig. 10.3.1) and transverse (Fig. 10.3.2) sonograms demonstrate hypoechoic mural thickening of the sigmoid colon. Note the surrounding hyperechoic, noncompressible tissue representing the inflammatory fat (*arrows*). Transverse sonogram at a different level (Fig. 10.3.3) reveals an inflamed diverticulum (*black arrow*), also with surrounding inflamed fat (*arrows*).

Case 4
■
Epididymoorchitis

A 33-year-old man presented with acute onset of right scrotal pain, without urinary symptoms or fever. With the suspicion of testicular torsion, a Doppler ultrasound scan was performed, revealing an enlarged right epididymis with hyperemia of testis and epididymis, asymmetric with the left side. After the diagnosis of right epididymoorchitis, the patient was treated with antibiotics and anti-inflammatory drugs and showed complete clinical recovery in a few days.

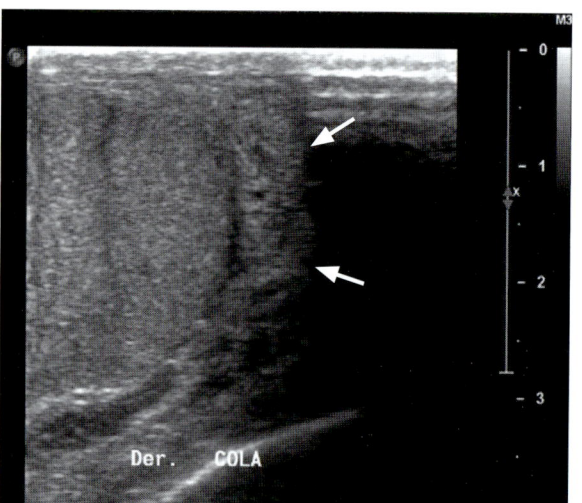

Fig. 10.4.1

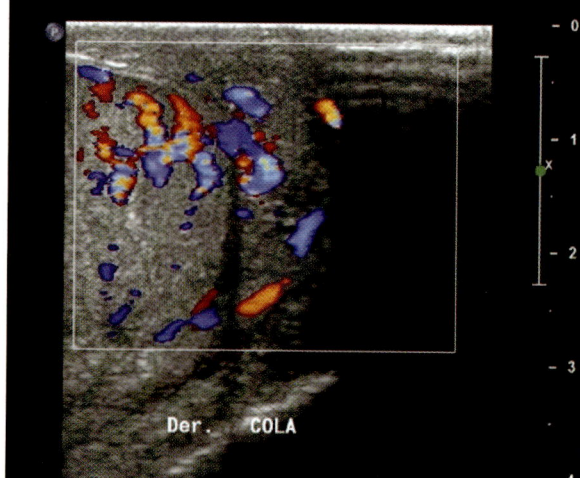

Fig. 10.4.2

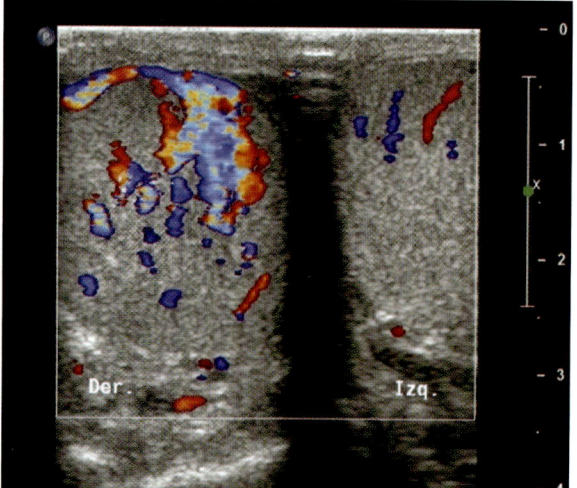

Fig. 10.4.3

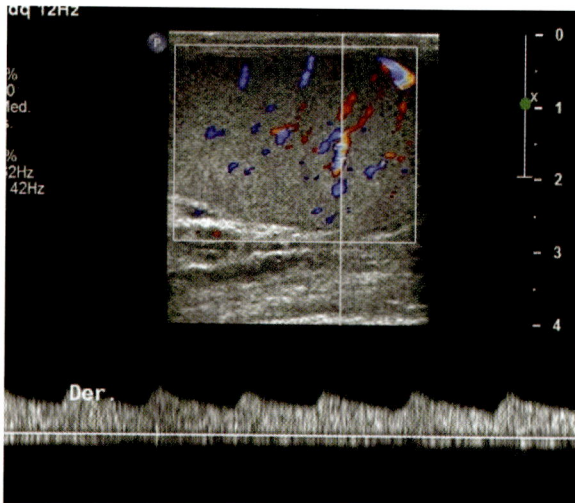

Fig. 10.4.4

The differential diagnosis for acute scrotal pain includes testicular torsion, infection (epididymoorchitis, epididymitis, or orchitis), torsion of the appendix testis, trauma, incarcerated inguinal hernia, hemorrhage in a testicular tumor, and vasculitis.

Acute epididymoorchitis and epididymitis are the most common causes of acute scrotum in adolescent boys and adults. Common pathogens are Chlamydia trachomatis, Neisseria gonorrhea, Escherichia coli, and Proteus mirabilis. Epididymitis first affects the tail of the epididymis and then spreads into the body and head. Orchitis develops in 20–40% of cases of epididymitis. Primary orchitis without associated epididymitis is relatively rare, but may be caused by HIV or mumps virus.

Patients with epididymoorchitis usually present with pain and swelling of the scrotum and its contents with systemic signs of infection. The clinical history, however, may be atypical, and relatively acute onset of symptoms may simulate torsion. Furthermore, many patients with testicular torsion often present without classical signs and symptoms, and this condition may mimic epididymoorchitis, with a nearly 50% false-positive rate for diagnoses of testicular torsion based solely on clinical findings. In patients in whom the history and physical examination do not reveal classical symptoms, ultrasound has been used to help differentiate between torsion and infection.

On gray scale images, the epididymis is enlarged and usually appears hypoechoic. Reactive hydrocele or pyocele with scrotal wall thickening are present in most cases. In cases of testicular involvement, gray scale may show testicular enlargement with diffuse hypoechogenicity. Later (sometimes within a few hours), the ultrasound appearance evolves from a diffuse pattern to increasingly well-defined patchy focal hypoechoic areas. These gray-scale sonographic findings are nonspecific. Torsion may present with similar sonographic appearances, and a heterogeneous echo pattern may be difficult to differentiate from neoplastic lesions. Because gray-scale findings are not specific, the Doppler component of the examination is essential.

The increased blood flow to the epididymis and testis on color Doppler examination is a well-established criterion for the diagnosis of epididymoorchitis. It is important to compare the vascularity in both epididymides, because blood flow can be seen in a normal epididymis. Increased vascularity in acute epididymoorchitis has a high-flow, low-resistance pattern. In normal volunteers, the resistive index in the testes is rarely less than 0.5, but more than half the patients with epididymoorchitis have a resistive index of less than 0.5.

With healing, the sonographic changes often resolve completely. In all cases of testicular inhomogeneity diagnosed as epididymoorchitis, the diagnosis should be reconsidered if there is no sonographic improvement with antibiotic treatment.

Complications arise in as many 50% of men with epididymoorchitis; these include abscess formation, necrosis, hematoma formation, and infarction with subsequent testicular atrophy.

Comments

Longitudinal gray-scale US image (Fig. 10.4.1) shows enlargement of the right epididymal tail (*arrows*). Color Doppler US image (Fig. 10.4.2) shows marked hyperemia. Transverse color Doppler US image of both testes (Fig. 10.4.3) shows hyperemia within the right testis (left side of screen), clearly asymmetric with the asymptomatic left testis (right side of screen). Pulsed Doppler imaging of the right testis (Fig. 10.4.3) shows testicular flow with resistive index of less than 0.5, typical of epididymoorchitis.

Imaging Findings

Case 5
■ Deep Venous Thrombosis

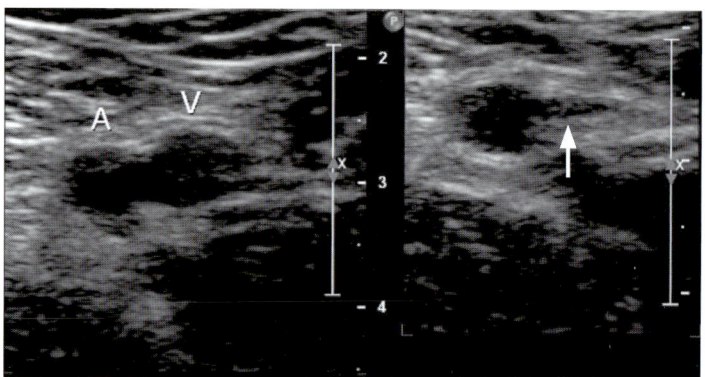

Fig. 10.5.1

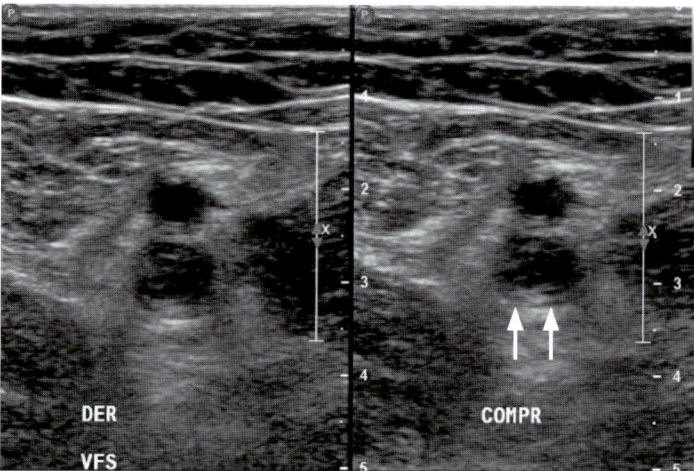

Fig. 10.5.2

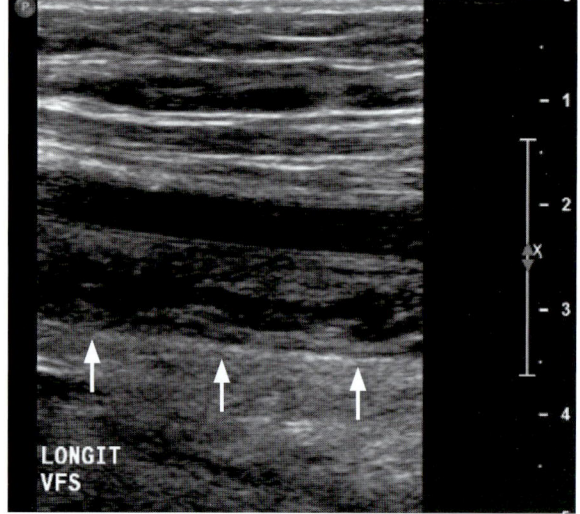

Fig. 10.5.3

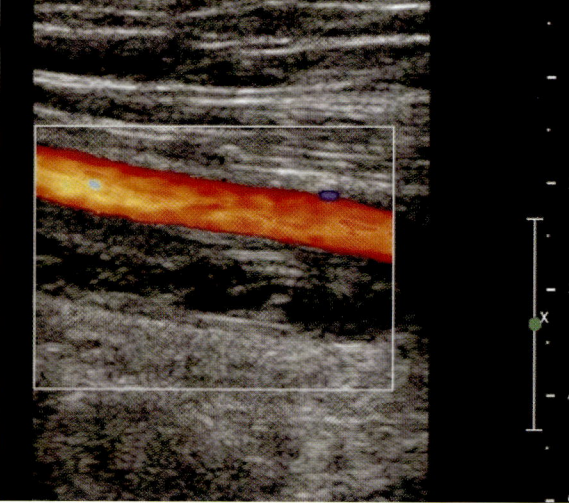

Fig. 10.5.4

A 51-year-old man experienced a gradual onset of pain and swelling in his right calf 5 days before admission. The patient had been immobilized for three weeks for an ankle sprain. A venous US scan of the right leg showed deep vein thrombosis in the femoropopliteal segment. Anticoagulant treatment was initiated and resulted in rapid improvement of symptoms.

Deep vein thrombosis (DVT) is a common problem in the acute care setting. Commonly, DVT begins in the veins of the calf and progresses proximally over time. Less than 20% of patients with confirmed DVT have thrombi isolated to the calf veins. While the thrombus is isolated in the iliofemoral region in only approximately 10% of patients with lower-extremity DVT, this is a common presentation of DVT during pregnancy, usually on the left side. The more central the thrombi, the greater the risk of pulmonary emboli. About 50% of patients with DVT develop pulmonary emboli, although many of these may be subsegmental and undiagnosed. Patients with acute calf-popliteal-vein thrombosis usually present with symptoms of unilateral pain and swelling in the calf and this condition may be associated with warmth, redness, and tenderness.

The signs and symptoms of DVT are notoriously unreliable, so a noninvasive screening test is usually necessary.

Compression ultrasonography (CUS) is the diagnostic procedure of choice for the assessment of patients with suspected DVT. It has been shown to be highly sensitive and specific for the diagnosis of DVT, particularly in the lower extremities in symptomatic patients. Sensitivity and specificity are near 100% in the femoropopliteal segment. Sensitivity decreases in isolated calf thrombi and in asymptomatic patients.

CUS of the deep venous system of the lower extremities is performed with the patient in the supine position, with the leg externally rotated and slightly flexed at the knee. Patients may be placed prone to assess the popliteal fossa and occasionally in the sitting position if there is difficulty in identifying the calf veins. A linear transducer with a frequency in the 5–12 MHz range is used. The transducer is placed transversely, moving down the leg following the common femoral vein, superficial femoral vein, and popliteal vein until it divides. Gentle pressure is applied to the vessels with the transducer at 1 cm intervals and, in the absence of DVT, the lumen of the vein should collapse. In the presence of DVT, the lumen does not collapse, and this is the most sensitive and specific sign of DVT. In acute DVT, the thrombosed vein is distended and clot echogenicity is variable. Duplex and color Doppler are not required but can be helpful. No spectral or color flow can be demonstrated at the site of total occlusion, and there is loss of phasic response in the segment distal to it.

The value of performing CUS of the calf veins when proximal veins are normal remains controversial.

US scan of a healthy volunteer (Fig. 10.5.1). Split screen transverse US image of a normal superficial femoral vein (V) and artery (A). Uncompressed (left side) and compressed (right side) images show that, in the absence of thrombosis, compression results in complete apposition of the walls of the vein (arrow) while the artery remains patent.

In our patient with femoral vein thrombosis split screen transverse US image (Fig. 10.5.2) shows a non-compressible superficial femoral vein (arrows). Longitudinal US image (Fig. 10.5.3) shows the distended vein (posterior to the artery) with intraluminal clot (arrows). Color Doppler longitudinal image (Fig. 10.5.4) shows normal flow in the superficial femoral artery and no flow in the superficial femoral vein.

A 47-year-old female patient presented with a 2-month history of a right neck mass, without fever or weight loss. Physical examination revealed palpable nodules in the right side of the neck. A cervical US scan showed multiple pathologic adenopathies located in the jugular and supraclavicular spaces and in the posterior triangle, suggestive of lymphoma. A right supraclavicular adenopathy was surgically excised and diagnosed as Hodgkin's lymphoma at histological examination. Staging computed tomography (CT) showed pathologic cervical adenopathies, without thoracic or abdominal involvement. The patient underwent chemotherapy.

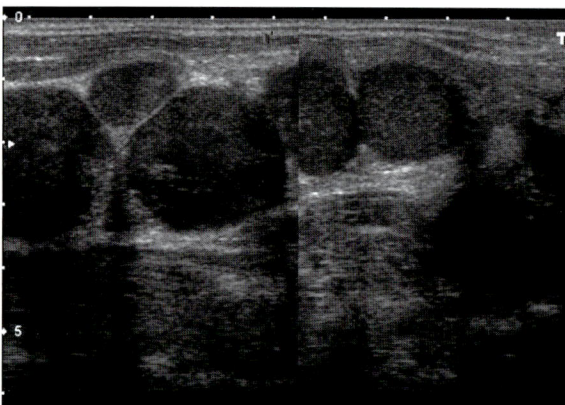

Fig. 10.6.1

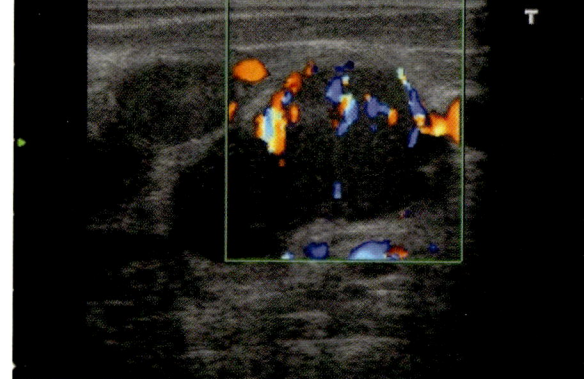

Fig. 10.6.2

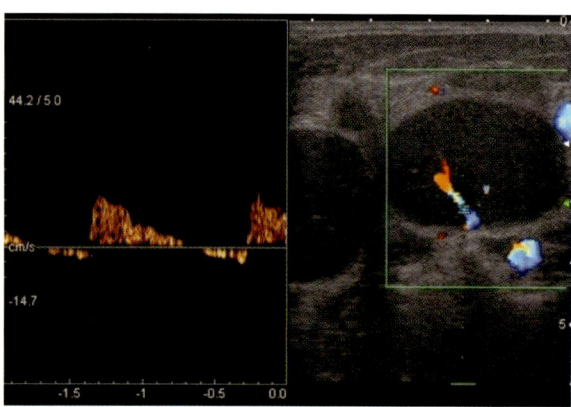

Fig. 10.6.3

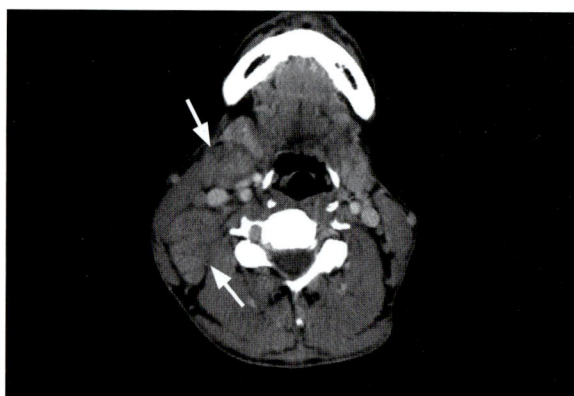

Fig. 10.6.4

Hodgkin's disease is a B cell lymphoma. In 80–90% of patients, the first manifestation of Hodgkin's lymphoma (HL) is lymphadenopathy, most frequently located in the neck. High-resolution sonography can be used as the first-line modality for evaluating cervical soft-tissue masses.

Sonography is a useful imaging tool in the assessment of peripheral lymph nodes. Gray-scale sonography is widely used in the evaluation of the number, size, site, shape, borders, soft-tissue edema, and internal architecture of lymph nodes. Spectral Doppler sonography with measurement of vascular resistance, color Doppler, and power Doppler may be helpful. High-resolution ultrasound is currently used in the diagnostic evaluation of lymph-node involvement in patients with head and neck carcinomas (cervical lymph nodes), breast cancer (axillary nodes), melanoma (regional peripheral nodes), and many other malignancies. Normal and reactive nodes tend to be oval and to have an echogenic hilum. The upper limit in minimal axial diameter of normal and reactive nodes varies with the location (5–8 mm for cervical nodes). Malignant lymph nodes (metastatic and lymphomatous) are usually round and without echogenic hilum; central necrosis (echogenic-coagulative or anechoic-cystic) is sometimes present. Eccentric cortical hypertrophy is a useful sign to indicate focal tumor infiltration in a node.

In both Hodgkin's and non-Hodgkin's lymphoma, lymph nodes tend to be round, hypoechoic, without echogenic hilum and to show intranodal reticulation.

Fine-needle biopsy and core biopsy are usually diagnostic for HL but may not yield enough material to enable the histological classification. Excisional lymph node biopsy is required to fully appreciate the architecture of the lymph node.

Staging in HL consists of determining the location and extent of disease, defining prognostic factors and manifestations that can be evaluated and will determine the choice of treatment. In essence, the staging is based on the number of sites of lymph node involvement, whether lymph nodes are involved on both sides of the diaphragm, whether there is visceral involvement, and whether B symptoms (fever, weight loss, drenching night sweats) are present.

Thoracic CT scanning is useful as it has a considerable potential to influence the initial treatment. Staging below the diaphragm is hampered by false-negative CT results due to CT's inability to detect HL in normal-sized nodes and the difficulties in detecting HL in the spleen by CT or ultrasound. Although bone-marrow involvement is relatively uncommon, a bone marrow biopsy is usually recommended. Magnetic resonance appears to be sensitive for the evaluation of bone and/or bone-marrow involvement. However, this modality has the disadvantage that only a limited area of the body can be investigated. Positron emission tomography is a very promising imaging modality for the staging of Hodgkin's patients.

Longitudinal gray-scale sonogram of the right posterior cervical triangle (Fig. 10.6.1) shows multiple rounded, enlarged lymph nodes. Nodes appear homogeneously hypoechoic and without echogenic hilum. Color Doppler sonogram (Fig. 10.6.2) shows nodes are hypervascular. Spectral Doppler sonogram (Fig. 10.6.3) shows a very high-resistance flow pattern with diastolic inversion, a feature that usually indicates malignancy. Cervical contrast-enhanced CT (Fig. 10.6.4) shows enlarged right-sided nodes with homogeneous density (*arrows*).

Case 7
■
Abdominal Wall Endometriosis

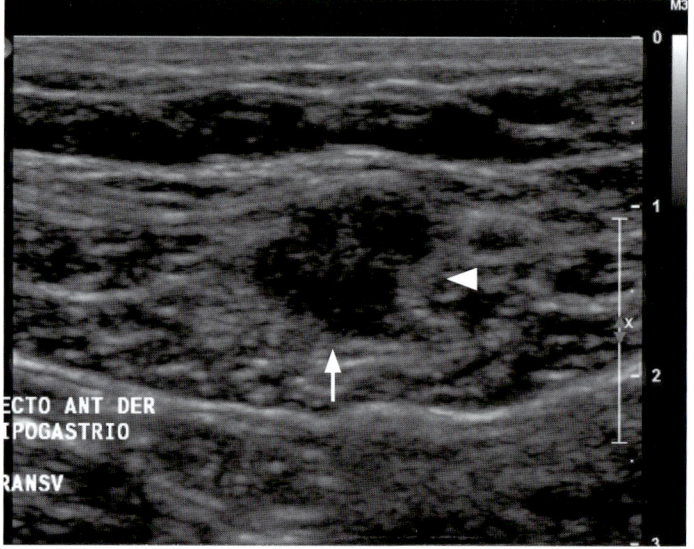

Fig. 10.7.1

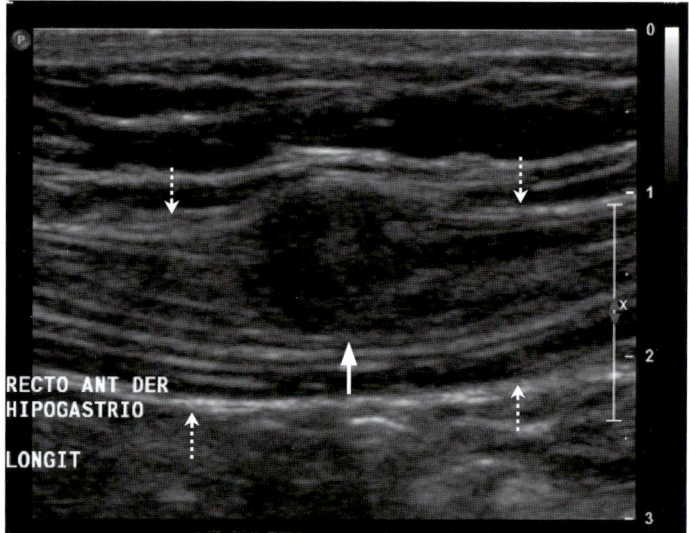

Fig. 10.7.2

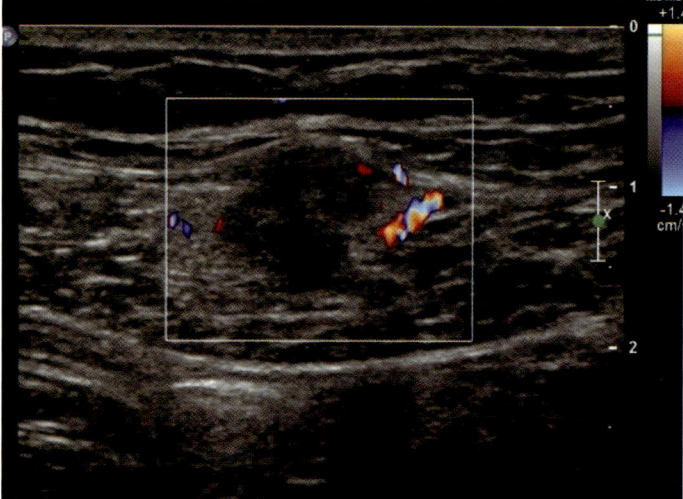

Fig. 10.7.3

A 37-year-old woman presented with right lower quadrant pain of two month's duration. Pain was cyclic, increasing during menses. She had a history of a cesarean section with Pfannenstiel's incision two years before. Physical examination found no palpable masses. US showed a focal solid nodule into the rectus abdominis muscle. US-guided core biopsy was inconclusive, showing fibrosis. The nodule was surgically excised. Histologic examination disclosed endometrial tissue infiltrating muscular tissue.

Comments

Endometriosis is classically defined as the presence of functional endometrial glands and stroma outside the uterine cavity. Endometriosis is a common and important clinical problem in women, predominantly affecting those in the reproductive age group. The most common site of involvement is the ovary, but virtually all pelvic organs can be affected and endometriosis can also occur in nongynecologic sites.

Endometriosis can occur within surgical scars, generally from prior gynecologic operations. Abdominal wall endometriosis may occur after pelvic surgery that violates the uterine cavity, such as a cesarean section, allowing endometrial tissue to be transplanted, and this usually occurs in the absence of any history of pelvic endometriosis. Other lesions, such as those of the umbilicus, are thought to occur spontaneously. Endometriosis of the abdominal wall may be difficult to diagnose, both clinically and with diagnostic imaging, and is often confused with other abnormal conditions such as a suture granuloma, incisional hernia, abscess, hematoma, sebaceous cyst, or malignant tumor.

Abdominal wall endometriosis can manifest clinically weeks to years after surgery as a palpable mass or focal cyclic pain associated with menses, both located near or under the surgery scar. However, many patients present with constant pain not associated with the menstrual cycle, and a palpable mass is not always present.

US features of abdominal wall endometriomas are variable. The most common appearance of these masses is solid, hypoechoic lesions with internal vascularity on color or power Doppler examination. An inflammatory reaction to the endometrial implant may be seen as a hyperechoic border. Cystic masses and complex cystic and solid masses have also been described, but these are uncommon. Lesions may be confined to the rectus sheath, located in the subcutaneous fat, or infiltrating both of these layers. Sonographic findings are nonspecific, but hernia, hematoma and abscess can be excluded in view of the solid appearance and Doppler-detected internal flow.

US-guided fine-needle aspiration (FNA) is a rapid and accurate diagnostic procedure, enabling malignancy to be excluded. If FNA results are inconclusive, as may occur because endometriomas are often fibrous in nature, an additional histological biopsy may be considered. Therapeutic options for abdominal wall endometriosis are pharmacologic therapy or surgical excision.

Transverse (Fig. 10.7.1) and longitudinal (Fig. 10.7.2) sonograms show a 13 × 7 mm hypoechoic solid mass (*arrow*) with irregular margins confined to the rectus abdominis sheath (*dotted arrows*). A hyperechoic rim partially circumscribes the nodule (*arrowhead*).

Imaging Findings

Color Doppler sonogram (Fig. 10.7.3) shows vascularity within the peripheral rim.

A 37-year-old woman presented with right lower quadrant pain of two month's duration. Pain was cyclic, increasing during menses. She had a history of a cesarean section with Pfannenstiel's incision two years before. Physical examination found no palpable masses. US showed a focal solid nodule into the rectus abdominis muscle. US-guided core biopsy was inconclusive, showing fibrosis. The nodule was surgically excised. Histologic examination disclosed endometrial tissue infiltrating muscular tissue.

Case 8

■

Carotid Artery Stenosis

A 66-year-old man presented with acute-onset dysarthria, postural instability, and disorientation. Urgent computed tomography (CT) detected no acute findings. Magnetic resonance imaging (MRI) of the brain on day 5 of admission showed small infarcts in both cerebral hemispheres. Doppler ultrasound revealed significant stenosis (>70%) at the right internal carotid (ICA) origin. Digital subtraction angiography confirmed 90% stenosis and an endovascular stent was implanted. The patient was asymptomatic after a one-year follow-up period.

Comments

Stroke is the third most important cause of death in developed countries and one of the most common causes of disability. The most well-known risk factor for the development of cerebrovascular events is high-degree internal carotid artery (ICA) stenosis. Three large-scale, multicenter, randomized trials, published between 1991 and1995 recommend carotid endarterectomy in symptomatic patients with >60% stenosis of the ICA and in asymptom-

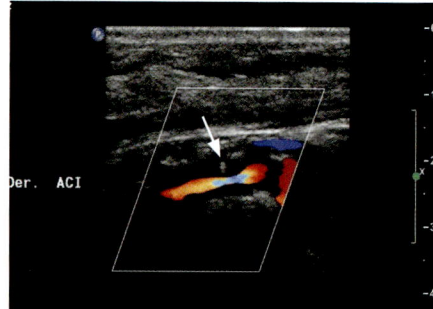

Fig. 10.8.1

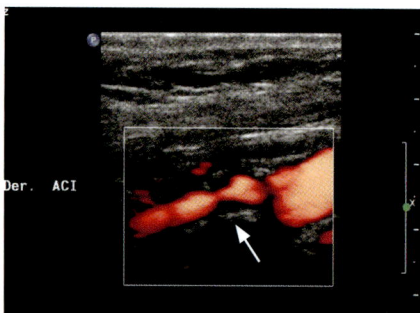

Fig. 10.8.2

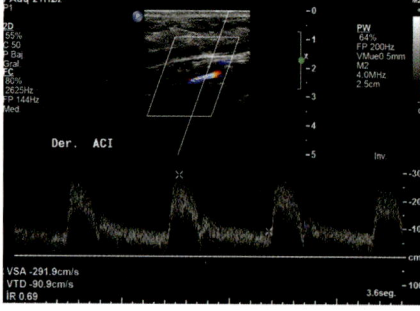

Fig. 10.8.3

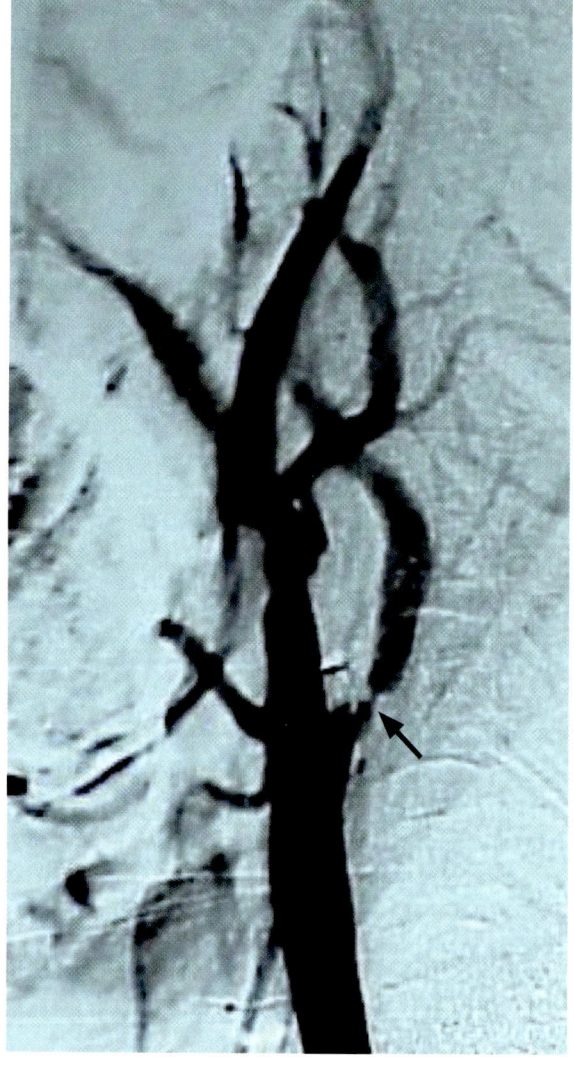

Fig. 10.8.4

atic patients with >70% stenosis. In recent years, stent implantation in the carotid artery has been shown to be safe and effective and seems to be a minimally invasive alternative to endarterectomy. Digital subtraction angiography is the standard imaging modality for quantifying the degree of stenosis but it is an invasive examination with a relatively high risk of mortality and morbidity. Duplex ultrasound is an excellent noninvasive examination for classifying above or below a certain degree of severity and is a widely accepted technique for screening patients with extracranial artery stenosis due to atheromatous disease. Other noninvasive tests are MR-angiography and CT-angiography. Ultrasound examinations of the ICA should be performed with gray-scale, color Doppler, and spectral Doppler in a standardized fashion. The Doppler waveform should be obtained with an angle of insonation less than or equal to 60°. As stenotic lesions increase in severity, they perturb carotid artery blood flow patterns. Stenosis over 50% of diameter narrowing will increase peak systolic velocity (PSV) and make the blood-flow profile more homogeneous at the point of maximal narrowing. Peak systolic velocities remain elevated for varying distances that typically extend for 1–2 cm beyond the stenosis. Care should be taken to position the sample volume within the area of greatest stenosis. Color Doppler serves as a guide for the sonographer: sites at which aliasing occurs are likely to have elevated peak velocities and correspond to areas of high grade stenoses that must be further evaluated with Doppler waveform analysis.

Doppler US cannot be used to predict a certain percentage of stenosis. Expert consensus recommends stratification of the degree of stenosis into the following strata: normal (no stenosis), <50% stenosis, 50–69% stenosis, > or equal 70% stenosis but less than near occlusion, near occlusion, and total occlusion. The diagnoses of near occlusion and total occlusion are usually not based primarily on the Doppler measurement of velocity but rather on gray-scale and color and/or power Doppler imaging. The ICA PSV and the presence of plaque are the parameters that should be used when diagnosing and grading ICA stenosis. Two additional parameters, the ICA/CCA – common carotid artery – PSV ratio and ICA end-diastolic velocity (EDV), are useful when ICA PSV may not be representative of the extent of the disease owing to technical or clinical factors (tandem lesions, contralateral high-grade stenosis, discrepancy between visual assessment of plaque and ICA PSV, elevated CCA PSV, or low cardiac output).

The ICA is considered normal when ICA PSV is less than 125 cm/sec and no plaque is visible sonographically. A <50% stenosis is diagnosed when ICA PSV is less than 125 cm/sec and plaque is visible. A 50–69% ICA stenosis is diagnosed when ICA PSV is 125–230 cm/sec. A 70% or greater stenosis but less than near occlusion is diagnosed when the ICA PSV is greater than 230 cm/sec, with visible plaque and luminal narrowing at gray-scale and color Doppler US. In cases of near occlusion the velocity parameters may not apply: this diagnosis is established primarily by demonstrating a markedly narrowed lumen at color or power Doppler US. Total occlusion should be suspected when there is no flow with spectral, power, and color Doppler US.

Imaging Findings

Longitudinal color Doppler (Fig. 10.8.1) and power Doppler (Fig. 10.8.2) US images of the proximal right ICA show heterogeneous plaque with apparent moderate-to-severe luminal narrowing (*arrows*). Duplex US image (Fig. 10.8.3) shows high pulsed wave Doppler PSV of 290 cm/s at the point of maximal stenosis. This velocity represents severe stenosis (more than 70% but less than near occlusion). Digital angiography (Fig. 10.8.4) shows a severe stenosis in the proximal ICA of about 90% (*arrow*).

Case 9
■
Carotid Artery Dissection

A 17- year-old male presented to the emergency department with a two-day history of left lower extremity weakness and paresthesia. Two weeks before he had had an accidental fall from an amusement park ride and, after this event, he had right-sided neck pain for one day. Physical examination revealed left hemiparesis. Cranial MRI showed some ischemic foci in the right cerebral hemisphere. Doppler ultrasound findings were strongly suggestive of internal carotid artery dissection with intra-mural hematoma. Digital subtraction angiography confirmed these findings. The patient was treated with anticoagulants and showed good clinical evolution.

Comments

Extracranial carotid artery dissection is a relatively uncommon cause of cerebrovascular symptoms and accounts for about 1% of all ischemic strokes; however, it accounts for 10–25% of strokes in young adults. Although the classification of internal carotid artery (ICA) dissection as traumatic or spontaneous may be apparent clinically, there are no angiographic differences between both groups. External trauma may be minimal in the former group, and spontaneous dissection may be linked in a few cases with an underlying arteriopathy such as fibromuscular dysplasia. The mechanism of dissection is thought to be either a tear in the intima, which allows intraluminal blood to dissect along the layers of the vessel wall or, alternatively, direct hemorrhage from the vasa vasorum of the media. The hematoma dissects longitudinally along the media. When the hematoma lies beneath the intima, luminal

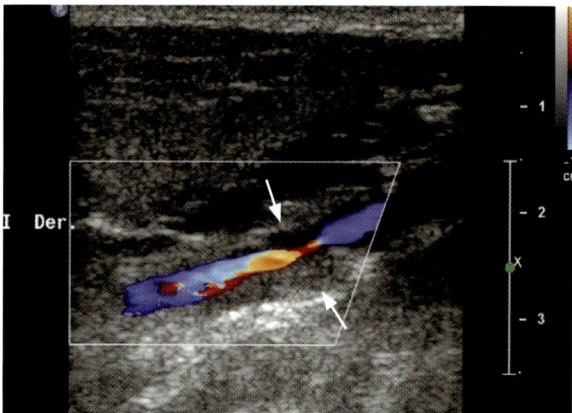

Fig. 10.9.1

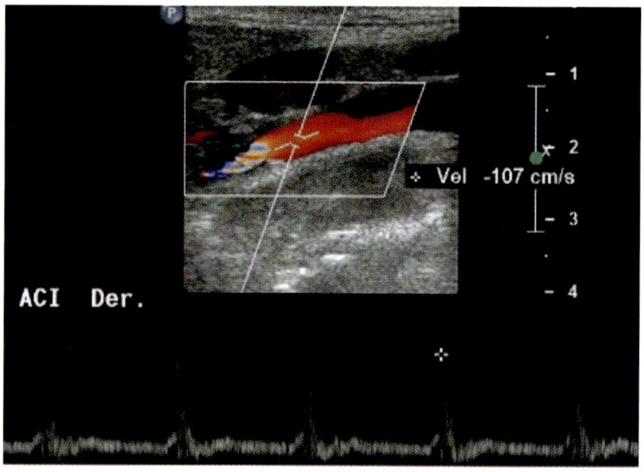

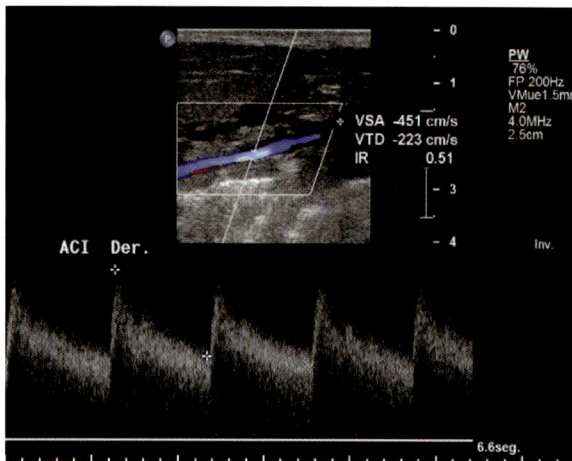

Fig. 10.9.3

Fig. 10.9.2

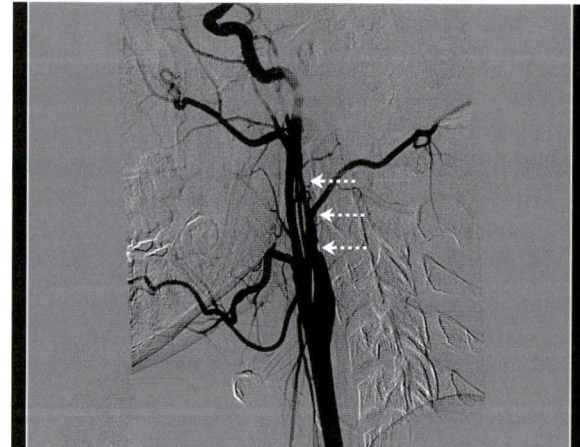

Fig. 10.9.4

narrowing or occlusion occurs. If the hematoma dissects beneath the adventitia, a pseudoaneurysm forms. A false lumen occurs if blood reenters the true lumen; this false lumen may remain patent, resolve completely, or thrombose and cause narrowing of the true lumen.

The typical patient with carotid dissection presents with pain on one side of the head, face, or neck, accompanied by a partial Horner's syndrome followed hours or days later by cerebral or retinal ischemia. This triad of symptoms is found in less than one third of patients. Cerebral infarcts are reported in 50% and transient ischemic attacks (TIA) in 20% of patients with ICA dissection.

The commonest location for a spontaneous ICA dissection is the cervical segment 2–3 cm distal to the carotid bulb. Dissections extend for a variable length but they rarely reach the point of entry of the ICA into the petrous temporal bone. In the absence of arteriopathy, recurrent dissection is rare.

Intraarterial angiography has been the gold standard in the diagnosis of dissections, but it is increasingly being replaced by noninvasive imaging techniques. The most common angiographic finding, reported in more than 50% cases, is an irregular stenosis starting about 2–3 cm distal to the carotid bulb. Other, less common angiographic findings (5–30% cases) are a flame-shaped occlusion, a tapered narrowing of the ICA ("rat's tail" or "string sign"), and pseudoaneurysm. All these appearances are indicative of dissection, but they are non-specific. The only pathognomic finding is an intimal flap with double lumen, but these flaps are detected in less than 10% cases. Angiography does not allow direct visualization of the vessel wall when there is a thrombus in the false lumen.

US provides direct visualization of the pathological findings, hemodynamic information, flow direction and velocity data, and enables evaluation of the vessel wall and lumen patency. The commonest gray-scale finding is the presence of a hypoechoic thrombus (corresponding to intramural hematoma or thrombosed false lumen) 2–3 cm cranially from the bulb, with or without true lumen narrowing. The presence of an arterial luminal flap (membrane) in the longitudinal and axial views is pathognomic, but this finding is uncommon.

The commonest spectral Doppler US finding in the affected ICA is a high resistance pattern or absence of signal in cases of total occlusion. Another, less common spectral pattern is a damped spectral waveform (lower amplitude with biphasic pattern). Visualization of intramural hematoma combined with high-resistance flow strongly suggests dissection. The diagnostic sensitivity of US decreases if an ICA dissection results in a low-grade stenosis, and gray-scale and spectral findings can be normal in these cases. US is less reliable for dissections located in the subpetrous segment and the carotid canal.

At present, the diagnosis of carotid dissection is essentially established with cervical MR and MR-angiography. The former can provide direct visualization of an intramural hematoma, which is the hallmark of a dissection, and the later allows noninvasive visualization of blood vessels. However, MR is not always available around the clock and many centers use ultrasound to assess carotid dissection. Furthermore, follow-up US studies can document recanalization, stabilization or progressive vascular occlusion.

Imaging Findings

Longitudinal color Doppler US (Fig. 10.9.1) of the right internal carotid artery (ICA) demonstrating a low-reflective intramural hematoma (*arrows*) compressing the true lumen of the internal carotid artery 2 cm cranially from the bulb. Color and spectral Doppler US of the ICA immediately prior to dissection (Fig. 10.9.2) shows a high-resistance triphasic waveform. Spectral Doppler at the point of maximal lumen stenosis (Fig. 10.9.3) shows a very high peak systolic velocity over 4 m/s. Digital angiography (Fig. 10.9.4) confirmed an irregular stenosis (*arrows*) starting 2 cm distal to the carotid bulb.

Case 10
■ Choroidal Melanoma

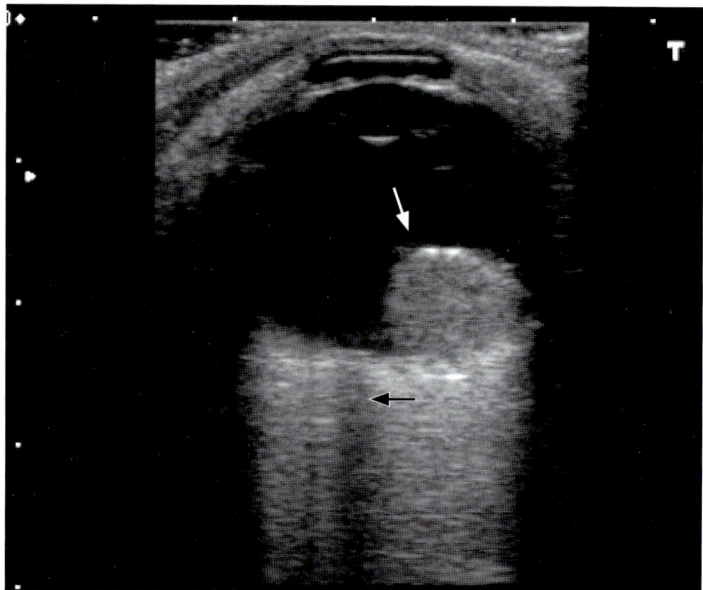

Fig. 10.10.1

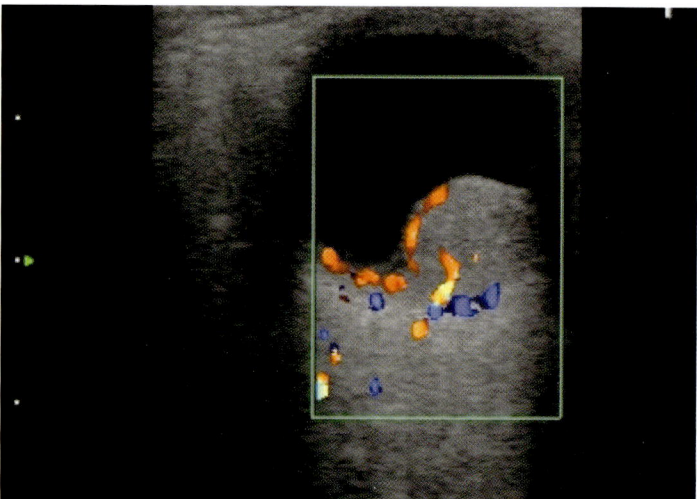

Fig. 10.10.2

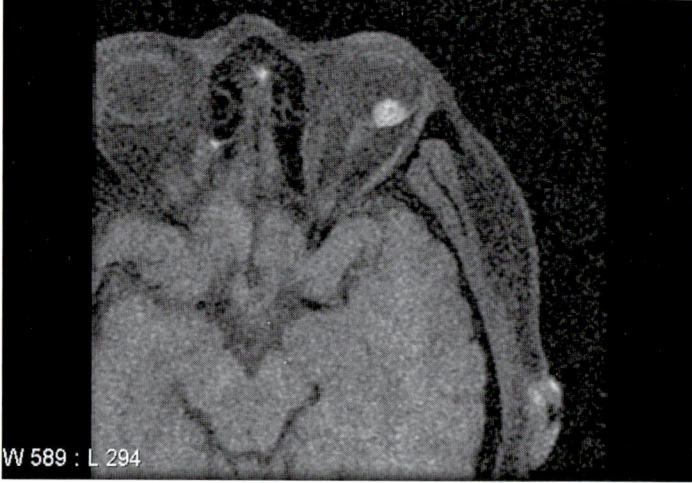

Fig. 10.10.3

A 57-year-old woman presented with decreased visual acuity. Ophthalmoscopic examination showed a brown mass suspected of choroidal melanoma. US scan and MRI showed a mass with typical features of melanoma with no signs of extraocular invasion or complications. No distant metastases were found. Enucleation was performed.

Malignant melanoma is the most common primary intraocular tumor in adults. It occurs more often in the choroid than in the iris or ciliary body. Some melanomas may originate from pre-existing nevi. The clinical appearance of malignant melanoma is variable, but it usually presents with decreased visual acuity and visual field defects. A circumscribed choroidal mass of varied pigmentation is identified on ophthalmoscopic examination. In some cases, the tumor may be amelanotic. Initially, the tumor is flat; later, it elevates resulting in the characteristic mushroom-shaped lesion growing towards the vitreous cavity. Choroidal melanomas can usually be diagnosed accurately by ophthalmoscopy, fluorescein angiography, or US. Misdiagnoses, however, are not uncommon. Lesions more than 3 mm in size are usually well visualized on CT and MR imaging. Smaller lesions are better studied with US. Extraocular extension of the tumor can be better diagnosed with MR.

Ultrasound typically shows a rounded or mushroom-shaped hypoechoic mass that sometimes is accompanied by marginal retinal elevation. A thin hyperechoic rim is usually seen, and this represents a combination of elevated retina and peripheral blood vessels. It is extremely easy to overestimate the extent of penetration of the layers of the wall of the globe with US.

Choroidal melanomas are very vascular tumors, and color Doppler shows vessels penetrating and encircling the lesion. This feature is useful to differentiate melanoma from nonneoplastic lesions such as large subretinal hemorrhages, which usually have no blood supply.

Melanomas of the eye can be complicated by retinal elevation and vitreous hemorrhage. These complications can be depicted with US.

Many benign and malignant lesions can be confused with malignant choroidal melanoma, including choroidal hemangioma, choroidal nevi, uveal metastasis, choroidal detachment, and retinal detachment, among others. Choroidal hemangioma has been commonly confused with malignant melanoma. Several authors have described the usefulness of MRI in evaluating and differentiating uveal melanomas from simulating lesions. Because of the paramagnetic property of melanin, uveal melanomas appear relatively hyperintense on T1-weighted images, making diagnostic differentiation possible with a high degree of accuracy.

The management of clinically and imaging suspected choroidal melanoma has been the subject of increasing controversy. Enucleation does not prevent metastasis. Choroidal melanomas of less than 10 mm in diameter and 3 mm in thickness have a relatively favorable prognosis. Clinically stable choroidal melanomas are usually managed with longitudinal observations. When tumor growth is evident enucleation may be indicated. A thorough search for metastasis is important to spare the patient an unnecessary enucleation.

Transverse gray-scale sonogram (Fig. 10.10.1) shows a rounded hypoechoic mass (*arrow*) with hyperechoic rim. Note the optic nerve, depicted as a hypoechoic band extending posteriorly (*black arrow*). Color Doppler sonogram (Fig. 10.10.2) shows blood vessels encircling and penetrating the tumor. Fat-suppressed T1-weighted MR image (Fig. 10.10.3) shows a hyperintense mass, typical of melanoma, without retrobulbar extension.

Further Readings

Books

Categorical course in diagnostic radiology: findings at US-what do they mean? Cooperberg PL (2002) Oak Brook (IL). Radiological Society of North America publications

Diagnostic Ultrasound. 3rd ed. Rumack CM, Wilson S, Charboneau JW, Johnson JA (2005) St. Louis (MO). Elsevier-Mosby. ISBN-13: 9780323020237

Introduction to Vascular Ultrasonography. 5th ed. Zwiebel W, Pellerito J (2004) Philadelphia (PA). Elsevier-Saunders. ISBN-13: 9780721606316

General and Vascular Ultrasound: case review series. 2nd ed. Middleton WD (2007) Philadelphia (PA). Elsevier-Saunders. ISBN-13: 9781416039891

Musculoskeletal Ultrasound. 2nd ed. van Holsbeeck M, Introcaso J (2001) St. Louis (MO) Elsevier-Mosby. ISBN-13: 9780323000185

Peripheral Vascular Sonography. 2nd ed. Polak JF (2004) Philadelphia (PA). Lippincott Williams & Wilkins. ISBN-13: 9780781748711

Practical Musculoskeletal Ultrasound. McNally E (2004) St. Louis (MO). Elsevier-Churchill Livingstone. ISBN-13: 9780443073502

Syllabus: A Special Course in Ultrasound. Bluth EI, Arger PH, Hertzberg BS, Middleton WD (1996) Oak Brook (IL). Radiological Society of North America publications

Ultrasound: A Practical Approach to Clinical Problems. Bluth EI, Arger PH, Benson CB, Ralls PW, Siegel MJ (2007) 2nd ed. New York (NY). Thieme. ISBN-13: 9783131168320

Vascular Diagnosis with Ultrasound. 2nd ed. Hennerici MG, Neuerburg-Heusler D (2006) New York (NY). Thieme. ISBN-13: 9783131038326

Web-Links

http://aium.org
http://auntminnie.com
http://emedicine.com
http://med-ed.virginia.edu/courses/rad/edus/index.htlm
http://radiographics.rsnajnls.org/cgi/collection/ultrasound
http://sonoworld.com
http://sru.org

Articles

Bartolotta TV, Midiri M, Quaia E, et al. Benign focal liver lesions: spectrum of findings on SonoVue-enhanced pulse-inversion ultrasonography. Eur Radiol 2005; 15:1643–1649

Basu S, Howlet DC. High-resolution ultrasound in the evaluation of the nonacute testis. Abdom Imaging 2001; 26:425–432

Beggs I. Pictorial review: Imaging of peripheral nerve tumours. Clin Radiol 1997; 52:8–17

Bennett GL, Balthazar EJ. Ultrasound and CT evaluation of emergent gallbladder pathology. Radiol Clin North Am 2003; 41:1203–1216

Bialek EJ, Jakubowski W, Zajkowski P, et al. US of the major salivary glands: anatomy and spatial relationships, pathologic conditions, and pitfalls. Radiographics 2006; 26:745–763

Bianchi S, Martinoli C, Abdelwahab IF. High-frequency ultrasound examination of the wrist and hand. Skeletal Radiol 1999; 28:121–129

Bianchi S, Martinoli C, Abdelwahab IF. Ultrasound of tendon tears. Part 1:general considerations and upper extremity. Skeletal Radiol 2005; 34:500–512

Bianchi S, Martinoli C, Bianchi-Zamorani MP, et al. Ultrasound of the joints. Eur Radiol 2002; 12:56–61

Bianchi S, Poletti PA, Martinoli C, et al. Ultrasound appearance of tendon tears. Part 2: lower extremity and myotendinous tears. Skeletal Radiol 2006; 35:63–77

Birnbaum BA, Wilson SR. Appendicitis at the millennium. Radiology 2000; 215:337–348

Boote EJ. AAPM/RSNA physics tutorial for residents: Topics in US: Doppler US techniques: concepts of blood flow detection and flow dynamics. Radiographics 2003; 23:1315–1327

Bottelli R, Tibballs J, Hochhauser D, et al. Ultrasound screening for hepatocellular carcinoma (HCC) in cirrhosis: the evidence for an established clinical practice. Clin Radiol 1998; 53:713–716

Boyse TD, Fessell DP, Jacobson JA, et al. US of soft-tissue foreign bodies and associated complications with surgical correlation. Radiographics 2001; 21:1251–1256

Brannigan M, Burns PN, Wilson SR. Blood flow patterns in focal liver lesions at microbubble-enhanced US. Radiographics 2004; 24:921–935

Brown DL, Doubilet PM, Miller FH, et al. Benign and malignant ovarian masses: selection of the most discriminating gray-scale and doppler sonographic features. Radiology 1998; 208:103–110

Brown ED, Chen MY, Wolfman NT, et al. Complications of renal transplantation: evaluation with US and radionuclide imaging. Radiographics 2000; 20:607–622

Bureau NJ, Chhem RK, Cardinal E. Musculoskeletal infections: US manifestations. Radiographics 1999; 19:1585–1592

Bushby LH, Miller FN, Rosairo S, et al. Scrotal calcification: ultrasound appearances, distribution and aetiology. Br J Radiol 2002; 75:283–288

Carr JC, Hanly S, Griffin J, et al. Sonography of the patellar tendon and adjacent structures in pediatric and adult patients. AJR Am J Roentgenol 2001; 176:1535–1539

Catalano O, Nunziata A, Lobianco R, et al. Real-time harmonic contrast material-specific US of focal liver lesions. Radiographics 2005; 25:333–349

Chau CL, Griffith JF. Musculoskeletal infections: ultrasound appearances. Clin Radiol 2005; 60:149–159

Chin EE, Zimmerman PT, Grant EG. Sonographic evaluation of upper extremity deep venous thrombosis. J Ultrasound Med 2005; 24:829–838

Cook JL, Dewbury K. The changes seen on high-resolution ultrasound in orchitis. Clin Radiol 2000; 55:13–18

Cornuz J, Pearson SD, Polak JF. Deep venous thrombosis: complete lower extremity venous US evaluation in patients without known risk factors. Radiology 1999; 211:637–641

Crossin JD, Muradali D, Wilson SR. US of liver transplants: normal and abnormal. Radiographics 2003;23:1093–1114

Davison BD, Polak JF. Arterial injuries: a sonographic approach. Radiol Clin North Am 2004; 42:383–396

Deurdulian C, Mittelstaedt CA, Chong WK, et al. US of acute scrotal trauma: optimal technique, imaging findings, and management. Radiographics 2007; 27:357–369

Dogra V, Bhatt S. Acute painful scrotum. Radiol Clin North Am 2004; 42:349–363

Dogra VS, Gottlieb RH, Oka M, et al. Sonography of the scrotum. Radiology 2003; 227:18–36

Durr-e-Sabih, Khan AN, Craig M, et al. Sonographic mimics of renal calculi. J Ultrasound Med 2004; 23:1361–1367

Esen G. Ultrasound of superficial lymph nodes. Eur J Radiol 2006; 58:345–359

Flis CM, Jager HR, Sidhu PS. Carotid and vertebral artery dissections: clinical aspects, imaging features and endovascular treatment. Eur Radiol 2007; 17:820–834

Fraser JD, Anderson DR. Deep venous thrombosis: recent advances and optimal investigation with US. Radiology 1999; 211:9–24

Fraser JD, Anderson DR. Venous protocols, techniques, and interpretations of the upper and lower extremities. Radiol Clin North Am 2004; 42:279–296

Frates MC, Benson CB, Charboneau JW, et al. Management of thyroid nodules detected at US: Society of Radiologists in Ultrasound consensus conference statement. Radiology 2005; 237:794–800

Gahn G, von Kummer R. Ultrasound in acute stroke: a review. Neuroradiology 2001; 43:702–711

Gaitini D, Soudack M. Diagnosing carotid stenosis by Doppler sonography: state of the art. J Ultrasound Med 2005; 24:1127–1136

Gore RM, Yaghmai V, Newmark GM, et al. Imaging benign and malignant disease of the gallbladder. Radiol Clin North AM 2002; 40:1307–1323

Grant EG, Benson CB, Moneta GL, et al. Carotid artery stenosis; gray-scale and Doppler US diagnosis – Society of Radiologists in Ultrasound consensus conference. Radiology 2003; 229:340–346

Hanbidge AE, Lynch D, Wilson SR. US of the peritoneum. Radiographics 2003; 23:663–685

Hangiandreou NJ. AAPM/RSNA physics tutorial for residents: Topics in US: B-mode US: basic concepts and new technology. Radiographics 2003; 23:1019–1033

Hensen JH, Van Breda AC, Puylaert JB. Abdominal wall endometriosis: clinical presentation and imaging features with emphasis on sonography. AJR Am J Roentgenol 2006; 186:616–620

Hermsen K, Chong WK. Ultrasound evaluation of abdominal aortic and iliac aneurysms and mesenteric ischemia. Radiol Clin North Am 2004; 42:365–381

Horrow MM, Stassi J. Sonography of the vertebral arteries: a window to disease of proximal great vessels. AJR Am J Roentgenol 2001; 177:53–59

Howlett DC, Alyas F, Wong KT, et al. Sonographic assessment of the submandibular space. Clin Radiol 2004; 59:1070–1078

Howlett, DC, Marchbank ND, Sallomi DF. Ultrasound of the testis. Clin Radiol 2000; 55:595–601

Inampudi P, Jacobson JA, Fessell DP, et al. Soft-tissue lipomas: accuracy of sonography in diagnosis with pathologic correlation. Radiology 2004; 233:763–767

Jacobson JA. Ultrasound in sport medicine. Radiol Clin North Am. 2002; 40:363–386

Jamadar DA, Jacobson JA, Theisen SE, et al. Sonography of the painful calf: differential considerations. AJR Am J Roentgenol 2002; 179:709–716

Kaakaji Y, Nghiem HV, Nodell C, et al. Sonography of obstetric and gynecologic emergencies: Part II, gynecologic emergencies. AJR Am J Roentgenol 2000; 174:651–656

Kessler N, Cyteval C, Gallix B, et al. Appendicitis: evaluation of sensitivity, specificity, and predictive values of US, Doppler US, and laboratory findings. Radiology 2004; 230:472–478

Khoury V, Cardinal E, Bureau NJ. Musculoskeletal sonography: a dynamic tool for usual and unusual disorders. AJR Am J Roentgenol 2007; 188:W63–W73

Kim EK, Park CS, Chung WY, et al. New Sonographic criteria for recommending fine-needle aspiration biopsy of nonpalpable solid nodules of the thyroid. AJR Am J Roentgenol 2002; 178:687–691

Koh DM, Burke S, Davies N, et al. Transthoracic US of the chest: clinical uses and applications. Radiographics 2002; 22:1e

Kono Y, Mattrey RF. Ultrasound of the liver. Radiol Clin North Am 2005; 43:815–826

Kruskal JB, Newman PA, Sammons LG, et al. Optimizing Doppler and Color flow US: application to hepatic sonography. Radiographics 2004; 24:657–675

Landwehr P, Schulte O, Voshage G. Ultrasound examination of carotid and vertebral arteries. Eur Radiol 2001; 11:1521–1534

Ledermann HP, Börner N, Strunk H, et al. Bowel wall thickening on transabdominal sonography. AJR Am J Roentgenol 2000; 174:107–117

Lieb WE. Color Doppler imaging of the eye and orbit. Radiol Clin N Am 1998; 36:1059–1099

Lin J, Fessell DP, Jacobson JA, et al. An illustrated tutorial of musculoskeletal sonography: Part I, introduction and general principles. AJR Am J Roentgenol. 2000; 175:637–345

Lin J, Fessell DP, Jacobson JA, et al. An illustrated tutorial of musculoskeletal sonography: Part 3, lower extremity. AJR Am J Roentgenol 2000; 175:1313–1321

Lin J, Jacobson JA, Fessell DP, et al. An illustrated tutorial of musculoskeletal sonography: Part 2, upper extremity. AJR Am J Roentgenol 2000; 175:1071–1079

Lin J, Jacobson JA, Fessell DP, et al. An illustrated tutorial of musculoskeletal sonography: Part 4, musculoskeletal masses, sonographically guided interventions and miscellaneous topics. AJR Am J Roentgenol 2000; 175:1711–1719

Madani G, Beale T. Inflammatory conditions of the salivary glands. Semin Ultrasound CT MR 2006; 27:440–451

Martinez-Noguera A, D´Onofrio. Ultrasonography of the pancreas. 1. Conventional imaging. Abdom Imaging 2007; 32:136–149

Martinoli C, Bianchi S, Gandolfo N, et al. US of nerve entrapments in osteofibrous tunnels of the upper and lower limbs. Radiographics 2000; 20:199S–217S

Martinoli C, Bianchi S, Prato N, et al. US of the shoulder: non-rotator cuff disorders. Radiographics 2003; 23:381–401

McGahan JP, Richards J, Fogata ML. Emergency ultrasound in trauma patients. Radiol Clin North Am 2004; 42:417–425

McGahan JP, Richards J, Gillen M. The focused abdominal sonography for trauma scan: pearls and pitfalls. J Ultrasound Med 2002; 21:789–800

McGahan JP, Richards JR. Blunt abdominal trauma: the role of emergent sonography and a review of the literature. AJR Am J Roentgenol 1999; 172:897–903

McGahan JP, Wang L, Richards JR. From the RSNA refresher courses: Focused abdominal US for trauma. Radiographics 2001; 21:191S–199S

McNamara MM, Lockhart ME, Robbin ML. Emergency Doppler evaluation of the liver and kidneys. Radiol Clin North Am 2004; 42:397–415

Miller FN, Rosairo S, Clarke JL, et al. Testicular calcification and microlithiasis association with primary intratesticular malignancy in 3477 patients. Eur Radiol. 2007; 17:363–369

Naik KS, Bury RF. Review: Imaging the thyroid. Clin Radiol 1998; 53:630–639

Nakamoto DA, Haaga JR. Emergent ultrasound interventions. Radiol Clin North Am 2004; 42:457–478

Nikolaidis P, Amin RS, Hwang CM, et al. Role of sonography in pancreatic transplantation. Radiographics 2003; 23:939–949

Paspulati RM, Bhatt S. Sonography in benign and malignant renal masses. Radiol Clin North Am 2006; 44:787–803

Puylaert JB. Ultrasonography of the acute abdomen: gastrointestinal conditions. Radiol Clin N Am 2003; 41:1227–1242

Rajiah P, Lim YY, Taylor P. Renal transplant imaging and complications. Abdom Imaging 2006; 31:735–746

Reeder SB, Desser TS, Weigel RJ, et al. Sonography in primary hyperparathyroidism: review with emphasis on scanning technique. J Ultrasound Med. 2002; 21:539–552

Ripollés T, Agramunt M, Martínez MJ, et al. The role of ultrasound in the diagnosis, management and evolutive prognosis of acute left-sided colonic diverticulitis: a review of 208 patients. Eur Radiol 2003; 13:2587–2595

Romero JM, Lev MH, Chan ST, et al. US of neurovascular occlusive disease: interpretive pearls and pitfalls. Radiographics 2002; 22:1165–1176

Rubens DJ. Hepatobiliary imaging and its pitfalls. Radiol Clin North Am. 2004; 42:257–278

Rutten MJ, Jager GJ, Blickman JG. From the RSNA refresher courses: US of the rotator cuff: pitfalls, limitations and artifacts. Radiographics 2006; 26:589–604

Saifuddin A, Burnett SJ, Mitchell R. Pictorial review: Ultrasonography of primary bone tumours. Clin Radiol 1998; 53:239–246

Schellong SM, Schwarz T, Hallbritter K, et al. Complete compression ultrasonography of the leg veins as a single test for the diagnosis of deep vein thrombosis. Thromb Haemost 2003; 89:228–234

Sheth S, Hamper UM, Stanley LB et al. US guidance for thoracic biopsy: a valuable alternative to CT. Radiology 1999; 210:721–726

Sidhu PS. Clinical and imaging features of testicular torsion: role of ultrasound. Clin Radiol. 1999; 54:343–352

Stewart VR, Sidhu PS. The testis: the unusual, the rare and the bizarre. Clin Radiol 2007; 62:289–302

Strauss S, Gottlieb P, Kessler A, et al. Non-neoplastic intratesticular lesions mimicking tumour on ultrasound. Eur Radiol 2000; 10:1628–1635

Stuart RM, Koh ES, Breidahl WH. Sonography of peripheral nerve pathology. AJR Am J Roentgenol. 2004; 182:123–129

Tahmasebpour HR, Buckley AR, Cooperberg PL, et al. Sonographic examination of the carotid arterics. Radiographics 2005; 25:1561–1575

Teefey SA, Roarke MC, Brink JA, et al. Bowel wall thickening: differentiation of inflammation from ischemia with color Doppler and Duplex US. Radiology 1996; 198:547–551

Tessler FN, Tublin ME. Thyroid sonography: current applications and future directions. AJR Am J Roentgenol. 1999; 173:437–443

Tublin ME, Bude RO, Platt JF. The resistive index in renal Doppler sonography: where do we stand? AJR Am J Roentgenol 2003; 80:885–892

Vourganti S, Agarwal PK, Bodner DR, et al. Ultrasonographic evaluation of renal infections. Radiol Clin North Am 2006; 44:763–775

Weber TM. Sonography of benign renal cystic disease. Radiol Clin North Am 2006; 44:777–786

Wernecke K. Ultrasound study of the pleura. Eur Radiol. 2000; 10:1515–1523

Wilson SR, Burns PN. An algorithm for the diagnosis of focal liver masses using microbubble contrast-enhanced pulse-inversion sonography. AJR Am J Roentgenol 2006; 186:1401–1412

Ying M, Ahuja A. Sonography of neck lymph nodes. Part I: Normal lymph nodes. Clin Radiol 2003; 58:351–358